HEALING WITH
CLINICAL NUTRITION

PROFESSIONAL EDITION

HEALING WITH CLINICAL NUTRITION

*A Guide to Nutrient-Rich Food
& Nutritional Supplements*

DR ABRAM HOFFER, PhD, MD, FRCP(C)
& **DR JONATHAN PROUSKY**, BPHE, BSC, ND, FRSH

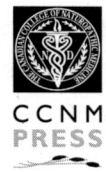

CCNM
PRESS

Copyright © The Estate of Abram Hoffer and Jonathan Prousky, 2011.

All rights reserved.

The publisher does not advocate the use of any particular treatment program, but believes that the information presented in this book should be available to the public. The nutritional, medical, and health information presented in this book is based on the research, training, and personal experiences of the authors, and is true and complete to the best of the their knowledge. However, this book is intended only as an informative guide for those wishing to know more about good health. It is not intended to replace or countermand the advice given by the reader's physician. The publisher and the authors are not responsible for any adverse effects or consequences from any of the suggestions made in this book. Because each person and each situation is unique, the publisher and the authors urge the reader to consult with a qualified professional before using any procedure where there is any question as to its appropriateness.

Previously published in a trade paperback edition as *Dr Hoffer's Laws of Natural Nutrition* (Quarry Health Books, 1996) and later revised as *Naturopathic Nutrition* (CCNM Press, 2006).

Cataloging in publication data is available.

ISBN-10 1-897025-42-4
ISBN-13 978-1-897025-42-0

Edited by Bob Hilderley.
Design by Sari Naworynski.

Printed and bound in Canada.

Published by CCNM Press Inc., 1255 Sheppard Avenue East, Toronto, Ontario M2K 1E2 Canada.
www.ccnmpress.com

CONTENTS

Preface   7

Our Health Dilemmas   11
    Beyond the High-Tech Diet   12
    Toward a Natural Diet   19

The Health Costs of the High-Tech Diet   25
    The Junk Food Era   26
    Dietary Diseases   48
    Public Malnutrition   74

The Health Benefits of a Naturopathic Diet   83
    Optimum Diet   84
    Optimal Absorption   99
    Naturopathic Healthcare   123

Nutritional Therapy   127
    Nutrient Deficiencies   128
    Nutrient Dependencies   135

Nutrient Supplements   139
    Vitamins   140
    Minerals   207
    Amino Acids   249
    Essential Fatty Acids   263

Nutritional Therapy Case Studies   271
Nutrient Content of Common Foods   299
References   330
Index   350

PREFACE

My grandmother died when she was 90 years old. Many friends and relatives at the funeral commented on how wonderful it was that she lived a full life and how lucky she was to have lived such a long life. Yes, I was blessed to have had her in my life for many years, but the last 20 years of her life were not wonderful. They were filled with severe chronic pain, cardiovascular disease, two bouts of cancer (thyroid and lung that eventually metastasized to her brain), muscle wasting, weight gain, osteoporosis, and diminished abilities to engage in a reasonable quality of life.

My grandmother was the perfect example of an elderly person whose chronological age was less "diseased" than her biological age. Chronological age is the age a person is in years, whereas biological age refers to the capacities of the different systems of the body to work as optimally as they can. Some people, for example, may be chronologically 50 years old, but biologically they function at a level comparable to those who are 30 years old. The majority of us are not that lucky. We tend to be biologically much older than our chronological age.

Even though there is nothing that can be done about chronological age, there is much that can be done regarding biological age. My grandmother could have lived a much better quality of life had she adopted the nutritional strategies presented in this book, with its focus on eating right and taking optimal doses of nutrients. These practices will ensure good health, regardless of your biological age, and prevent diseases associated with poor lifestyle and eating habits. I am convinced that if we all adopted these strategies, there would be significant reductions in the major causes of death (heart disease, cancer, diabetes, lung diseases, and kidney diseases) and significant improvements in difficult-to-treat medical conditions (mental illnesses and neurological diseases).

Individuals who have followed these strategies have proved its validity. One such example is Dr Abram Hoffer himself, my co-author. He is 88 years old. Only recently did he retire from full-time psychiatric practice after having served his patients for 55 years, though he is still a much sought after expert on orthomolecular psychiatry. He eats well, exercises regularly, and supplements with optimal doses of nutrients every day. He walks and moves well; he is free of disease. His mind is sharper than most. He has published more than 500 scientific papers and more than 15 books. He still writes books and lectures at medical conventions. I cannot recall many other elderly people his age as healthy as he is who have not adopted naturopathic nutrition strategies.

I have had the great privilege of working with Dr Hoffer on this book as his co-author – and of learning how to help others improve their health through eating a natural diet and taking optimum amounts of nutrient supplements.

Our message is simple: read this book, then incorporate this information into your life each and every day, and you may also live a long and fulfilling life free of major diseases and infirmity.

– Dr Jonathan Prousky

During my adult years, I have seen an enormous increase in the number of people who become sick. In 1950 when I started my education in psychiatry, we saw very few children with learning and behavioral disorders. We did see children who could not learn and who were said to be 'retarded', but the combination of hyperactivity and learning disorder so common today was very rare. I believe that pediatricians who can still remember what their practices were like in the 1950s will support this conclusion. Today, these problem children are so numerous, many pediatricians look upon this as normal behavior that they will outgrow. Other disease conditions are also on the rise. Breast cancer has increased from 1 in 20 women to 1 in 9 women in the past 20 years, and may still be increasing. In the United States a few years ago, there were 750,000 cardiovascular deaths, 164,300 cerebrovascular deaths, and 465,000 cancer deaths. I have estimated that every second Canadian has one or more chronic disease. This figure is easily arrived at by adding up the number who are very obese and suffer the consequences of the diseases caused by their low-fiber, high-sugar diet; the alcoholics and addicts; the mentally sick, especially the Alzheimer's sufferers and schizophrenics; the victims of muscular degenerative diseases and some of the modern plagues, such as the viral influenza and AIDS.

Obviously, advances in drug research and surgical skill have not led to better health. Poor eating and nutritional ignorance have, however, led to an increase in chronic disease. This dilemma is caused by the combination of the persuasive power of high-tech food processing industry and the poor quality of the nutritional education given to our children. It follows that there will be no solution to the problem of chronic illness until we become aware that only by eating foods that can nourish us properly will there ever be a decrease in the growth of chronic disease.

All good food to which anyone has adapted is both preventive and therapeutic. It prevents the diseases that will inevitably occur if the food is deficient in quantity or quality, and if the diet that had made the people sick is corrected, it will help restore their health. However, even the best diet is not always adequate because the nutrient content of our food has been depleted, degraded, and contaminated by modern agricultural and food processing practices. As a result, we may need to supplement our diet with vitamins, minerals, amino acids, and essential fatty acids. In this book, Dr Prousky and I offer a convenient guide to eating nutrient-rich food and taking nutritional supplements for optimum health. We trust you will find the book not only informative but also practical. Individually and collectively, good health and lifelong well-being are within our reach if we improve our nutrition.

– Dr Abram Hoffer

Naturopathic Nutrition is defined as the therapeutic or clinical use of nutrient-rich foods and nutritional supplements to improve health and prevent disease. The diet should be modified first to be as ideal and health promoting as possible. Nutritional supplements are then added to correct any dietary insufficiencies that remain.

The clinical application of naturopathic nutrition must adhere to the principles and practices of naturopathic medicine when addressing the specific needs of the individual patient:

- First, do no harm
- Support the self-healing potential of the body
- Address the fundamental causes of disease (whenever possible)
- Heal the whole person through individualized treatment
- Teach the principles of health living and preventive medicine

Dr Jonathan Prousky is a practicing naturopathic doctor, who teaches naturopathic clinical nutrition at The Canadian College of Naturopathic Medicine.

Orthomolecular Medicine is defined as the therapeutic or clinical use of nutritional supplements to treat or prevent disease by optimizing the concentrations of substances (for example, vitamins, minerals, amino acids, and essential fatty acids) normally found within the human body. Each person has unique biochemical needs for these substances. Individuals may be deficient in these substances or dependent upon them. Orthomolecular medicine understands that dietary modifications are paramount for achieving optimum health, but the addition of nutritional supplements is also required. The term orthomolecular was first defined within the context of mental disorders, but has been expanded to include all medical conditions and diseases.

Dr Abram Hoffer, medical doctor and psychiatrist, founded the *Journal of Orthomolecular Medicine*.

OUR HEALTH DILEMMAS

1 | BEYOND THE HIGH-TECH DIET

The three basic elements of good health are our genetic inheritance, our education, and our chemical environment, of which food and how we use it to construct our diet is a major component. We cannot yet change our genetic inheritance, although this is an objective pursued by some scientists, but we can and must know how health is connected with food and nutrition so that we can extract the maximum benefit from available food and nutrients. And we must pass this information on to our children at home and in our schools, beginning in the earliest grades.

What's to Eat?

Before the development of food technology, not counting the introduction of fire and cooking, we only needed to know what foods were safe and what ones would make us sick or kill us. This information was developed by personal experiences passed on by example and instruction to our offspring. We did not have to depend upon reading and teaching.

Fortunately, we did have good instincts based upon our sense of taste, smell, and touch. These are the senses that guide animals in their selection of food. Plant or animal food that did not taste good was avoided. Usually, this meant that these products were too bitter. Foods that taste bland, salty, or sweet were preferred and, as a rule, are not poisonous. If any food made us sick, this would soon be recognized and thereafter avoided. We used other clues, such as the appearance and the tactile feel of the food, to decide whether or not to eat it. From the small number of safe foods, it was normal healthy practice to eat what was available without knowing anything about the composition of those foods. These were all whole foods, which in themselves were well balanced and could maintain health. Whole wheat, for example, can nourish animals for long periods of time, while white flour will soon cause the same animals to die if this is their only food source.

Modern high-tech food processing, however, has robbed us of the use of our senses in determining whether a food is or is not good for us. Modern foods are designed to appeal to the senses. Visually, they are packaged in appealing containers and painted with interesting colors. They are usually sweet, some much sweeter than others, contain some salt (usually too much), and are thus made attractive to the mouth. These cosmetic attributes are given to all the overly processed foods, ranging from those that will make us sick because they are so inadequate in their nutrient composition to those that are more nourishing. It is no longer possible to depend upon our senses to determine how nourishing food will be.

The three basic elements of good health are our genetic inheritance, our education, and our chemical environment, of which food and how we use it to construct our diet is a major component.

For this reason, we now have to depend upon our education to select foods that will serve us as well as they did before these high-tech processes became so common. This will be very difficult because an enormous advertising industry drives home the message that all these foods are good for you. They emphasize that sweet is healthy. Public education will have to displace all that commercial advertising. We would recommend that advertising for junk foods should be placed in the same category as advertising for tobacco, alcohol, and addicting drugs.

Modern high-quality nutrition depends upon the combination of good nutritional education and an adequate supply of foods, so that the education can be applied to the selection of a healthy diet. But we do not think that the education needs to be of the caliber required of nutritionists, dietitians, and physicians. The majority of people do not have to know the amount of vitamins, fat, or carbohydrate present in foods. They do not have to be so skillful with nutrients that they can construct a diet entirely derived from the 50 or so nutrients. It is enough to know which food products available to them are healthy and which are not. This book is written for the majority of people who do not want to spend much time on food tables, but who wish to have a few simple guidelines they can follow to ensure they will become healthy and remain well.

Why Aren't We Getting Healthier?

The loss of our senses as a good guide for selecting our food is the main reason for one current dilemma in the field of disease and health. Stated briefly, this dilemma is the close parallel development between the rise in the amount of chronic disease in our society and the improvement in the technology of medicine and surgery. Medicine and surgery have made enormous strides in curing a number of diseases, such as infections, in preventing deficiency disease, such as scurvy or beri beri, and in surgical and anesthetic methods for doing superb surgery with a minimum of pain and other discomfort. In fact, it was commonly believed in 1949, when Dr Hoffer graduated in medicine, that we were on the threshold of the wonder era in medicine when we could look forward to a society free of disease and enjoying an optimum state of health. The antibiotics had at last been fully accepted, the corticosteroid drugs, such as cortisone and ACTH, were curing almost everything, and surgery was being rapidly perfected. The financial development of government-run health plans in countries, such as Canada, depended upon the assumptions that the number of people requiring care and treatment would decrease as a result of new drug treatment and surgical methods. But parallel to the remarkable advances in medicine and surgery, we have seen an equally remarkable increase in chronic cardiovascular disease, cancer, diabetes, and so on.

Nevertheless, some physicians and public health officials persist in talking about the overall state of improvement of our health, using the fact that many more people today reach retirement age than did people 100 years ago. The real test of general health is not how many reach the age of 65, but how closely can we push the average age of death to the theoretical limit of 110 to 120 years. We have improved a little. A 55-year-old man in 1900 could expect to live another 17 years on the average. Today, that same man can expect to live about 20 more years. Our grandparents could expect almost the same additional years of life as we can.

The loss of our senses as a good guide for selecting our food is the main reason for one current dilemma in the field of disease and health. Stated briefly, this dilemma is the close parallel development between the rise in the amount of chronic disease in our society and the improvement in the technology of medicine and surgery.

J.D. Beasley and J.J. Swift, in their classic book *The Kellogg Report: The Impact of Nutrition, Environment and Lifestyle on the Health of Americans*, observe that "adults today may be living a couple of years longer than our ancestors, but we're still being cut down before our time." We are not "doing better than ever" – we are simply being killed off by disease at slightly later points in our lives. The irony is that these diseases are a product of our own living patterns. To quote former U.S. Health, Education, and Welfare (HEW) Secretary Joseph Califano, "I can compress what we have learned about the causes of these modern killers in three summarizing sentences: We are killing ourselves by our own careless habits. We are killing ourselves by carelessly polluting the environment. We are killing ourselves by permitting harmful social conditions to persist – conditions like poverty, hunger, and ignorance – which destroy health, especially in infants and children." He also reported, "while death from the major acute infections and diseases plummeted between 1900 and 1970, the proportion of mortality from major chronic disease, such as heart disease, cancer and stroke, increased more than 250%."

Panacea or Bioindividual Diet?

In this book, we provide the kind of information we think most people want in order to select foods that are good for them, but not necessarily good for everyone. This will not be a panacea diet in the sense that one diet will be good for every person.

Diet books often become bestsellers. We have no quarrel with any diet books, even with panacea diets, except when these diets are prescribed to be followed by everyone. They ignore the most important principle or law of nutrition: we are all different. Most diet books advise us what to eat and the various combinations of food we can try. These diets may be very specialized, very restrictive, and often feature how the authors respond to the foods they prefer. There are high-fat and low-fat diet books. There are high-protein and low-carbohydrate diet books. There are diet books featuring high fiber and low fiber intake. Acid-base and blood-type diets. Vegetarian diet books and meat lovers diet books. But these diets often ignore individuality – and they ignore the presence of food allergies or toxic reactions.

The diet we recommend will be discovered by each person in a scientific way, a diet which is, therefore, individualized or tailor-made and which, once discovered, will need only minor adjustments with changing circumstances. It will be a panacea *method* that can be applied by almost everyone. We have found it very useful in advising thousands of patients how to determine their own optimum diet. It can be mastered fairly easily. After that, patients are armed against the cure-all diets appearing on the scene at regular intervals, and they are able to maintain their health with little need to consult physicians. We are dependent on food all of our lives, so it is best if our food is enjoyable and leaves us feeling not only full but also good.

Triangular or Square Meals?

Very few popular diets stress that the most important objective of eating is to provide the calories needed for us to function, to grow, and to repair. Many diets restrict calories or concentrate calorie intake in one meal. This is not healthy, as registered dietitian Miriam Hoffer has shown in her book, *Fuelling Body, Mind and Spirit: A Balanced Approach to Healthy Eating.*

Hoffer distinguishes a 'triangular' diet from a 'square' or 'rectangular' diet. In the triangular diet, little is eaten at breakfast, with most calorie intake concentrated at dinner and in evening snacks. Prolonged eating in this ways often results in the triangular or pyramid body shape characteristic of very obese individuals. Triangular people are much heavier around the waist and hips. Men are often apple shaped and women pear shaped.

In a triangular diet, breakfast is at the apex. Food intake is slight or nonexistent. During the day food intake increases, reaching its maximum at dinner, when the most calories are consumed, and continues until bedtime. Nature surely must find this ironic: the individual consumes no food when it is most needed in getting ready for daily expenditure of energy, then eats the most when it is least needed for energy in the evening. Nature is eminently more sensible, having had billions of years during which to erect its laws, and surely wants a steady source of energy. An even supply of calories from food spread over the day is essential for optimum health.

> **By following a rectangular diet plan, you can actually eat more and lose weight at the same time, a happy conundrum for people wanting to manage their weight.**

The more sensible diet plan is rectangular. Healthy men and women fit more comfortably into a rectangular form than do the overweight and obese. In the rectangular form, most men are slightly larger around their shoulders compared to their hips, suggesting the consumption of a hearty breakfast, and most women are slightly larger around their hips, suggesting the consumption of three balanced meals. About one-third of the total daily need for calories should be provided by each of the three meals.

The key meal for optimum health is breakfast, the meal that is most neglected in modern Western culture. In North America, the popular 'continental' breakfast consists of coffee or tea with sugar, served with sweetened white flour baked into an appealing and tasty pastry. Toast and coffee does not constitute a healthy breakfast, yet it is the most common breakfast among our patients. A good breakfast should be more like the old style English breakfast with juice or fruit, cereal and milk, some bread and some high protein food, like ham or bacon.

By following a rectangular diet plan, you can actually eat more and lose weight at the same time, a happy conundrum for people wanting to manage their weight. When you eat a good breakfast to start the day, you will not be as hungry as the day progresses and will likely eat less at dinner and before bedtime. When placed on the rectangular diet, many of our overweight patients are surprised to find they are not nearly as hungry as they formerly were. Eating more frequently also increases calorie consumption. People consuming a diet of 2,000 calories daily in one meal at dinner will gain weight, whereas the same calorie intake spread over three meals will not result in the same weight gain. It appears that the body is more effective at processing food when it does not get overloaded at one meal.

When otherwise healthy patients want to reduce their weight, we always counsel them that being fit is more important than weight loss – and then advise them to become rectangular in their eating habits. Most are surprised how much better they feel.

Feast or Famine?

When the day starts with no food at breakfast, the body goes into a famine mode in order to preserve life, seeking to compensate with a feast. When the body gorges on a feast at dinner, it stores fat for the next famine. And so the feast or famine cycle turns. The effects of this cycle on our health are significant, especially so when the food we feast on is predominantly 'empty' calories.

Our modern diet is characterized as a continuous feast, but largely on calories, not on the essentials nutrients needed for these calories to be used efficiently in our body. This is another dilemma we face in our current healthcare system. While living in Western society we are seldom subject to the malnutrition from starvation that our ancestors experienced or third-world societies still suffer, but we are prone to malnutrition from a deficiency of essential nutrients. We need a diet that not only supplies adequate calories over the course of the day, but also provides adequate vitamins, minerals, amino acids, and essential fatty acids. In a word, we need a nutrient-rich naturopathic diet for optimum health.

② | TOWARD A NATURAL DIET

There are many people who are well and, therefore, do not need to modify their diet. They, obviously, have found the diet to which they are adapted. Any modification of their diet would likely reduce their state of health if it were continued for a long time. So the question is, how can you find out for yourself if you have good health or whether your health can be made better by changing the food consumed? There are two sides to this question, one short term, the other long term. Are you well now? Will you be well many years from now? In our view, your state of health ought to be so good that there is no deterioration toward the end of your life.

Are You Healthy?

Most people know when they are in good health. They are able to feel rested and relaxed after 6 to 8 hours of sleep. They awaken in the morning feeling well and looking forward to the day. They enjoy the food they eat. At work or at home, they have enough energy to do what they want to do, and they do not become excessively tired even in the evening. They will carry on with the day without becoming excessively sleepy or tired in the mid morning or mid afternoon, an indication that food allergies are not present. During the day and later on at home, they will remain in good humor, free of depression, unless there is something that would depress any other normal person, such as the loss of an idea, loss of a job, death of a friend or family member, or any other major disappointment. When they do feel sad, this will in time clear as it does for normal people. They will not suffer prolonged deep depression long after the event that precipitated it has passed. They will enjoy their work or profession, or if it cannot be enjoyed, they will tolerate it and find other activities to make up for what they are not getting from their work. They will make decisions that are rational most of the time. They are able to deal with stress. When they get sick, they recover in fewer days than do most people who are not well. If this is their state of health, they are, in our opinion, in good health.

Criteria for Evaluating Your Health

We use four main criteria for evaluating the state of health of our patients:

1. Are they free of signs and symptoms of ill-health or disease?
2. Are they getting on reasonably well with the family?
3. Are they getting on reasonably well with the community?
4. Are they working, either at home or on the job?

We define work as any activity that a person does, whether or not they are being paid to do it. If our patients fail to achieve even one of these four main points, we do not consider them well.

Evaluating Your Health

To evaluate your own health, you should consider the following questions:

1. Do I have enough energy to do what I want to do or am I suffering from too much fatigue? Am I tired too much of the time, especially when it is not appropriate to be tired?
2. Is my mood fairly stable with swings into depression or cheerfulness appropriate to events? Is my mood considered appropriate by other people in similar circumstances?
3. Do I have symptoms that indicate I might be suffering from any disease?

If you do not have any known health condition, you should then determine whether you are suffering from one of the many forms of malnutrition, from a defect arising from poor diet, from a vitamin or mineral deficiency, or from any one of the nutrient dependencies.

If you are well, not much needs to be done. Either you are already on a good diet, to which you have been adapted, or you have such a marvelous constitution and biochemistry that you can remain well even on a less perfect diet. Your only concern is for the future. It would be wise to tighten up the diet by following the nutritional laws and principles described in this book and to supplement this by taking the optimum amount of vitamin C and a good B-complex vitamin preparation. Many people are surprised after they have been following this vitamin program for several months how much better they feel.

In our view, your state of health ought to be so good that there is no deterioration toward the end of your life.

Many years ago a high-school teacher came to our office with his identical twin schizophrenic brother. His brother had been ill for many years and was not able to work. We prescribed vitamin B-3 and vitamin C for him and arranged to see him regularly to follow his progress. Several months later the 'normal' brother asked us whether he could take the same vitamins. We assured him that he could. He had seen great improvement in his schizophrenic twin and wondered what the supplements might do for him. A few months later, he told us that he had always considered himself well, but when he realized how much better he felt on the vitamins, he knew that he had not been as well as he had thought he was.

We have seen the same realization in families where the mother and/or wife became our patient. We would advise her to follow a good diet, usually by eliminating sugar and junk and very often milk plus any other food she might be allergic to. We would outline which vitamins she ought to take. Very often the husband, who was well, did not want to give up sweets and desserts, and our patient did not want to deprive him of these. However, after many months of preparing two sets of meals, one for herself and one for the rest of the family, she would decide to place the whole family on her diet, primarily because she was now well. In most cases, she would gradually decrease the sweets program and eventually would have the whole family on her diet. We would then hear from her how much healthier the whole family was. The husband was more energetic, less irritable, and more relaxed. If the husband were with her, he would cheerfully admit the change in himself and how he had resisted changing. Our patient would often tell us that the whole family had the flu or a severe cold and she had remained well. In the past, she had developed the same virus infections as they had.

If you are not well, be sure to see your family doctor for a medical check up, especially if you suspect you are experiencing the symptoms of any disease. Anything you and your doctor find must be corrected. After that, you should follow a procedure of improving your diet and adding the correct supplements. It is desirable to do this with medical supervision, but you may find it very difficult to find a physician or nutritionist able to advise you. If you cannot find a physician, read everything you can about how to do so.

Four Steps to Optimum Health

Every person, no matter how well they feel, can determine very easily how well they really are by placing themselves on the natural diet recommended in this book, with or without supplements. To discover your optimum diet, we recommend the following 4-step program:

Step 1. Eliminate all the junk from your diet, especially all the free sugars, and any food you suspect you might be allergic to. Take vitamin C, 1 gram after each meal. Stay on this diet for at least 1 month. If by then you feel well, this is your diet. If you are not any better or have gained only a little, examine your diet again for other possible food allergies, including allergies to dairy products and processed protein. Then eliminate them and carry on for another month. If you cannot find any other food allergies, go to step 2.

Step 2. Supplement your diet with a good vitamin B-complex tablet or one of the stress tablets. We recommend the B-complex 50 or 100 preparations. You can take as many as you wish, but in most cases 1 to 3 tablets per day will be adequate. These all contain riboflavin or vitamin B-2, which will color the urine yellow. This is a good test whether or not the vitamins are being absorbed in the gastrointestinal tract. Stay on this program for several months. If you have not reached the state of well being you want, then start to add other individual vitamins, minerals, and fatty acids. The main objective of this book is to describe these nutrients and how to use them well enough so that you can use them with safety. All these nutrients are compatible and can be taken together, usually with food in the stomach. Nutrients are compatible with all medication and with each other.

Step 3. For the rest of your life keep reviewing both your diet and the supplements you are taking because requirements change with age, with sickness, and with degree of stress. Be aware of the changes in you and adjust your diet accordingly. There is a constant need to maintain the adjustment between your needs and the food you eat.

Step 4. If you are still not well, you probably have very serious problems and will have to consult specialists in the field of naturopathic or orthomolecular medicine.

From this book, you should be able to determine if you are suffering from one of the many forms of malnutrition, from a health defect arising from poor diet, from a vitamin or mineral deficiency, or from any one of the nutrient dependencies. You should be able to discover a diet that will lead you out of our current dilemmas in nutrition into a new age of optimum health.

THE HEALTH COSTS OF
THE HIGH-TECH DIET

③ | THE JUNK FOOD ERA

The reason why we need to eat for the best health is so obvious it should not have to be restated. Nature has spent millions of years perfecting animals and plants so that they can extract the best from other plants and animals that make up our food. The primary objective of life is to perpetuate itself; survival is essential, at least until the species has passed reproductive age and the genes of the elderly are no longer needed for species survival. Animals are, therefore, endowed with senses that help them to identify potential food and with enough logic to decide when they should try to obtain these foods. These foods must be harmless and also must be nourishing if the animal is to live and reproduce.

Vomit Reflex

But how can animals decide which foods are the ones best for them? Obviously, they have done a better job of this than we have in the modern age of high-tech food. They have done this by judging the quality of the food by the impact it has on their health. The effect of eating the food may be immediate, within a few minutes or hours, or it may require weeks or months before it becomes evident. The immediate effect of toxic food has been examined by scientists, who have found that there is a powerful gag and vomiting reflex. When animals eat something that is highly toxic for them, and if it can be identified by its bad taste or by some other attribute, the animal will no longer eat that particular food.

Attempts have been made to manipulate this natural reflex to control the appetite of natural predators for farm animals. Lithium salts have been placed in sheep's meat and scattered in areas where natural predators live. The encounter between the predator, a fox or coyote, and the salted meat has been filmed. The animal ate the meat with relish but shortly after became violently ill with retching and vomiting. Thereafter, the predator would no longer eat sheep's meat. When the same animal found other sheep's meat, it would turn away apparently in disgust. It was hoped that this would produce the same aversion to living sheep as it had to their poisoned flesh. Conventional wisdom says that if you are going to poison rats, you had better put in enough poison so that they are killed the first time. The survivors will not eat the same bait again if it can be identified by taste or smell or some other attribute.

> **The survival or vomiting reflex may be written as a rule or law of natural nutrition: Avoid any food that makes you sick or that is psychologically disgusting to you.**

Human beings have the same survival reflex, though the creators of our modern high-tech foods have so successfully masked potentially poisonous products with flavors and other additives that this reflex is often delayed or deadened. Many years ago, a mother brought two of her sons to see us. One was adopted. Both were 7 years old, both suffered from severe hyperactivity, and both were having learning difficulties. We suspected that the amount of sugar and junk food they were eating was a factor and advised the two children and their mother that they should go onto a sugar-free diet.

The two children were horrified. A month later, one child was well and the other remained as hyperactive as he had been before. The boy who was well had been following the diet, while the other refused to do so. He told us in no uncertain terms that he would never ever stop eating sugar and stamped his foot to emphasize his decision. We then advised them to go on to plan B. They both asked us what was plan B, expecting something even worse. We asked them, "Would you follow the no sugar diet on week days if you could have all the junk you wanted on Saturday?" They both agreed. When they came back after another month, both boys were well. Their mother then told us what had happened.

In preparation for 'junk-food' Saturday, they had gone to a store. The boy who had been cooperative before was very upset because his brother was going to get all those sweets. His mother agreed he could also go onto the same program. But then the five other children in the family complained that they were being left out. Mother finally said the whole family could do so. The following Saturday, one of the children became violently ill with nausea and vomiting after consuming sweets. Pretty soon every child in that family was sick with headaches, nausea, or vomiting. After that, the little boy who had been so determined he would never give up sweets told me, adamantly, that he would never ever eat sweets again.

The survival or vomiting reflex may be written as a rule or law of natural nutrition: Avoid any food that makes you sick or that is psychologically disgusting to you.

Food Sense

We use our senses to identify potentially offensive food, and our experiences and beliefs determine whether we will vomit when we consume that food. Smell and taste are the most important senses involved in this survival reflex. Smell forewarns the person that the food may be toxic. Bad smelling foods are generally not liked unless long experience with that bad smell has convinced the person that the food is not toxic. This would apply to very ripe cheeses and other odoriferous foods. Smell warns one even when the food is many feet away. Smell will, of course, also foretell that good food is available, if that smell is associated with food a person has enjoyed. If the food passes the odor test and is placed in one's mouth, taste becomes the next arbiter. But taste also depends to a large degree on the sense of smell. That is why people with plugged noses, with colds or allergies, will not have the same sense of taste as when they are well. In the same way, people deficient in zinc will lose their ability to both taste and smell foods.

The four basic tastes are bitter, sour, salty, and sweet. Usually foods that are bitter are not liked. Alkaloids tend to taste bitter and are poisonous. Animals have learned early on that these foods are best avoided. Plants defending themselves against being consumed will form these bitter tasting substances. Nicotine was developed by the tobacco plant to protect itself against predators, not for the enjoyment and destruction of people.

The sour (acid) and salty tastes are accepted or rejected, depending on the concentrations of compounds present in the food and therefore on the intensity of the taste. Very sour foods will be rejected, but lesser degrees of acidity may make the food very desirable. Many people love very sour pickles, for example. Excessive sourness is a warning sign to which people pay attention. The same applies to salty foods. Some love excessive amounts of salt. This is one of the factors in the current high incidence of high blood pressure and hypertension.

The almost universally liked taste is sweetness. These foods are usually safe to eat because they contain no bitter and poisonous compounds. There is an optimum concentration of the sugars, which varies tremendously. Some love excessive amounts. It is not uncommon for many people, especially alcoholics, to add enough sugar to their coffee to make it a saturated solution with crystals left in the bottom. Others cannot tolerate this much. People who have been on a sugar-free or low-sugar diet long enough generally develop a dislike for too much sweetness in their foods. Even a quarter teaspoon of sugar in coffee or tea is cloyingly sweet.

Foods that are bland are also acceptable and preferred by many. Bland foods include breads, potatoes, rice, and all the cereals. A bland food can be consumed in large amounts without satiating the person, and they can be used as carriers for other foods, such as gravy, jam, and butter. When bland foods taste bitter or salty or sour, they will be quickly rejected unless it is known that products have been added to impart this quality to the food.

Sugar Addiction

Almost all the overly processed foods contain sugar. The amount present in some foods will surprise many. Thus, catsup contains 30% sugar. Some breakfast cereals have more sugar in them than do chocolate bars, containing more than 50% sugar. The love for sweetness is so great it makes sugar the best addicting drug we have today.

Overly processed food contains lots of sugar for two reasons: sugar masks the bland taste of overly processed foods (tends to remove the natural flavors of the original raw food) and is addicting. If there are two competing pea soups made by different companies, the one with the most sugar in it will sell the best. There is an advantage to the bottom line if one can sell sugar in the product at the price of beans or peas when the price of sugar is low enough.

There are a number of sugars. Food additives ending with "ose" are sugars, such as sucrose (table sugar), lactose (milk sugar), fructose, glucose, maltose, and so on. If companies want to avoid the intent of labeling laws, they will use several different sugars so that these sugars can be printed further from the beginning of the label. By law, if sugar is the major ingredient, it must be listed first. If, however, one uses three different sugars, each one will be listed further on. It is thus possible to have a product that is 60% sugar, but none of the sugars will appear first since individually these are not the major components.

> Once people see and feel the connection between what they eat and how they feel – once the original survival mechanism has been reactivated – there is very little further difficulty in following what we call the No Sugar Law: Eliminate foods with sugar additives from your diet.

Sugar is the pervasive food additive, present in almost all processed food, which also contains a number of other food additives to create 'desirable' properties of taste, color, odor, consistency, stability, or ability to be emulsified. They are *not* added to enhance the nutritional quality of the food. Indeed, food additives, especially sugar, can be harmful to good health. When given an additional amount of sugar, a person eating large amounts of sugar of one type or another daily will not react adversely to it, but the sugar may be causing a large number of pathological reactions in the body that are chronic. Excessive eating of sugar causes sharp reactions in many people when they have become allergic to it. They will consume a quantity of sugar or even binge on it. This is followed by a feeling of well-being, which may last several hours, and this in turn is followed by a major or minor slump into depression and fatigue. We have seen patients who would go into a hypomanic state for 3 to 4 days after a sugar binge, followed by a major depression lasting many days. When they eat large amounts every day, this effect upon their mood is masked by the general ill health from which they suffer.

In order to reactivate the connection between the intake of the substance and the reaction of the body, it is necessary to eliminate the product from that person's diet for at least 5 days, sometimes for up to 1 month. At the end of that time, the immune system has recovered to the extent that if one then consumes the sugar, there will be a sharp reaction. This will be apparent to the person and certainly to family members in close proximity. It is especially notable with children. Once people see and feel the connection between what they eat and how they feel – once the original survival mechanism has been reactivated – there is very little further difficulty in following what we call the No Sugar Law: Eliminate foods with sugar additives from your diet.

Other Addictive Additives

Overly processed foods are rich not only in sugar but also in fats, salt, and other additives with xenobiotic or foreign flavors. It is important to make the final product taste and smell good, but the original appetizing characteristics of the food are destroyed by the processing. The manufacturers give a new flavor to that food by adding all these additives. Many people can only recognize the sensations of sweetness or saltiness. When they are placed upon a sugar-free diet, which usually also removes the other additives, they will remark many months later how good other food tastes again, something they had forgotten over the years.

Foods to which an animal has not adapted or foods containing toxins that do not kill immediately produce chronic ill health. An example would be the placing of arsenic in one's food in small amounts. Arsenic tastes sweet and is, therefore, not detectable by taste or smell. Over weeks and months, it will make the person quite ill. This was at one time a favorite method for poisoning enemies. These toxic or poisonous foods do not alarm us since there is no way the senses can alert them to the danger. Modern high-tech food removes the natural ability of our senses to warn us about the lack of nutrition of the food because all these foods are made too sweet, too salty, and too flavorful with xenobiotic flavoring agents. This is why the majority of people have no idea that the food they buy and consume does not nourish them and is mainly responsible for a large number of chronic diseases.

Infants learn basic nutrition from their parents as they graduate from milk to solid foods as soon as their digestive apparatus is capable of dealing with them. They learn by observing what their parents eat and by eating food brought to them by their parents. They will also experiment with food tastes, avoiding the ones that taste too unusual or taste bitter. They will learn by being made sick by eating certain foods. However, they will not draw the connection between taste and health when eating toxic food that has a low level of toxicity, but will make them just as sick over a period of months or years. Only from their parents, teachers, or doctors can they learn this connection and thus eliminate low-level toxic food from their diet.

> The major problem with modern food technology is that it has destroyed our senses as good indicators for what foods are safe and nutritious and for what foods are not.

Man has been pretty good at discovering the 100 or so different plants we can use as food from the many thousands of plants that could have been food but are either poisonous, toxic, or not nourishing. Until the beginning of modern food technology about 10,000 years ago, we did pretty well. All the foods culled from the much larger total potential supply were nourishing. We did not have to worry about balanced diets, since all these foods, no matter in what combination they were used, were inherently well balanced. The balance was destroyed from foods after the introduction of food technology, especially its development over the past 50 years. Until the dawn of agriculture, we did not have to use our intellect to eat well. Our main problem was to obtain enough food. What was available was nutritious. We suffered food shortages and often starvation, and as we moved to colder climates began to suffer from annual epidemics of scurvy. Fruits and fresh vegetation were not available in those times. Today, we have too much food. We no longer are worried about starvation in highly industrialized nations, but we now have a major problem deriving good nutrition from the depleted quality of our food. We live with an abundance of low quality food which we eat indiscriminately and which makes most of us chronically sick. We have arrived at the time in our evolution when we can no longer depend upon our senses and have to depend upon our intelligence and knowledge to select only those foods to which we have been adapted and which will keep us well as long as we are alive. The major problem with modern food technology is that it has destroyed our senses as good indicators for what foods are safe and nutritious and for what foods are not.

Raw, Cooked, Refined, and Processed Foods

Our modern high-tech diets have been developing over the past 10,000 years, but the pace of change has accelerated sharply over the past 50 years. We have the same genetic structure our ancestors had 10,000 years ago, but the food supply today is totally different from what it was then. The change in our food supply has been so rapid that it has been impossible for evolution to keep pace. Most of the diseases endemic to high-tech societies arise from this maladjustment between our long-developed adaptation to our environment and our contemporary nutritional habits, between ourselves and our food.

Our relationships to our food can be divided into four major eras. Each succeeding era is shorter than the preceding one. The last one, the junk-food era, is probably 100 years old, merely a second in the time required for our culture to develop. Each era represents an accelerated transformation of our diet, completely outstripping our ability to adapt.

The 'Raw' Era

During this era, man must have had the same foods as any other primates. We were hunters and gatherers, depending primarily on vegetable food and supplementing this with animal foods that could be caught. It is unlikely we lived in the cold polar regions since fire had not been discovered. This means we had access to vegetables year round and so did not suffer from spring scurvy so common more recently in Europe. Nor did we suffer from vitamin D-3 deficiency due to lack of exposure to the sun. Starvation was more of a problem than malnutrition. Obesity must have been extremely rare.

The 'Cooked' Era

With the discovery of fire, man began to cook food, especially the animals that could be dismembered and cut up with newly-discovered cutting utensils or knives. The advent of cooking was on the whole beneficial to health. It made it easier to digest certain vegetables and softened animal food, thus requiring less work in eating. It also destroyed insects and parasites, thus decreasing infectious diseases.

Cooking did not necessarily make food more palatable, for palatability is a matter of experience. Excluding the bitter tasting foods, people enjoy food that tastes like food they have enjoyed in their infancy and youth. People who are used to eating raw, fresh meat will continue to enjoy this meat. We, who are accustomed to cooked meat in appearance, texture, and taste, find raw meat repulsive. But it cannot be concluded that cooking has made our food more palatable.

An old documentary compared the eating habits of native people in the South Pacific to our modern Western habits. Two teen-aged girls were walking along the beach. Suddenly, one girl pounced on the sand, drew out a long wriggling worm, and with obvious relish ate it on the spot, much as a North American teenager might enjoy a hamburger or an ice cream cone.

There are many disadvantages to cooking. Heat alters the natural state of food and makes it less nutritious, less able to support life. Proteins are denatured. Their structure is altered so that enzymes designed to digest living protein tissue now must work on denatured tissue. Amino acids recombine into new peptides, which may be harder to digest, or they may combine with sugar to form brown substances. The outside of a broiled or fried steak or a roast is brown for this reason. Unsaturated fats are oxidized by heat and essential fatty acids are destroyed. Starches are made more digestible, but sugars are oxidized. Heat labile vitamins, such as vitamins C and E, are destroyed. Cooking is usually a combination of heat and water. Hot water dissolves more of the water-soluble constituents, such as sugar, vitamins, minerals, and amino acids. These are usually lost as the cooking water is often discarded.

On balance, cooking was probably beneficial during the 'prechemical' stage of nutrition, for chemical additives were not available and thus could not react with food during the cooking process.

The Agricultural Era

About 10,000 years ago, the introduction of herding and cropping secured a stable supply of large quantities of food and made man less dependent on gathering and hunting in the wild. There was no change in food technology except for storage. It was now possible to store grain for several years. In the bible, Joseph advised the Pharaoh to store a 7-year supply of grain in preparation for the 7-year drought he predicted.

Agriculture forced a change in social habits, from a wandering, nomadic existence to the development of large cities. Territorial needs were changed from sparsely occupied areas with few interactions with others to huge, over-crowded, over-concentrated areas we know as modern cities.

Increasing food supply did not decrease our workload; likely the opposite came about. Agriculture is not an easy occupation. Farmers work hard and require a lot of food, probably much more than did the earlier gatherers and hunters. Did the story of Adam and Eve and their banishment into the real world signify the transition from hunting and gathering to agriculture? It has been estimated that hunters and gatherers were able to obtain enough food for their needs by working only 2 hours a day.

Primitive agriculture probably did not reduce the variety of food available; on the contrary, newer varieties of foods were probably selected and cropped. Modern agriculture has, of course, done the opposite because of its heavy reliance on single, high-yielding varieties. Another consequence of agriculture was the increased use of yeast in food. Man has domesticated yeast for production of alcoholic beverages and making bread. Or has the yeast species domesticated man to become a supplier of sugar and simple carbohydrates, both inside and outside of the body?

The Chemical Era

Agriculture provided a stable supply of meat and cereals – barley, rice, wheat, corn, oats. It is impossible to visualize the huge populations on earth without this remarkable supply of food. People have lived primarily on whole-grain foods supplemented with small amounts of fish and meat. Cereals are easily grown, yield reliably, are easy to harvest, transport, and store. They retain the most important quality of foods – they are whole and alive. They can be ground, baked, cooked into a variety of foods, and sprouted. Of these, breads and cakes are the most important.

White Bread

Ground grain has been used for making bread for thousands of years. These breads have ranged in quality from heavy whole-grain bread to whiter, less heavy breads, but the technology for developing the pure white, fluffy, cottony, modern bread had not been invented. Grain could

> Today, the majority of people eat the poorest fraction of the wheat in their bread and pasta and feed the most nutritious parts to their animals.

be ground, but only after the invention of the modern steel roller mill and accurate silk screens was it possible to separate wheat into coarse bran and germ, less coarse middlings, and the pure, fine, white flour, the endosperm, from which we make our white bread. Grinding and separating cereal components is the basis for much of our present food technology.

Grinding was an important discovery because it made it possible to digest foods that formerly could not be digested. Sifting out the most nutritious portion of the grain to create while flour became fashionable for the wealthier classes. The poor, slaves, and peasants had to be content with whole-meal grain. They were, of course, lucky and must have been healthier than their masters and superiors. But even the whitest of flour was still not as white as is modern flour because the sieves to screen out the bran and germ particles were discovered only about 300 years ago. Today, the majority of people eat the poorest fraction of the wheat in their bread and pasta and feed the most nutritious parts to their animals.

Fermentation

Fermentation was also discovered several thousand years ago and was used to make alcoholic beverages. By the time the Old Testament was written, wine was a staple of many diets and drunkenness was described. Pure sugar was unknown, but honey was liked and harvested when it was located. The crystallization of sucrose from sugar cane juices became established about 300 years ago. Pure white sugar was very expensive during the rule of Queen Elizabeth. Average annual consumption in England was 5 lb per person per year. The Queen was a sugar junky, and this probably rotted her teeth, making it essential for her to have iron plates. This could have accounted for her irritable personality later on in life. Today, in England the consumption of all the sugars (sugar cane, sugar beet, and the syrups) runs close to 130 lb per person per year. This is an average figure, including infants. Therefore, 50% of the population eats much more than 130 lb. The diet of some teenagers is 50% pure sugars.

Fractions

As chemists became more skillful, they discovered how to break foods down into its major components or fractions – carbohydrates, fats, and proteins. In 1900, it was believed that knowing the composition of foods in terms of these three major components was the basis for fashioning a 'perfect' diet. Many doctors thought that infant foods made only from carbohydrate starches, fat, and protein would be adequate to ensure good health. This notion was so popular in England that many of children died when they did not breast-feed or have wet nurses to supply other nutrients. By 1900, white bread and pure sugar had massively displaced whole grain cereals as food staples in high-tech societies.

This trend accelerated in the 20th century. Dr Ross Hume Hall, in his book *Food for Naught: The Decline in Nutrition*, estimates that since the Second World War, consumption of overly processed food has increased from 25% of the total food intake to more than 75%. This provides an estimate of the invasion of our food by chemistry, which has made our food less nutritious, if not harmful to our health.

Chemical Additives

Besides the nutritional disadvantages of cooking and refining foods, the modern high-tech diet is less nutritional because of chemical additives. Of the deleterious factors in overly processed foods, the use of additives is among the worst. Additives are small quantities of chemicals used to impart special properties to the final food preparation. They are designed to impart taste, to preserve, to color, or to emulsify. The number of chemicals used for these purposes runs into the thousands. Governments allow them to be used on the basis that when tested on animals individually they appear to be non-lethal and non-toxic. But Dr Hall has shown that toxicity tests of individual chemicals do not provide a true measure of the toxicity of a large number of chemicals present in food consumed for many years. An animal may survive one or two chemicals, but each additional one throws an additional burden on the body's defense systems.

The body defends itself against chemicals by converting them to less toxic substances – by eliminating them in expired air, in urine, in feces, in sweat or by depositing them in skin and its appendages, hair and nails. The so-called theory of a toxic dose means that a dose below this level is non-toxic, that there is a 'safe' level. This is no longer considered true for many compounds, and even when it is true, the safe level may be so narrow it is meaningless. Also the safe levels will depend on the presence of other additives that are negative factors and on nutrients protecting the body. Thus, fiber and ascorbic acid protect animals against the toxic effect of cadmium. A diet deficient in fiber and low in ascorbic acid will enhance the toxic effect of additives. Another problem is that additives will combine with food under the influence of heat to form new, unnatural compounds. The toxicity of these has not been studied carefully.

We can minimize the amount of trace additives in our food by avoiding overly processed foods whenever it is possible and by using processed foods that have undergone the least amount of processing.

Negative additives may be divided into two main groups: cosmetic additives and trace additives. Cosmetic additives include all the additives known to be present and permitted by law. They are used to alter taste, color, consistency, or stability and often include sugar as a bulk additive, which is used because it perpetuates the addiction to sugar. These cosmetic additives do not enhance the nutritional quality of the food; on the contrary, they undoubtedly diminish it. We may need a simple law that treats every processed food product as a drug. Before a drug can be released on prescription, it must be shown to be safe and effective for what is claimed it can do. If we applied the same idea to overly processed foods, we would have a much healthier society.

Assume the product was the ubiquitous French fries. According to this non-existent law, French fries would be fed to one group of growing animals, fresh potatoes to another. If the rate of growth on both sets of animals was identical, one could claim that commercial French fries are as nutritious as whole fresh, living potatoes. If animals on French fries grew half as fast, they would be labeled as having 50% of the nutritional quality of the original food. Each overly processed food would carry in the label this mark of quality, as well as a list of the additives. This living test of food quality is the only way to measure the impact of processing on the product.

Trace additives are not listed on the food label because the manufacturer either does not know they are there or because there is no legal requirement that they be listed. Every organic chemist knows that it is impossible to synthesize an absolutely pure compound. One of the most expensive chemicals is pure water. Whenever any chemical is made, it contains traces of the other chemicals that were used in making it. Sugar is made from cane or beet, and the final product is remarkably pure, perhaps 99.9% pure. Yet that 0.01% which is not sugar does contain traces of every chemical used in making it, as well as traces of the natural products present in the original food. The same principle applies to every synthesized compound. Every chemical that enters any plant in the food production line, from the farmer to the store, is present in trace amounts somewhere in the food.

A manufacturer who buys sugar to make a syrup or a pastry may know the product contains these traces and may not like it, but there is no requirement that it be listed or even detected. These trace additives are not added for any special reason. They are the contaminants from the process converting natural food into overly processed food.

Toxicologists believe that these trace quantities are too low to be significant, but they have not proven this. If a person consumes 200 g of sugar per day, he will also consume 0.02 g (20 mg) of these contaminants per day. We have drugs that are highly active in these quantities; this amount of Haldol, a major tranquilizer, would keep most people totally incapacitated, and one-tenth of one milligram of LSD will incapacitate most normal people for up to one day. We know Haldol and LSD are not present in sugar, but the principle remains – we must not assume these small quantities are inactive.

We can minimize the amount of trace additives in our food by avoiding overly processed foods whenever it is possible and by using processed foods that have undergone the least amount of processing. Thus, rolled oats is nearly as good as whole oats and is much healthier than any sugared cereal with an oat base.

There is also a class of additives that can be said to be helpful. The added substances enhance the nutritional quality of the final product. These positive additives are primarily nutrients, such as minerals and vitamins. Enriched white flour is better than ordinary white flour, but is not as nutritious as whole-wheat flour. The use of nutrient additives allows companies to make claims for the nutritional value of their products, which are dubious, if not false. Chemically treated food is also claimed to be less expensive, easier to store, and less time-consuming to prepare. The first claim is, on close examination, seldom true. Today, a pound of wheat costing less than 10 cents to the farmer, perhaps 25 cents to the purchaser, will yield many more breakfasts than the same wheat converted into a cereal for over one dollar. The second advantage is real. Overly processed food can be stored much longer and can be used to provide food when natural supplies are low. There are significant detrimental effects of storage on the nutrient content of the food, however. Less work is required to prepare the food. It is easier to buy bread than to bake it, easier to heat up a prepared meal than to make it from scratch. Convenience foods have made it easier for women to join the workforce and for both parents to hold down jobs. The nutrient quality of the food prepared for their children and themselves has deteriorated, however.

Dead, Stale, Toxic . . .

Another way to understand the differences between a 'primitive' or pure diet and a modern or high-tech diet is to compare them using this table:

Primitive	High-tech
Whole	Artifact
Alive	Dead
Fresh	Stale
Varied	Monotonous
Non-Toxic	Toxic
Scarce	Abundant
Endogenous	Exogenous
Natural Flavor	Synthetic
Simple	Complex

Artifact

Much modern high-tech food is *artifact*. By this we mean that foods are broken down to their constituent fractions, such as starch, sugars, fats, oils, and protein, and these are then recombined to make preparations that have the appearance of natural food but are not. For example, it is possible to buy tomato soup that contains no tomatoes, but, in appearance and flavor, would lead one to believe that it is really tomato soup. It is possible to buy overly processed cheese that has little of the original cheese in it, and overly processed fish or crab that appears to be crab. Only the bad odor before it is fried will give it away. It is possible to buy overly processed turkey that is turkey protein pressed out to look like slices of real turkey meat but isn't.

These artifacts are dangerous because they are made to look and to taste like food. The average person eating these foods would naturally assume that they are what they appear to be, yet they would not contain the nutrient quality that was present in the original food. Overly processed foods not only fool the senses of taste and smell, but they also make it impossible to judge the quality of the food by using the subterfuge of appearing to be real food. Artifacts are pseudo foods, preparations that are made up from a combination of artifacts or fractions of the original foods.

Dead

Much modern high-tech food is *dead*. Alive food does not store well. Animal products very quickly deteriorate due to oxidation, enzymatic activity, and decomposition by bacteria and fungi. These changes can be inhibited by freezing, drying, or cooking the products. Cooking will slow down the rate of decomposition. The food is also preserved by the addition of chemicals, which retard the growth of bacteria and fungi and which are antioxidants, thus retarding the oxidation of the food. Milk can be heat treated at such a high temperature that it is stable even at room temperature for a long time. It does not turn sour because the lactobacilli that ought to be present to sour the milk are destroyed. Modern bread has many chemicals that prevent it from aging and turning hard. Bread without these additives will be fresh one day and will be stale the second day. Canned foods can be stored for years, as can frozen foods. The least damaging way of storing food is to freeze it, followed by canning.

Removing the enzymes and the reducing compounds will decrease the rate at which these foods oxidize. Removing vitamins and minerals will discourage bacteria and fungi, which must also have these nutrients to grow. The more a food is deprived of nutrients, the more apt is that food to be stable. This is why starch extracted from wheat or potatoes is much more stable and can be stored much longer than the original plant material. But the price for the increase in stability is an equal decrease in the nutritional quality of those products. The price, however, is paid by the consumer, not by the high-tech industry that creates these long-lived stable foods. One of the aims of processing good food, such as wheat or oats, is to convert it to a final product that costs a lot more, is much more stable, tastes sweet – and is much more dangerous to our health. We increase the commercial value of products by converting good food into junk. In economic terms, this is considered to be value-added.

Stale

Stale is another quality of high-tech food. Most of what we have said about dead applies as well to this term. As a rule, overly processed food is both dead and stale.

Monotonous

The term *monotonous* refers to the limited variety of foods available to us. This will be surprising to shoppers who have not thought about it, especially when they are cruising around a supermarket with 15,000 to 20,000 different items on the shelves. They must think that we have an enormous variety of foods. But consider this: if the prepared breakfast section carries 50 different products, are we in fact having access to 50 different foods? We are not because they are all artifacts made from oats, wheat, rice, sugar, flavors, and other additives packaged in attractive boxes. Even if we eat a wide variety from each of the 50 items, we are still eating the same three grains and sugar.

A monotonous diet is responsible for many of the health problems present in high-tech societies. There are two reasons for this. First, there will be a shortage of vitamins, minerals, and essential fatty acids. A diet containing a variety of cereals, vegetables, fruit, and animal products is much more apt, even if only because of chance, to provide an adequate amount of these essential nutrients. Second, a monotonous diet increases the probability of developing allergic reactions to foods.

Nutrient Shortage

For over 99% of man's existence on earth, there was no need to apply intelligence toward food selection. The only important fact was whether the food was poisonous or not. Among the foods found not to be poisonous, it was good enough to eat everything else provided there was ample variety available. Since there was no abundance of any one food, it was necessary to eat what was available from all the foods. Thus, primitive tribes living as hunters-gatherers would eat everything in their path that was edible. The variety depended on what was available in their community and varied from morning to night, from week to week, from season to season. Variety, combined with the absence of high-tech food products, was adequate to maintain a reasonable state of health.

> A monotonous diet is responsible for many of the health problems present in high-tech societies.

Studies of the natives of the Kalihari desert show this process. Previously nomadic, these people have been forced into villages, their lifestyle has been altered, and they have been introduced to the limited monotonous high-tech diet. There has been a remarkable deterioration in their health.

We have seen the same phenomenon closer to home. About 50 years ago the average grocery store contained few items, often in bulk, chiefly vegetables, grains, and fruit. A person ignorant of nutrition could by chance purchase what would be needed to sustain good health. Suppose one were instructed to purchase 12 different items. The number of good items would be greater than the number of poor items nutritionally. That person could be healthy using those 12 items that had been selected at random, without any intellectual knowledge of which foods should be eaten or not. This is no longer possible in the modern supermarket. It was easier for the naive shopper to buy food that would maintain health 50 years ago than it is today. Out of the 15,000 items available, about 50 would be suitable to maintain health. The vast majority of items would not be nourishing since they are the product of the high-tech industry. About the only safe place in which to shop is around the walls of the supermarket, for that is where the vegetables and fruits, the meat and fish, the dairy products, much of the frozen goods, and the breads are found.

A combination of variety and good food is all that is needed for us to remain well. Our appetite will ensure that we eat a variety of food, for we tend to become satiated with too much of one food at one time. The body seems to have an instinctive revulsion at eating too much of anything unless, of course, that food has been corrupted by the addition of sugar, salt, and other additives so commonly used.

Allergic Reactions

The second reason for the ill effects of a monotonous diet is that the probability of developing allergic reactions to foods is directly related to the proportion of our diet occupied by that food. That is why most allergic reactions are to foods that are staples for that region. In England, tea allergies are more common than they are in the United States. In countries where rice is the main staple, there are more allergic reactions to rice. In wheat countries, wheat products are common allergens, and in countries where corn is used extensively and corn by-products are incorporated into prepared foods, corn allergy is common. In our practice, we have estimated that between 25% and 40% of patients have one or another type of dairy product allergy.

Allergic reactions to food can become evident at any time in life. Infants fed on formula (milk and sugar) often become allergic to both milk and sugar. They then may have symptoms like colic, frequent colds, runny noses, rashes, itches, and so on. Later these somatic symptoms may subside only to be replaced by behavioral changes and learning disorders. Many hyperactive and learning disordered children have dairy allergies. Wetting the bed is a very common milk allergy. Later in life, by the time they are adult, they may have developed an aversion to milk, but may be excessively fond of cheese.

Young people with a violent nature and who are often in trouble with the law have been found to eat excessive amounts of sugar and milk products. They are often very immature in their behavior; we have considered them as infants who have not yet been weaned from their milk. One such individual had for breakfast each morning a quart of Coca Cola and a quart of milk. Another middle-aged man, who had been in prison several years for assaulting a police officer, carried a quart bottle of concentrated sugar with him all the time. When he became tired, he would drink that solution. This indicates a food allergy is present. One of the treatments for food allergy is to rotate the diet, which means introducing variation into the diet.

Toxic

Modern high-tech foods are often *toxic*. By toxic we do not mean they contain poisons that will kill rapidly, but taken over long periods of time, years and decades, they produce a state of chronic ill health. Before additives can be incorporated into foods, they have to pass certain toxicity tests. The test may simply be one where the additive has been used for a long time and has apparently not made anyone ill. The modern test is to add the chemicals to the diet of animals and to determine the toxic dose, the so-called LD_{50}. This is the amount that will kill half the animals given the chemical over a period of time. The chemicals are also tested to determine whether they have any effect on the growth of young animals and whether they interfere with pregnancy or the development of the fetus.

These are usually short-term experiments. They are seldom given to animals over a major fraction of their lives, so they do not accurately test the effect of chronic use. A second objection is that additives are tested singly. When given in combinations, the toxic properties of these chemicals can be additive and probably are. Most high-tech foods contain more than two additives. Seldom is the exact mixture of the food used in tests to determine its long-term effect. The third objection to testing is that the additives are tested on animals that are fed properly. Laboratory animals are given nutritious food of the type they have adapted to. A healthy animal is better able to resist the toxic effects of chemicals. However, the diet for most people is inadequate and they are less able to cope with the chemicals present in their food. The major additive is sugar, followed by salt, but each person also consumes 5 lb of other chemicals each year in their food.

Abundant

Modern diets are *abundant;* more accurately, they are *excessive*. Before high-tech foods became available, the common problem facing mankind was starvation. We had adapted to this problem by developing mechanisms for storing extra calories that could be drawn on during these periods of inadequate food supply. It is much like the camel's ability to store water to be used when none is available. Usually, what food was available was of good quality. There simply was not enough.

Today, there is no starvation in high-tech societies, unless it is created by war and other man-made activities. There are many people who believe they are not getting enough food, but the proportion of our population that is too thin, suffers from protein-calorie deficiency, or from marasmus is very small. On the contrary, perhaps 25% of the population is overweight, even among people seeking extra food from community agencies. The problem in modern times is that there are too many calories and the foods carrying these calories are lacking in nutritional quality. They are short of vitamins, minerals, and fiber – and excessive in sugars, fat, and oils. The diseases generated by the over consumption of high-tech food will be described further on when we deal with the saccharine disease.

Exogenous

Our modern diet is *exogenous*. This refers to foods that are gathered, grown, or raised in areas of the world that are climatically much different. An example would be the consumption of fruit native to the tropics in cold countries like Sweden or Canada, or the importation of apples grown in Canada to the tropics. The essential fatty acid composition of these exotic foods will differ significantly from the composition of the vegetables and fruits raised in the same areas. Cold climate animals and vegetables contain a higher proportion of unsaturated fatty acids relative to the saturated fatty acid. The essential fatty acids make living organisms more cold tolerant.

Artificially Flavored

High-tech processed food is *artificially flavored*. Chemical flavor additives have no value in nutrition, except for cosmetic purposes, and over the long haul will be found to be toxic. More and more additives are being removed from the market, usually after many complaints, after some testing, by government decree. Flavor additives also destroy the ability of our senses to distinguish good food from bad food, and in this way add to the general burden of ill health caused by these high-tech diets. The major flavoring substance is sugar, followed by salt.

Complex

The last adjective we can apply to the modern high-tech diet is *complex*. High-tech foods are composed of a large number of items. For example, one breakfast cereal lists the following ingredients: "whole oat flour, degermed yellow corn meal, wheat starch, sugar, salt, dextrose, vitamins, reduced iron, calcium carbonate, color, trisodium phosphate." This is one of the better cereals, containing less than a gram of sugar per serving. There is a reason for each ingredient. The major item is the oats. De-germed corn is used since germ would make this product more unstable and it could not be stored as long. The sugar, salt, and dextrose (another sugar) are flavoring agents. Color is added with phosphate to stabilize the color. The vitamins and iron enhance its nutritional quality and try to restore what has been lost in the processing.

The main problem with complex foods is that the consumer does not know what is present in the food. It may contain ingredients to which we are allergic. Many patients have a multiple allergy syndrome and are reactive to almost every chemical. The presence of so many chemicals increases the likelihood that they will have an additive effect in causing toxicity and ill health. The foods we have adapted to contain a combination of nutrients that can be dealt with by our digestive apparatus. If we were given the 50 or so pure nutrients and asked to provide the proper balance for all our needs, there would be great difficulty. The combination of ingredients placed in these complex foods has not been worked out by nutritional tests. They have been worked out on the basis of economics, cosmetic properties (taste and smell and appearance), and the need to prepare mixtures that will not deteriorate over time.

It is claimed that the complexity of the label on processed foods should not be a deterrent since a label on natural foods would be even more complex if every ingredient were listed. The difference is that in whole natural food none of the ingredients are in a pure state. They are all part of a very complex series of molecules. And they have been around for so long that the body is accustomed to them and knows how to deal with them. They are 'orthomolecular' products. The synthetics added to food are xenobiotic or foreign and therefore they present major problems to the body.

④ DIETARY DISEASES

More than 75% of our current diet consists of processed food. This diet is deficient in fiber, too rich in processed fats, too rich in simple sugars, and deficient in vitamins, minerals, and essential fatty acids, especially the omega-3 type. It is also too rich in additives.

This unnatural diet is responsible for the large number of sick people today. When they give up this diet for a naturopathic diet, the majority of patients become well. When they revert back to the high-tech diet, they again become ill. We have seen this effect on thousands of our patients over the past 40 years, as have other naturopathic and orthomolecular physicians.

The diseases caused by the modern unnatural diet may be classified into a few simple causal groups for convenience, but remember that these are all diseases caused by inadequacies of the diet and that the treatment for each one of these diseases will be almost the same – restore the natural diet and thus the adaptation.

A logical way to relate the inadequacies of the diet with the various diseases is to work with the compositional changes in the food supply due to high-tech processing. The modern diet is a high-sugar, low-fiber, high-fat, high-additive, high-calorie diet, which at the same time is deficient in micronutrients, such as vitamins and minerals. Let's consider how each of these factors plays a role in making people sick and the kind of diseases suffered as a result.

High-Sugar Diet

All carbohydrates are broken down or hydrolyzed during digestion into the simple sugars. These simple monosaccharides are then absorbed through the intestinal wall and enter the bloodstream. This sugar provides energy for all the cells of the body.

Two common sugars circulate in the blood – glucose, which is essential and safe when the concentration is not too high, and fructose, which is not safe. If the concentration of glucose in the blood drops too far, cells become starved for food energy, and the brain may suffer enough deficiency that the person will faint and go into a coma. This is what happens when a diabetic takes too much insulin. This drives the blood sugar too far down by increasing the amount of glucose the cells take up. Glucose released by digestion and absorbed into the blood will not cause any harm if the food being digested is the whole food, such as whole wheat, carrots, brown rice, and so on. The rate of entry into the blood is slow, controlled, and accompanied by the nutrients in the whole grain. Each molecule of sugar released in this way comes with a package of other nutrients, vitamins, and minerals, and these are available to the body for the processing of the sugar molecules into energy and other products.

> This unnatural diet is responsible for the large number of sick people today. When they give up this diet for a naturopathic diet, the majority of patients become well. When they revert back to the high-tech diet, they again become ill.

In sharp contrast are the so-called free sugars that have already been refined, liberated from every nutritional component of the foods in which they were made. They can be eaten very quickly, so that in addition to the quantities consumed, which are excessive, they are absorbed too rapidly. This throws an enormous burden on the body to deal with all the sugar.

Whole foods contain very little free sugar. Even ripe fruit will contain less than 20% sugar, and fruits that have not been altered by plant breeders contain even less. Natural fruit tends to be less sweet, but plant breeders have selected for sweetness since this appeals to the taste of the public. The major source of sugar before the advent of the chemical age was the honey that our ancestors gathered. With the development of cane and beets as good sources of sugar, it became possible to consume large amounts of free sugars. This has had a major impact on the health of the populations that follow the high-tech diet. When combined with a low-fiber diet, diabetes and candida yeast infections may result.

Saccharine Disease

Overloading with sugar throws an extra burden on the pancreas to release enough insulin to deal with the amount absorbed, which is stressful to the pancreas. There is a direct association between the annual consumption of all the sugars and the incidence of diabetes mellitus. T.L. Cleave, in his book *The Saccharine Disease,* pointed this out some time ago. Dr Cleave formulated the 20-year rule: It takes about 20 years after any group of people go onto the high-sugar diet before its health effects begin to show up in population statistics. In Canada, the incidence of diabetes has risen during the past 50 years from around 1% of the population to about 4% today. In some countries, for example in Mexico, the incidence is very much higher – some epidemiologists have claimed that about 40% of the population is potentially diabetic.

The combination of high sugar and low fiber in the diet creates the condition called the saccharine disease. The symptoms are peptic ulcer due to a deficiency of protein when gastric juice is secreted while eating. Drinking a sugared, carbonated drink stimulates secretion of acid, which finds no protein it can attach to. This excess of sugar, along with excess fat and lack of exercise, are factors causing obesity and diabetes mellitus, especially the late maturity or adult onset type. It is probably more accurate to consider this type of diabetes a variant of hypoglycemia. Relative hypoglycemia afflicts nearly two-thirds of all psychiatric populations and 100% of all addict populations. Out of several hundred tests, we have yet to find one alcoholic with a normal 5-hour glucose tolerance curve.

Excessive intake of sugars is much more closely related to relative hypoglycemia. This is measured by the standard 5-hour glucose tolerance test.

The normal curve present for healthy people is distorted for people on high-sugar diets, usually by going too high in the first 2 or 3 hours and then dipping down too quickly and too far over the last 2 or 3 hours. People with this problem often note an exacerbation of symptoms, such as drowsiness, sleepiness, nausea, and headache, a few hours after meals rich in the sugars.

> Dr Cleave formulated the 20-year rule: It takes about 20 years after any group of people go onto the high-sugar diet before its health effects begin to show up in population statistics.

This is found in almost every person who is obese. Many doctors do not read the last 2 hours, however, and if the first 3 hours are normal, they will conclude that the entire test curve is normal. They will advise patients that they do not have this condition of hypoglycemia and may also advise them to control their low blood sugar by taking more sugar. This is inappropriate advice since it is the sugar intake that was responsible for the drop in sugar. Other foods will also yield similar low blood sugars if the person is allergic to these foods. Hypoglycemia is found most frequently in middle-aged, obese patients and may be confused with diabetes. They usually respond well to dietary control and do not require insulin.

The intake of sugars is not the only factor in causing diabetes. Evidence is accumulating that viral infections can destroy the Islets of Langerhans in the pancreas; this can be a main problem, even for people who do not eat much sugar. The genetic make up of some families may be causal for diabetes type II, but there is striking evidence that taking vitamin B-3 (niacin or niacinamide) will protect them from getting diabetes. Unfortunately, few people receive adequate levels of vitamin B-3 in their diet.

Arteriosclerosis

Too much sucrose and other sugars in the diet may also be a factor in the development of arteriosclerosis. Dr I. Shine studied the incidence of heart disease on the island of St. Helena. On this island in the South Atlantic Ocean, 1,200 miles west of Africa, the land is hilly and there are no cars, so the islanders have to walk a lot. Very few smoke. They are relaxed and their fat intake is fairly low. Still, they have a very high incidence of heart disease.

Their intake of sugar since 1900 has increased to the level in England and in Canada, about 125 lb per person per year.

Yeast Infections

Excess sugar also provides a medium for yeasts that inhabit our gastrointestinal tract. The combination of too much sugar, antibiotics (which destroy normal bacterial flora and allow yeast overgrowth), and birth control medication (which encourages vaginal overgrowth of yeast) is largely responsible for the candida yeast infection that troubles so many people. In addition, chemotherapy or steroid therapy decreases the immune defense system. A combination of yeast overgrowth and decreased immune defense may be responsible for a number of autoimmune diseases, such as multiple sclerosis, lupus, muscular dystrophy, and rheumatoid arthritis.

Low-Fiber Diet

Fiber is mainly carbohydrates and passes through the gastrointestinal system because it cannot be completely digested. There is much more fiber in plant food than in animal food. Plant fiber can be divided into three different types: cereal fibers, vegetable fibers, and fruit fibers. A person consuming whole foods need not worry very much about adding additional fiber to the diet, but a person living primarily on overly processed foods will probably experience health problems due to fiber deficiency.

Constipation

Constipation, sometimes alternating with diarrhea, is the hallmark of a low-fiber diet. In constipation, bowel movements occur less frequently than one per day with stools that are hard, small in volume, and require much effort to expel. Ideally, one should have one to two movements per day with large bulky stools that are semi-fluid and expelled with minimal effort. Diarrhea is present when the stools are very watery and very frequent. The best rule is: hard food in, soft stools out; conversely, soft food in, hard stools out.

Normally, the contractions and relaxations of the small and large bowel propel the food toward the large colon and rectum, from where it is expelled. However, if the food lacks fiber, there is little material for the bowel to grab on to. Low-fiber foods are so thoroughly digested in the stomach and in the small intestine that when the contents reach the colon, there is little fiber present. As the bowel contents travel onward, nutrients

> A person consuming whole foods need not worry very much about adding additional fiber to the diet, but a person living primarily on overly processed foods will probably experience health problems due to fiber deficiency.

released by the digestion and water are absorbed. At the same time, the bacteria and fungi present in the colon become more active. By the time the feces are expelled, the bulk may consist entirely of the dead bodies of yeast, bacteria, and other organisms that have converted the fiber to other insoluble material.

Other Low-Fiber Related Diseases

People living on a diet low in fiber-rich foods tend to have many diseases not present in people who consume whole foods that are rich in fiber. A low-fiber diet can lead to colitis, diverticulosis, hemorrhoids, gall bladder disease, appendicitis, and cancer of the colon. The combination of too much sugar and too little fiber is a factor in causing hypercholesterolemia and atherosclerosis. Coronary disease is one outcome, as is stroke. There is little doubt that if we reverted back to a high-fiber, low-sugar diet, coronary disease would almost disappear and heart surgeons would have little to do. The lack of vitamin C is another main factor in causing hardening of the arteries, but other vitamins, such as niacin and pyridoxine, also are involved. The low-fiber, high-sugar diet is low in many essential nutrients, including the key vitamins.

In his studies of low-fiber diets, Dr Burkett has observed that among different nations there is an inverse relationship between the size of the stools and the size of the hospitals. With small stools, he found that large hospitals were needed. While his arguments for the value of a high-fiber diet have been accepted by the medical community, this same community has been so accustomed to working with fractions of foods that it ignored his finding that the fiber was needed as a constituent of whole foods, not as a form of bran or pure fibers. They soon found that these pure fibers by themselves were not nearly as helpful as the whole foods. Bran and other high fiber foods are useful in many circumstances, but they should not be used to replace the whole foods rich in fiber.

High-Fat Diet

Life would be impossible on a diet with no fat. Hardly any food is totally devoid of fat. In natural food, it is present in an intricate complex mixture of protein and carbohydrates with their essential vitamins, minerals, and enzymes. There are very few natural foods that contain too much fat, but the free availability of fats and oils in the high-tech diet creates a major problem. Most people now consume too much fat. The North American diet contains about 40% fat, whereas the optimum amount of fat expressed as calories probably varies between 10% and 20%, depending on the climate.

Fat is an important source of energy, providing much more energy per gram, 9 calories, than sugar and protein, which provide about 4 calories. Fat is also the main storage depot for calories. If we had to depend upon carbohydrates to store our energy, we would be over 200% as bulky. Movement would be impossible.

When our consumption of calories is greater than our use of energy, the extra energy is stored in the body in the fat depots. For our ancestors, this ability to store excess calories was a marvelous device for balancing food intake and expenditure. During famine or milder food shortages, our ancestors would draw upon the fat they had accumulated during periods when food was abundant and intake was excessive. Nature also made allowance for nourishing fetuses and babies by providing women with more storage capacity for calories, which could be drawn upon during pregnancy and lactation.

Too Little Fat

Too little fat is can be a problem because it will be impossible or very difficult to maintain weight, to have enough energy for physical activity, to fight cold weather, to absorb fat soluble vitamins, and to provide the essential fatty acids. On a low-fat diet, people will be hungry, and this will tempt many to increase their intake of sugars in order to replace the missed calories. However, our major problem today in high-tech diets is too much fat, not too little. Fat artifacts are readily available – butter, milk, cream, cheeses, margarine, and liquid oils are all staple items used in cooking. The favorite companion is sugar. Sweets consist of a mixture of sugar and fat. The sweet taste and the composition of the fat make this a very attractive food item. The doughnut represents the acme of the high-tech diet, for it consists of white flour, pure free sugar, and pure fat.

Too Much Fat

Too much fat is much more pathological since it causes overweight, obesity, and their health complications. This high-fat, high-cholesterol diet contributes to cardiovascular disease, coronary occlusion, and strokes. The usual advice given to patients who want to know how to decrease the chance of getting heart disease is to exercise, stop smoking, learn to relax, and decrease their intake of fat.

There is no doubt that fats are involved in atherosclerosis, that high blood cholesterol and high blood triglycerides increase the risk of developing atherosclerosis. We also believe that there is no relationship between consumption of whole foods and atherosclerosis. These foods will prevent elevation of blood fats, except in familial hypercholesterolemia. But we would expect that consumption of pure fats is related. Thus, there should be no fear of eating eggs, a whole food, but we should be concerned over utilization of butter, margarine, and the commercial oils. If epidemiologists would report total fat intake, fat intake from whole foods, and fat intake from butter, cream, margarine, and oils, they would have a much clearer view of the relationship of fats to atherosclerosis, coronary disease, and strokes.

We are convinced that high sugar intake is a greater risk factor for heart disease than is the fat level of the food. Low-fat diets, rich in complex carbohydrates and low in sugar, should be the best diet for preventing arteriosclerosis.

Vascular disease caused by arteriosclerosis is a very common and serious outcome of the high-sugar, low-fiber, high-fat diet. Fat intake is believed to be the main factor in causing elevated cholesterol levels with the resultant increase in hardening of the arteries. High sugar intake, especially high sucrose, is also a factor. People on a low-fat diet will increase their sugar intake unless they are advised not to do so. If they do, any gain they might obtain by lowering fat will be overcome by the increased pathological effect of sugar on cholesterol levels. This area of research will have to be studied much more carefully. We are convinced that high sugar intake is a greater risk factor for heart disease than is the fat level of the food. Low-fat diets, rich in complex carbohydrates and low in sugar, should be the best diet for preventing arteriosclerosis.

Poor Quality Fat

Not only is too much fat being eaten, the quality of that fat has been deteriorated by processing. Whole foods are seldom very rich in fat, and what is present is not destroyed by heat or by oxidation. Not many whole foods contain as much as 20% fat. However, when the fats are separated from the food, it becomes possible to consume very large quantities. These processed fats include butter, cream, margarine, and all the oils. The problem with butter and cream is that it is too easy to eat large quantities and so overload the body with calories. The problem with commercial oils and margarines is they are heat treated and oxidized. The natural fatty acids are changed by heat into unnatural fatty acids. This creates problems for the body, hastening atherosclerosis.

Another consequence is the destruction of essential fatty acids (EFAs). These fatty acids are highly reactive and easily become rancid when stored and, therefore, must be removed. This deprives us of essential fatty acids, which creates a variety of pathological conditions. There is also a displacement of foods rich in EFAs by sources that contain very little. Crops grown in warm areas do not need protection against cold and, therefore, have little unsaturated fatty acids. Temperate crops, such as wheat, oats, and flax, require more; unsaturated fatty acids have lower melting points. Flax and its oil, linseed oil, were used as staples many years ago. They have been replaced by corn, coconut, canola, and other warmer-crop oils. As a result, we now consume only 20% of the EFAs that we did before 1950.

High-Additive Diet

We are just becoming aware of the impact food additives and trace elements have on health. They are a factor in diminishing our immune defenses.

They also play a role in causing learning and behavioral disorders in some children.

The average person consumes about 140 lb of food additives per year. Of this, 102 lb is sucrose, 13 lb is dextrose, 15 lb is salt, 8 lb is pepper, mustard, baking soda, citric acid, and 26 other common kitchen substances. The remaining 2.1 lb comes from about 2,400 synthetic cosmetic additives. Trace additives coming from processed products used to make food mixtures are additional.

Environmental Contaminants

During the past few decades, scientists have detected the presence of a wide variety of chemical contaminants in our food and water supply. At the Wingspread Conference Center, Racine, Wisconsin in the early 1990s, scientists studied the effect of man-made chemicals, such as pesticides, PCBs, and dioxins, on human development. Four general points were made: these chemicals may have entirely different effects on the embryo, fetus, or perinatal organisms than on the adult; the effects are most often manifested in offspring, not in the exposed parent; the timing of exposure in the developing organism is crucial; and although critical exposure occurs during embryonic development, obvious manifestations may not occur until maturity.

Some of these chemicals, such the PCBs and dioxins, persist in the environment and bio-accumulate in the food chain. In addition, most of our food has been treated with pesticides, designed to kill small organisms, but capable of affecting our health in larger concentrations. These are trace elements found in our food and water.

Autoimmune Diseases

The majority of cases of cancer are due to environmental factors – chiefly, the chemical pollutants in our air, water, soil, and food. These contaminants break down or block our natural immune defenses. To compound the problem of the toxins borne in our food, the nutrient-poor high-tech diet does not supply the nutrients needed to bolster our immune system. For example, the only substance known to increase cancer-fighting interferon production in the body is ascorbic acid, often deficient in the high-tech diet. Leukocytes deficient in ascorbic acid are not able to engulf bacteria. Dr O.

Truss has suggested that chronic yeast (candida) infection caused by a high-sugar diet may lead to an immobilization of the natural defense system and a distortion of the relationship between various types of leukocytes.

These nutrient deficiencies and excesses compound the symptoms of autoimmune diseases (the immune system attacks normal tissues), including rheumatoid arthritis, multiple sclerosis, lupus, and perhaps muscular dystrophy. Treatment for these conditions is largely palliative, using steroid hormones and immuno-suppressants. When they do help, improvement is temporary and partial.

Children's Learning and Behavior Disorders

Not only sugars but also phosphates present in many of our processed foods, especially in the soft drinks, are a major cause of hyperactivity. The soft, astringent drinks so very popular are loaded with several of the most causal factors in hyperactivity – sugar, phosphates, and a variety of chemicals, including dyes.

Modern high-tech food additives have the same impact on children who experience learning and behavioral (hyperactivity) disorders as on adolescents who exhibit antisocial and criminal behavior. We have seen how addiction to sugar has paved the way to violent behavior in adolescents and adults. These addicted children invariably begin to steal money from their parents and from others in order to buy sweets. They may not be caught for a long time, for parents find it difficult to believe their children will do this. They may be caught only occasionally. If they are punished 10% of the time, this is a small price to pay for having gotten the desired sugar. Once the pattern has been established, it will continue into adolescence, where the wants are different but the method of achieving them the same. Now they steal for cigarettes, for alcohol, or for drugs until the criminal pattern of behavior is well established.

Several years ago, the New York Public School System (803 schools) introduced a diet policy that lowered sucrose, synthetic food colors, and two preservatives over 4 years. This was followed by a 15.7% increase in mean academic percentile rating above the rest of the nation's schools that used the same tests. It has also been shown that behavioral problems decreased 48% in a detention facility involving 276 delinquents during the year the diet was changed. Many other institutions discovered the same facts. Decreasing sugar and additives lowered the incidence of bad behavior. Anyone who doubts this need only see what happens when their children are placed upon a sugar-free diet for at least 2 weeks. It is important to do this before advising children to avoid sweets permanently and totally.

Mental and Emotional Disorders

Food additives may also cause mood disorders. The symptoms include fatigue, depression, and anxiety, in various mixes. Most sufferers of the very severe and manic depressions do not fall into this category, but there is evidence that they are suffering from severe allergic reactions, perhaps to foods. We have seen many patients with mood disorders recover when the proper nutritional supplements were used.

The relationship of the schizophrenias to nutrition is not as clear. But since the most effective treatments include modification of the diet and the use of vitamin B-3 and vitamin B-6 as the main supplements, it must be a major factor. There are patients who are allergic to foods as well as to other chemicals. We have treated over 100 patients who had not responded well enough to our program of drugs and vitamins by having them do a 4-day fast. The majority was well by the fifth day. When the food they were allergic to was re-introduced, they promptly became psychotic again.

Vitamin and Mineral Deficient Diets

Although the classic deficiency diseases are not necessarily produced by the modern high-tech diet, for we rarely see scurvy (vitamin C deficiency), beri beri (vitamin B-1 deficiency), pellagra (vitamin B-3 deficiency), or rickets (vitamin D deficiency), this diet does cause modern deficiency diseases with vague, diffuse symptoms. These patients share in common the fact that usual clinical examination and laboratory tests do not reveal a cause for their fatigue, distress, and malaise. Most are eventually labeled as psychosomatic or psychiatric. For this reason, it is more appropriate to call them subclinical deficiencies. Medical literature contains reports of subclinical deficiencies, especially among residents of hospitals and nursing homes.

Zinc Deficiency

For example, in elderly people, the senses of taste and smell can be diminished due to a deficiency of zinc and perhaps by an accumulation of copper. There is nothing that destroys appetite as fast as a distorted taste and smell. Foods become tasteless or bitter or flat. The taste becomes so objectionable that a person cannot eat and may become very depressed. A rapid test of the sense of taste can be conducted by administering a solution of zinc sulfate. Normal people find this solution very sharp and bitter, but when they have lost their sense of taste due to a deficiency of zinc, they will not find any unusual taste in this solution.

A blood test for zinc and copper will help establish the diagnosis. An elderly woman who was very depressed because she could no longer taste her food was referred to us for care. She had seen more than 10 different doctors trying to get help, but nothing they could do was effective. We started her on tablets of zinc sulfate, which she took for over 2 years without any improvement. Then we started her on zinc sulfate solution, giving her 100 mg of zinc per day. Within a few months, she began to recover and has been well for more than 10 years. Her sense of taste is not fully normal, but has improved so much that she can enjoy her food and she is not depressed.

B Vitamins Deficiency

Patients who suffer from eating disorders, such as obesity or bulimia, probably have an abnormal appetite for carbohydrates and sweets because of a need to obtain enough of the essential nutrients. In 1949, a medical research scientist ran a very interesting experiment with rats that proved this relationship between carbohydrate appetite and vitamin deficiency. The rats were kept in a running cage, a device that allowed the rats to run and measured the distance they ran each day. Normal rats fed a good healthy rat diet would run a certain number of miles each day, around 3 miles. When the same animals were given a diet low in calories, they would double the amount that they ran. This is understandable since in nature it is hunger that motivates animals to wake up and start hunting. A lion after a feed will sleep for many hours until aroused once more by hunger. This is a life saving reflex, probably present in all animals.

When the same rats were given a diet that had enough calories, but was deficient in the B vitamins, they ran as much as the fasting rats, even though they were not starving. Apparently, the bodies of these rats were not satisfied due to the vitamin deficiency: they had an established reflex that equated enough food (calories) with enough other nutrients, and they were hungry since they were not able to metabolize their food as well without the B vitamins.

Whenever we have an agitated, hyperactive child in our office, we are reminded of this experiment. The child's body, due to the deficiency of certain B vitamins, is compelled to respond, as did the rats kept on a B vitamin deficient diet. We think it is a reasonable hypothesis that patients with eating disorders are trying to obtain enough nutrients by increasing the amount of food they eat, but the major increase in calories, which

> Patients who suffer from eating disorders, such as obesity or bulimia, probably have an abnormal appetite for carbohydrates and sweets because of a need to obtain enough of the essential nutrients.

drives them to obesity, forces them to seek ways of controlling the food intake by vomiting or using laxatives. With vomiting they do not get any extra nutrients, but with the laxatives they may obtain a few more of the essential nutrients they would otherwise not obtain. It is probable that all the addictions are caused by similar factors – by the excessive intake of sugars and starches combined with the deficiency of essential nutrients.

Combined G.I. Diseases

Now that we have seen the diseases caused by the modern high-sugar, low-fiber, high-fat, and high-additive diet, we can look at the combined affects of these unnatural dietary practices on the digestive system. To do this systematically, let's begin from the mouth and teeth and follow the gastrointestinal (g.i.) tract to the anus. This comprises one organ system, not a series of individual and separate organs. If the mouth is sick, so is the rest of the g.i. tract.

Mouth

The modern diet causes dental caries. Deposits of sugar from the food are not properly swept away from the teeth by the food and by the saliva because of an excess of sugar and a deficiency of fiber. Foods rich in fiber must be chewed, and in this process, the teeth are cleaned.

Esophagus and Stomach

The main diseases of the esophagus and stomach are hiatus hernia, dyspepsia, peptic ulcer, and cancer. With respect to hiatus hernia, there are two main symptoms, discomfort after meals (which is often confused with dyspepsia) and actual bulging of the esophageal-gastric juncture through the diaphragm, which is caused by constipation and frequent straining to have bowel movements. Additional pain and discomfort comes from the high-sugar, low-fat diet, especially if the patient is allergic to these foods. Many patients diagnosed as having hiatus hernia lose their discomfort when the foods they were allergic to are eliminated from the diet.

Ulcer is caused by eating foods that are too low in fiber and in protein. When we start to eat, the stomach prepares to do its job of secreting hydrochloric acid needed before pepsin can digest protein. When the food enters the stomach, the acid is absorbed onto the protein and cannot do any harm to the walls of the stomach. The acidity in the stomach can be very high, so high that if you put your finger into stomach contents it will be burned. The stomach wall can resist the acid it secretes, but not if it lies about in the stomach too long. If one drinks a soft drink containing no protein and high in acid, there will be nothing there to absorb the acid, and it will damage the stomach wall.

Not all high-protein foods are useful. If the high-protein food in itself stimulates the extra secretion of acid, it will have a detrimental effect. This is one of the problems with dairy products. Many years ago the favorite treatment for peptic ulcer was the high milk diet, called the Sippi diet. It is now known that people with peptic ulcers ought to avoid milk. Antacids decrease the secretion of acid and are useful in the treatment of peptic ulcers. Niacin may also increase the secretion of acid, but it can also absorb some acid. A few patients with ulcer cannot tolerate it, but most of the patients with ulcers we have treated were able to take niacin with no difficulty. It did not increase their pain and discomfort. Fiber can also absorb acid and prevent it from attacking the stomach wall.

The most recent clinical evidence indicates that most cases of peptic ulcer are caused by a bacterium, *Helicobacter pylori*. Specific treatment with a proper antibiotic regimen and a naturopathic diet will cure most ulcers.

There is recent evidence that the chronic infection – that is, chronic peptic ulcer – is a predisposing factor for stomach cancer. The actual cause of cancer of the stomach is not as clear. Malnutrition is a major factor because of the deficiency of antioxidants, such as vitamin C, vitamin E, selenium, and others. It is known that chronic irritation of any tissue is also one of the factors. For this reason, a chronic peptic ulcer in a person also suffering shortages of essential micronutrients is more susceptible to the development of cancer.

Small Intestine and Colon

The major stage of the digestive process, the breaking down of the food into its primary components, occurs in the small intestine and partially in the large intestine or colon. For this process, there was must be an adequate supply of enzymes from the pancreas and from the intestinal walls. There also must be enough muscular movement to propel the intestinal contents slowly towards the rectum. This movement, called peristalsis, consists of alternate contraction and dilation, like squeezing a toothpaste

> There is an increased likelihood of getting cancer of the colon due to the combination of poor nutrition and back-pressure.

container to expel the contents. When the foods remain undigested and when there is too little bulk or fiber, the intestine and colon have great difficulty in performing their main function. This results in a number of pathological changes that have been considered separate diseases but are really various expressions of the one disease, the saccharine disease.

The main symptom arising from lack of fiber is constipation because the intestinal walls are not challenged by the lack of bulk in the food. The muscular walls apparently need some stimulus that comes from the extension of the diameter of the bowel by the accumulation of food therein. As a result of the constipation, which is usually chronic and may be very severe, other symptoms develop. Because of the need to strain to eliminate the stools, there is more back-pressure on the veins around the anus; this will result in hemorrhoids if the problem is there for a long time.

With chronic constipation, there may be a large amount of fecal material in the colon, which exerts pressure on the large veins leading from the legs to the heart. When this is present long enough, it may lead to varicose veins in people who are, for reasons not known, more susceptible to this vascular problem. The increased back-pressure may also lead to small bulges in the wall of the intestine, called diverticulosis, and if these become infected, they are called diverticulitis.

Appendicitis is also considered one of the consequences. In South Africa many years ago, only people who spoke English ever got appendicitis. This was because they were eating a low-fiber diet. The increased back-pressure may also lead to gall bladder disease. There is an increased likelihood of getting cancer of the colon due to the combination of poor nutrition and back-pressure.

When too much sugar is present, it will be absorbed into the blood stream too quickly and compromise the ability of the body to deal with these amounts. The body is used to absorbing the sugar slowly as it is released from its foods by digestion. If the sugar cannot all be absorbed, it will find its way down to the colon, where there should not be any, and provide food for organisms that should not be there, such as the yeasts.

Undigested sugars too far into the colon will create serious problems. A good example is the lactose in milk, milk sugar. This is a double sugar, a disaccharide, consisting of a union between one glucose molecule and one galactose molecule. In infants and to a lesser degree in children and adults, the stomach provides the enzyme lactase, which splits this sugar in the intestine. But when it is lacking, as it is in many adults, the original sugar passes down until it can be fermented by the fungi and yeast in the colon, creating serious symptoms of diarrhea, gas, and pain. This problem is solved by swallowing lactase tablets (the enzyme) at the same time one drinks the milk. If sucrose (common table sugar which is also a double sugar made from glucose and fructose) is not split, a similar problem will develop.

Ulcerative colitis and Crohn's disease are also symptoms of the high-sugar, low-fiber diet, according to T.L. Cleave. We have treated many patients with Crohn's disease and find that many of them are allergic to wheat and other grains and to dairy products. Dairy foods, considered by many physicians and nutritionists to be an essential food group, are in fact the cause of allergies and disease in many people.

When only whole foods are consumed, the masticated food, the enzymes and fluid added to it, and the products of enzymatic digestion are propelled through the gastrointestinal (g.i.) tract, clearing the system in less than 24 hours. However, in a high-sugar and low-fiber diet, this transit time increases.

In the absence of sufficient fiber, peristalsis is decreased, leaving food in the intestinal system much longer. As a result bacterial content of the feces is much higher in areas of the intestine where this normally does not occur. The longer the food remains in the gut, the higher is the bacterial and yeast cell count, for these organisms thrive in a warm, wet medium containing partially digested food. There normally is a gradient of bacterial count, which is lowest in the duodenum and highest in the colon. The whole g.i. tract functions to keep bacterial yeast count low in the small intestine, where most of the nutrients are absorbed, while allowing bacterial count to rise in the colon, where there is little absorption. The products of bacterial metabolism, which are harmful, are thus retained in the colon and excreted with the feces. But the longer the food is stored, the greater the contamination.

The small intestine must be kept bacteria free. When too much sugar is present, it stimulates overgrowth of yeast. The saccharine inducing diet also leads to bacterial and yeast overgrowth in areas of the intestine where this should not occur. Fasting, with or without enemas, has been used for many decades to treat a variety of diseases, ranging from cancer and arthritis to serious psychiatric problems. Perhaps the common factor is the elimination or marked reduction of candida or yeast infection from the gastrointestinal tract. A 4-day fast (96 hour) would eliminate yeast from most people. But for a person with a fast transit time, 1 or 2 days might be enough. A water diet would be more therapeutic than a juice diet, because the sugar in the juice would provide nourishment for the yeast. A combination of enema and fasting would be more effective than a simple fast, especially for people with sluggish bowels.

Food Allergies

Allergic reactions tend to develop against staple foods in various regions. Thus, in wheat consuming regions of the world, wheat allergy is much more common than it is in rice consuming regions, where rice is a greater problem. In tea drinking countries, tea will more often cause allergic reactions than coffee, while the converse is true in coffee consuming countries. Cow milk is a major staple of the North American and European diet. Almost everyone is introduced to milk as an infant, either directly through a bottle or indirectly though their mothers who drink milk. It is consumed for a long time, often for a lifetime. However, many people are allergic to cow milk. Even people who can consume dairy products with few immediate allergic reactions, such as diarrhea or upper respiratory problems, are subject to more silent adverse reactions to milk, such as nutrient deficiencies, tooth decay, multiple sclerosis, atherosclerosis, cancers, and psychiatric and behavior disorders.

Dairy Products

Milk and its many derivatives are the most widely promoted and advertised food product in North America and Western Europe. According to Dr Frank Oski, in his book *Don't Drink Your Milk*, 14% of all food dollars go to buying milk and dairy products. This is the second major food expense, following the combined costs of meat, fish, poultry, and eggs. Milk is big business.

Milk products are promoted by the majority of physicians, by almost every dietitian and nutritionist, by most professors of nutrition and biochemistry when they teach nutrition in medical schools, by Public Health departments, and, of course, by the most powerful group of all, the various national, provincial, and state dairy organizations. It has become an article of faith that unless children are given copious quantities of milk, at least 3 glasses each day, they will not grow and they will not develop. Mothers are told their babies will not get enough calcium unless they are fed cow milk. Women are told they will get osteoporosis after menopause if they don't drink milk.

> Milk causes gastrointestinal and respiratory disturbances arising from lactose intolerance and from milk allergies, as well as nutrient deficiencies due to these gastrointestinal reactions.

However, Dr Oski and a growing band of supporters maintain that milk is not a perfect food, that it is not even a good food, and that milk must be used with extreme caution. We would support the idea that all dairy products be labeled with the warning sign applied to cigarette packages, something like *Warning, This Product May Be Hazardous to Your Health*.

The public is confused about the various mammalian milks. We believe we should have different names for human milk and for cow milk so that they will not be equated as equivalent good products. Cow milk is good for calves but has never been shown by any independent experiment to be good for human babies or for adult women to protect them against osteoporosis. Most mammals feed on their mother's milk until they have tripled their birth weight. In human infants, this takes about 1 year. Among all the mammals, the human species alone never gets weaned from milk. Since formula is rich in sugar and milk is rich in lactose (another sugar), it is more accurate to say that only humans never get weaned from milk and sugar, the two of the most common and most injurious food allergens.

Americans and many Europeans have developed a taste for milk that is not natural, while most people in East Asia, Africa, and South America regard cow milk as not fit for human consumption. They are in better tune with the rest of our mammalian cousins. We have broken the adaptation between our need and the food by depending so much on cow milk. Nature never intended that children should forever be dependent on their mother's milk, and the loss of the enzyme lactase is a reflection of this adaptation.

Milk causes gastrointestinal and respiratory disturbances arising from lactose intolerance and from milk allergies, as well as nutrient deficiencies due to these gastrointestinal reactions. It plays a role in the development of atherosclerosis. Milk may play a role in the development of childhood leukemia, multiple sclerosis, and tooth decay in infants. It plays an epidemiological role in cancer. In adults, peptic ulcer is another reaction. Milk allergy causes nephrosis, eczema, growing pains, rheumatoid arthritis, appendicitis, and predisposes one to Group A beta-hemolytic streptococcus infection. It is involved as one of the causal factors in antisocial and criminal behavior in children and adults.

Lactase Deficiency

Several gastrointestinal disorders may be caused by lactose intolerance or lactase deficiency. After infancy, many people no longer make enough lactase, the enzyme that splits lactose into galactose and glucose. The lactose cannot be absorbed and stays in the intestine, where it is fermented by bacteria, creating gas and intense bowel discomfort.

The frequency of lactase deficiency varies enormously among different populations. More than 80% of Filipinos, Japanese, Taiwanese, and Thais lack this enzyme. Over 60% of Black Africans, Afro-Americans, Arabs, Jews, and Greek Cypriots also lack this enzyme, while less than 10% of Danes, Swiss, and American Whites have the same problem. Dairy allergy is present in a considerably high percentage of the North American population. Dr J. Gerrard, Professor of Pediatrics at the Medical School, University of Saskatchewan, after a series of careful studies, concluded that 59 infants out of 787 were milk allergic, or 7.5%. He reported that the frequency depended upon how soon the infants were started on milk. One quarter of the babies started on milk before they were 3 months old became milk allergic.

Peoples who had to depend upon milk to survive have by a process of natural selection retained the ability to create lactase long after it was natural for the same people who did not have to consume so much. Thus in Nigeria, tribes that did not raise cattle had a 99% deficiency of lactase, while other tribes, where milk was a traditional food, had only a 20% lactase deficiency. This is good news for the dairy industry, for if milk consumption can be maintained long enough, no matter what the cost, most groups will have developed the ability to retain lactase production.

It is now possible to swallow lactase tablets before the milk is drunk or to drink lactase treated milk and thus avoid most of the symptoms of lactase deficiency. However, this will not solve the problem for the milk allergic individual. Allergic reactions to dairy products are very common and can cause an amazing variety of allergic reactions anywhere in the gastrointestinal tract and very often in the upper respiratory system.

Dr Hoffer is an expert in dairy allergy, one among many, because he has a fixed allergy to these foods. Many years ago when he got a common cold – at least that is what he thought it was – he did what he should have done to bring it under control, including taking large quantities of vitamin C and vitamin A, but there was no relief. For 2 years, he had a constant nasal drip, which was so bad that when he gave a lecture, he would have to hold a Kleenex in one hand and his notes in the other. He always carried pockets full of Kleenex. After 2 years, he had given up hope. At that time, for other reasons, he did a 4-day water fast. To his amazement, he was well by the fourth day. On a retest with a little milk, his drippy nose promptly returned in about 15 minutes. For the next few years, whenever he was exposed to dairy products, whether he was aware of it or not, he would get another 4-day cold. Since then, for about 35 years, he has not had any colds and has been inadvertently exposed to dairy foods on only a few occasions. His dairy allergy expressed itself as a runny nose, congested sinuses, sore throat, with difficulty in clearing the ears with changes in air pressure.

Diarrhea and Iron Deficiency

The most common gastrointestinal reaction is chronic diarrhea, ranging from frequent soft stools to numerous, watery, and explosive stools, occasionally showing traces of red blood. The diarrhea impairs the absorption of nutrients. If there is chronic slow bleeding, a protein deficiency will develop, leading to swelling of the abdomen, hands, and feet. It will also lead to iron deficiency. Half the iron deficiency in infants is a result of feeding infants cow milk. Iron deficiency will make many babies irritable with impaired attention span. This has caused a common problem called the blue bottle syndrome. The child walks about with a plastic bottle of milk, from which he drinks now and then. When only glass bottles were available, they would drop these so often and break them that mothers would stop giving them bottles. With plastic bottles, there is no relief for the child. Blue bottle babies are usually iron deficient. Colic is also a common manifestation of milk allergy.

Other Nutrient Deficiencies

As well as causing iron deficiency due to chronic bleeding in the gut, excessive intake of milk also is associated with other nutrient deficiencies. Excessive intake of dairy products crowds other foods out of the diet, foods that are richer in vitamins and minerals. Chronic inflammation of the intestine can result because of decreased absorption of nutrients. Another common deficiency is zinc and pyridoxine. We have been surprised at the large number of children we have seen who had white areas in their fingernails. This is due to a deficiency of pyridoxine and zinc. Most often these children are heavy consumers of dairy products. In some cases, 50% of their calories came from this source. Milk tends to be low in zinc and in pyridoxine. Milk inhibits the absorption of zinc in the digestive tract.

Atherosclerosis

There are many nutrient deficiencies involved in the production of atherosclerosis, including deficiencies in ascorbic acid, nicotinic acid, and pyridoxine. Excess intake of sugar and excess consumption of fat are also important factors. The major source of excess fat in the human diet comes from dairy products.

Early consumption of milk is associated with atherosclerosis. A pathologist examined the coronary arteries from 1500 children and adolescents who had died as a result of accident. Some of the children had normal blood vessels, others did not. The single characteristic that distinguished them was that the children whose arteries were not normal had been fed cow milk or formula based on dairy products.

Cancers

The Lancet, a British medical journal, reported some years ago that unpasteurized milk fed to six baby chimpanzees caused two of them to develop leukemia. The milk had come from infected cows with bovine C-type virus. Later *Science* carried a report written by three doctors from the University of Pennsylvania, School of Veterinary Medicine. They concluded that there was an association between human and bovine leukemia, that there was a significant increase in the number of humans with acute lymphoid leukemia in areas with a high incidence of bovine leukemia. They suggested that there must be further investigation of this relationship. Very few people drink unpasteurized milk in high-tech societies. This will be a problem for countries that do not pasteurize their milk.

Of all the possible connections between cancer and diet, the one most readily accepted by the cancer research agencies is the relationship to fat. There is almost a linear relationship between the average fat consumption of the diet of various countries and the incidence of breast cancer. In the United States and Canada and many European countries, 40% of calories come from fat. These countries have the highest incidence of breast cancer. Countries where fat intake is below 10% have a much lower incidence. There is also a direct link between fat consumption and estrogen secretion. Women eating high-fat diets secrete more estrogen.

Multiple Sclerosis

Two scientists from the University of Michigan began to look for links between multiple sclerosis and environmental factors. They found a striking correlation between the incidence of multiple sclerosis and low per capita milk consumption in the United States. The correlation was 0.82. In

Europe, a similar relationship was found. Patients with MS do very much better when they are on a low-fat diet. A low-fat diet means that dairy products are eliminated from it, as they are the major source of fats. Dr R.L. Swank and his colleagues have found that patients with MS who adhered to his low-fat diet regimen, as described in his *The Multiple Sclerosis Diet Book,* experienced good results. Patients who started on the program early had the best results.

Swank also saw a cultural and demographic pattern linked to the incidence of MS. As he explains, "two parallel and little mixed cultures based on food have evolved. These are the beer-butter and the wine-oil cultures. The first extended across northern Europe (Scandinavia, Germany, Holland, Belgium, northern France, northern Switzerland, and the British Isles) and has become the mode of life in the United States and Canada. The second predominates in the Mediterranean area (Spain, Italy, southern France, southern Switzerland, and Greece) and stretches to the Middle East and North Africa. The beer-butter culture corresponds geographically to the area of high incidence of multiple sclerosis and vascular disease; the wine-oil culture corresponds to the area where these conditions have a low incidence." Of course, there are other factors as well. MS is caused by environmental factors in genetically susceptible individuals. It is important that these various factors be isolated and their relative importance in the cause and in the treatment be examined.

In the meantime, the optimum diet for patients with multiple sclerosis is the Swank diet. A combination of this diet, plus vitamins, has been very successful for our patients, and we have seen many who have gotten well, or if they have not, they have stopped deteriorating and are neurologically stable. Vitamin C is a natural booster of interferon production in the body and has been shown to double its concentration. A deficiency of vitamin D-3 is also being studied as a cause of MS.

Tooth Decay
Dr F. Castano, a research dentist, has evidence that milk will increase tooth decay. Many mothers use milk to get their babies to fall asleep. The baby sucks at the bottle and dozes off. The baby stops swallowing the milk, which then stays in the mouth and begins to eat away at the teeth. During sleep, saliva production is decreased. The milk on the teeth turns sour because of the same

bacteria that causes dental caries. Dr Castano has observed that decay has been so rapid that the teeth appeared to be melting away, especially if the milk drinking practice is continued after age 12 months. Juices in bottles are just as bad. Babies should not be put to bed with a bottle in their mouth.

Psychiatric and Behavioral Disorders
The psychiatric and behavioral changes caused by milk are also numerous. Any food allergy can cause almost every known psychiatric syndrome from infantile autism and schizophrenia to mood and behavioral disorders. Milk is no exception.

> Another youngster diagnosed with infantile autism by a clinic specializing in these disorders became normal on a diet free of dairy and sugar products in 1 month.

The first dramatic case we saw of milk allergy was in a teenaged girl who was typically schizophrenic with visual and auditory hallucinations, many paranoid delusions, and severe depression. She had not responded to any previous treatment. But after a 4-day water fast, she was normal. One day later, after one glass of milk, she was psychotic again in 1 hour.

We have also seen a chronic paranoid schizophrenic who had been resident in a mental hospital for years. He suddenly could not urinate. He was brought to City Hospital in Saskatoon from the mental hospital and came under our care when it was found he was physically normal. After a fast, he was psychologically normal. The next day after a test dose of milk, he became violently ill with nausea, vomiting, severe diarrhea, headache, and more. He had been mentally normal after the fast, but after milk he was once more the same psychotic person we had known for many years. The case ended sadly. He refused to keep away from dairy products because, he told us, if he remained well he would have to get a job and try to make his way outside the hospital. He was too old for this and preferred to remain in a mental hospital, where he would be looked after. He died there 2 years later from leukemia.

We had one young boy as a patient who was at the bottom of his class of 20 in the fall term. On a milk-free diet, he was at the top by the following spring term. Another youngster diagnosed with infantile autism by a clinic specializing in these disorders became normal on a diet free of dairy and sugar products in 1 month. His mother had placed him on this diet against the advice of his therapists, who laughed at her when she first discussed it with them.

Over a period of 3 years, we fasted over 200 patients who had not responded or had responded only partially to the treatment we were using. More than 75% were much better after the 4-day fast. Of these, many were milk allergic. The syndromes produced by these allergies included learning and behavioral disorders, depressions, and schizophrenias. One female had been depressed for over 20 years. She had not been helped by medication or even one series of electro-convulsive treatment. She went on a dairy-free diet on a Friday and by the following Monday her depression was gone. When we take a medical history, we never forget to take an allergy history in the hunt for clues. With children or young adults, it is vital to examine for the presence of the common allergic diseases as a factor in causing their psychiatric problems.

Processed Protein

For many decades, protein has been looked upon as something we should all have in ample quantities. Like motherhood, little bad could be said against protein. But the term should be applied only to protein-rich foods, not to the pure protein extracted from food and then used to make artificial products or artifacts. Foods prepared from processed meat and fish are not as nutritious as the original food and ought not to be used as food. This includes extruded proteins, whether of animal or vegetable origin. It also includes imitation fish, such as processed lobster or other artifacts that look like and try to taste like the original fish but seldom succeed. Several years ago there was some interest in converting oil to protein and then using this as food. Maybe one day when we know much more about nutrition and our needs, it may be possible to make synthetic food identical to the food to which we were once adapted. But that time has not yet come.

Few people need more protein than a simple natural diet provides. Although high-protein diets can be tolerated (provided this means high protein-rich foods), there is no advantage to this diet. There may be a number of disadvantages, though. A high protein diet increases the demand for calcium and thus may be one of the factors leading to osteoporosis.

⑤ PUBLIC MALNUTRITION

A report in the *Proceedings of the National Academy of Science*, reviewed in a syndicated newspaper article in 1993, described life inside Biosphere 2, an experimental environmental project. The residents lived there for 2 years, sealed so that only sunlight, electrical energy, and heat were exchanged with the outside environment. This was a model of a closed ecosystem. Their diet consisted of fresh fruits, cereals, peas, peanuts, beans, greens, sweet and white potatoes, with small quantities of goat milk and yogurt, goat meat, pork, chicken, fish, and eggs. Vitamin and mineral supplements were taken as well. Their fat intake was 10% of their total calorie intake.

After 6 months, their nutritional needs had changed and their health had improved markedly. They discovered that they needed only 1,780 calories per day instead of the usual 2,500 North Americans consume. They exercised a lot and worked 3 to 4 hours each day. Their weight decreased by 12 kg for the men and 7 kg for the women. Their mean blood pressure dropped 20%, mean blood sugar dropped 18%, and mean blood cholesterol dropped 36%.

"This is astounding," Dr Colin Rose, cardiologist and Associate Professor of Medicine at McGill University, remarked. "Conventional Western medical wisdom dictates that only 5% to 10% of blood cholesterol can be influenced by diet, and that only rare 'salt sensitive' people will change their blood pressures minimally on a low-salt diet. Most physicians we know believe that these parameters are genetically determined and can be altered only with drugs, if at all."

Maintaining a state of public malnutrition with a high-tech diet has become highly profitable for food and drug manufacturers.

Dr R. Walford, one of the "citizens" in the Biosphere, made the point that if all Americans were to follow this natural diet, the United States would save $50 billion per year from the remarkable caloric reduction, about $100 billion per year from the decreased need of packaging for processed foods, and $200 billion per year from savings gained through the decreased incidence of diseases caused by the typical high-tech diet, combined with the decrease in the amount of drugs needed to treat these diseases. Oral hypoglycemics, cholesterol-lowering drugs, blood pressure lowering drugs, and treatment for obesity account for billions of dollars in the American economy. Preventing these conditions, rather than waiting to treat them, would eliminate their complications, such as blindness, renal failure, heart attacks, heart failure, blocked leg arteries, and strokes.

In short, the Biosphere scientists discovered exactly what naturopathic nutritionists and orthomolecular doctors have been claiming for years. Of course, such a radical change in the national diet toward what the citizens of the Biosphere consumed would produce a major disruption of the entire food and agricultural complex. This would be resisted by the agricultural industry and laborers alike, not to mention the medical and pharmaceutical establishment. Maintaining a state of public malnutrition with a high-tech diet has become highly profitable for food and drug manufacturers.

Malnutrition Studies

The amount of disease caused by poor nutrition has been studied in institutions, primarily hospitals and nursing homes. These are the last places in the world you would expect nutrition to be neglected. In one study, it was found half the surgical patients suffered protein-calorie malnutrition, and the general medical patients were even worse off. In another study, 20% of the patients studied were deficient in each nutrient examined. For example, while diabetics, who generally are more nutrition conscious, had fewer deficiencies, peptic ulcer patients had the lowest vitamin C levels. In general, malnutrition was widespread.

Here are some other surprising statistics from these studies:
- 31% of 200 consecutive patients were malnourished on admission
- 65% of 1,000 surgical patients in an affluent suburban hospital had moderate to severe malnutrition
- 100% of the malnourished patients experienced further deterioration of their nutritional status after spending 3 weeks in a modern hospital
- 75% of well-nourished patients showed a decline in their nutritional status after spending 2 weeks or longer in hospital
- Malnourished patients stayed 90% longer in hospital than other medical patients
- Malnourished patients had 75% higher costs of care than the overall hospital average

The amount of malnutrition is just as bad in nursing homes. In one home with 232 patients, 59% of the patients showed some protein-calorie malnutrition. Seventeen had bedsores – they were all in the severely malnourished group. Another study showed that 60,000 deaths each year in the United States came from skin destructive bedsores.

The first major population studies of the link between health and nutrition arose out of food rationing in England during the Second World War. Due to trade blockades, England was not able to provide the accustomed diet to its citizens. The per capita consumption of sugar decreased from about 120 lb per person per year to half that amount. There was also a major decrease in the use of white flour and meat. White flour was replaced by a more nutritious brown flour, containing more wheat germ and bran. The government carried out a massive educational campaign to teach the people how to make nourishing meals from their vegetables instead of using meat.

Physicians, especially psychiatrists, had predicted with great confidence that there would be a major *increase* in disease in England due to the stress of war – the bombing, the dislocations of people, the loss of homes, the deprivations. It was predicted there would be a major increase in the psychosomatic diseases, such as peptic ulcer, ulcerative colitis, arthritis, and thyroid disease. But after the war, to everyone's surprise, it was found that none of the predictions had come true.

> Epidemiological studies of people who have forsaken their native diet have invariably found an increase in ill health.

On the contrary, the people as a whole had never been healthier. There was a major decrease in disease, even in psychiatric disease. For the first time, there was a decrease in the incidence of schizophrenia, as well as a decrease in heart disease and peptic ulcer. After the war, the government discontinued the educational program, removed the wartime restriction on the importation of sugar and white flour, and the intake of sugar quickly returned to the previous 120 lb per year.

Other countries with similar drastic changes in their food consumption experienced similar vast improvement in their overall health. Denmark enforced a major rationing of animal food and sugar. The Danes became much healthier.

Epidemiological studies of people who have forsaken their native diet have invariably found an increase in ill health. In South Africa, the prevalence of diabetes and cancer of the colon was very low as long as the inhabitants lived on their native high-fiber, low-sugar diets. As these people adopted the modern high-sugar, low-fiber diet, they have become very ill. In Israel about 40 years ago, Jews from North Africa were examined and found to be physically healthy, free of modern disease. Today, the same people are suffering from as much disease as their fellow citizens. It takes about 20 years of the high-tech diet for the high-tech diseases to develop.

Animal studies have shown that once a population of animals is placed on an inadequate diet, the health of the animals decreases for eight generations until it reaches a steady state of *poor* health. When the diet was restored to the level that had maintained good health in the past, it required another four generations before the original state of health was achieved.

Let's place this in the context of human populations eating a poor diet. One generation is about 20 years. If our current high-tech diet is maintained, our health will continue to deteriorate for eight generations or 160 years. The start of this deterioration in health needs to be backdated to 1950 or so, to the advent of the high-tech diet. We might expect to achieve a steady state of miserable health by the end of this century. Perhaps we will reach a state where 90% or more of the population has one or more chronic disease. If, however, we return to a natural diet, we should be able to achieve general good health among the population within four generations or 80 years. This process of recovery can be greatly accelerated by supplementing a natural food diet with ample quantities of the nutrients on which our high-tech diets have made us dependent.

Healthcare Crisis

Public healthcare programs have not been able to keep up with the costs of the consequences of this kind of malnutrition. Since the 1950s, there has been a real increase in the number of people who become sick, despite the ever-increasing amount of money spent to make them well. Today, every second Canadian has one or more degenerative disease. The costs of improved methods for diagnosing and treating the increase in disease conditions has not been rewarded with a reduction in disease or an increase in lifespan.

We no longer have major epidemics of pellagra, scurvy, or previously common infectious diseases. Surgical methods and drug treatments are vastly improved. Our society should be much healthier and our citizens should be living much longer – and the public cost of health care costs should be going down substantially. Why, then, has just the reverse occurred? On the average people live longer – that is, many more live into old age – but the expectation of additional years by the time one reaches 50 has not changed in the past 100 years. What has gone wrong? Why did we not foresee these changes in 1960 when our health plans were being formulated?

Universal healthcare programs were introduced many years ago in Canada and several European nations, before there was enough information on which to base the future cost of disease. No consideration was given to the impact of the high-tech diet on the production of ill health. If the prevalence and incidence of disease had remained constant at the 1960 level, there would be no economic crises in health care today.

This economic crisis afflicts not only public healthcare plans but also private programs. Neither Canada nor the United States has been able to control the growth of healthcare costs. Brian Ferguson, Associate Professor of Economics at the University of Guelph, has shown that the healthcare system of both countries yield similar results if measured by the usual measures, such as infant mortality.

The planners did not foresee the impact on health of the major technological changes in our food supply. The rapid deterioration of the quality of our food is the major factor in causing our health crisis today. Twenty-five years ago the evidence connecting the quality of our food and health was not as well known. There were many individual physicians and people interested in nutrition who did understand and warned us but few of us listened. Today, the evidence is available to a much larger degree: it is clear and striking. Yet, it is still consistently ignored by the medical profession and governments responsible for administering public health and food quality measures. North American medical schools neglect to teach their students the importance of good nutrition in treating disease and maintaining health. When they do attempt to teach nutrition, it is left to biochemists, who are not clinicians – they have never seen the impact of poor food in causing disease and of good food in restoring health.

Irresponsible Medicine

Any healthcare system that ignores the profound effect of nutrition on health and disease is going to make little appreciable difference to the general health of the population. Modern medicine has gone about as far as it can with its present methodology and therapeutic measures, and there it will stay until nutrition is brought into the body of medicine, taught in medical schools and used by the profession.

Dr D.C. Hemingway has recently examined the relationship of good nutrition to health costs. He proposes that we "must improve the nutritional status of Canadians to lower our healthcare costs. Governments can demonstrate the effectiveness of nutrition by promoting better nutrition for our hospital patients. Governments could recognize nutrition therapy fees under 'medicare' and as income tax deductions. This would encourage doctors and patients to use nutrition instead of drugs. Governments on behalf of the people of Canada must take the initiative to finance studies to show the effectiveness of Nutritional Therapy and Nutrition as a method of disease prevention. Industry cannot finance nutrition research because their shareholders demand profits. Nutrients cannot be patented and therefore there is no way to recover the costs of the research. Insurance companies, governments and citizens are the people that pay medical bills and they are the ones that can benefit from lower health care costs. We as health professionals and concerned citizens must continue to encourage our politicians to take a more active role in Health Maintenance."

This is not a new call to action. In the 1950s, Dr T.D. Spies, one of the foremost nutritional physicians of the times, an expert pellagrologist and clinical nutritionist, published an article in the *Journal of the American Medical Association* on the central role of good nutrition in achieving good health. "I have discussed with you a few of the many advances which have been made in nutrition in recent years," he explained. "You have seen that what patients eat has much to do with their health and with their recovery from ill health. Primary or secondary nutritional disorders produce or complicate all the problems of the sick. I have stressed that we should be concerned with the prevention and with the earlier stages of disease when the disturbances are almost imperceptible and that we should not wait until these disturbances bring tremendous burdens and stark tragedies."

> **There will be no relief from the enormous psychosocial, physical, and economic costs of this imbalance until it is corrected, until we return to the whole living diets of our ancestors – or until we adopt the feeding principle and practices of any good zoo.**

This statement is as applicable today as when it was written. It is sad that we learn so slowly, that pride keeps us from accepting the discoveries and teachings of our colleagues. We cannot change the past, but we can use the information gleaned from the past to change our ways of promoting health today. Tomorrow is our responsibility.

Modern food technology has become food chemistry. We know a good deal about the chemical structure of food, but in the process of developing the chemistry of food, we have neglected to study the physiology of food. There is thus an almost total imbalance between our needs and what we eat. It is almost as odd as feeding lions only on grass. Our needs are the type of whole foods to which our ancestors had adapted 10,000 years ago. Since then we have remained the same physiologically, but our food supply has been altered until it is only a caricature of what food should be. This imbalance is the main factor in causing most of the physical and psychiatric disease we must deal with.

There will be no relief from the enormous psychosocial, physical, and economic costs of this imbalance until it is corrected, until we return to the whole living diets of our ancestors – or until we adopt the feeding principle and practices of any good zoo. We know more than did our ancestors 10,000 years ago. We know about nutrient supplements. We should use the best food available and for those with special needs provide the extra quantities required. We should practice the principles of naturopathic nutrition and orthomolecular medicine.

THE HEALTH BENEFITS OF A NATUROPATHIC DIET

⑥ OPTIMUM DIET

Most people are convinced that modern high-tech food provides the best in nutrition. This is the message put forward by the food industry in their advertisements and by many nutritionists and doctors of the old school. However, most doctors know very little about clinical nutrition and have no experience in treating patients whose illness arises from their malnutrition. Between 1999 and 2005, 41 medical students each spent 2 days in training with us. They came from various schools in Europe, Australia, and Canada. We asked each student how many hours of clinical nutrition education they had received; on average, they had 1 hour (not year) of instruction.

Epidemiologists have claimed that our society is healthier than it has ever been, using the infant mortality rate and the increasing number of people living to retirement age as their key criteria. Some conclude that the high-tech diet has been the main factor in bringing about this apparent high state of good general health. However, the high incidence of chronic disease (every second Canadian, for example, has one or more chronic disease) contradicts this claim, as does the ever-increasing cost of medical care.

Individual Adaptation

One of the chief factors in generating chronic disease is the mismatch between the food that we have become adapted to and the food that we now consume. The adaptation developed over evolution has been destroyed by the changes in our foods that have come about so quickly it has been impossible for our digestive apparatus to accommodate them.

Maladaptation and Survival

All living organisms live within an environment they have to adapt to. The environment may be relatively constant over enormous periods of time or it may shift very rapidly. Organisms, plants, or animals that cannot adapt to their environment cannot survive. Obviously, the rate of adaptation will depend upon the rate at which the environmental changes occur. When the environment changes slowly, there is ample time for the organisms within that environment to adapt and to change. When the environment changes rapidly, there may not be sufficient time, and species of living beings may be wiped out very quickly simply because there has not been enough time. Dinosaurs were wiped out over a relatively short period of time by a rapid change in the atmosphere caused by the collision of a large object with earth. This is one of the theories being examined to account for their disappearance after having successfully inhabited this earth for over 100 million years.

> One of the chief factors in generating chronic disease is the mismatch between the food that we have become adapted to and the food that we now consume.

Animals may adapt to the change in their environment by changing their habits without needing much if any change in their genetic structure. Genetic changes in animals, excluding insects, tend to be very slow and require long periods of time. Changes in habits may occur very quickly. Modern examples are the invasions of cities in North America by animals, such as raccoons, rabbits, deer, and even cougars in Vancouver Island. Rats have survived in the presence of people for thousands of years. These animals have learned to live within environments that would have been intolerable for them a long time ago.

Genetic changes occur very slowly, requiring millions of years. Darwin discovered that the pressure to survive created species of animals that favored fitness. Animals best able to survive in the changed environment would be more apt to reproduce and gradually their offspring would become the predominant species. Species that became too rigid in structure, form, or physiology would be less adaptable, and although they could survive, they would not be able to change. Some animals appear to be the same as they were millions of years ago. They have learned how to survive in environments that are fairly stable. Thus evolution does not necessarily go along with survival. Survival also plays a role only during the reproductive periods.

> Lack of recognition of the need to match our food supply with our inherited needs underlies the health crises about which we hear so much today.

For humanity, what happens after age 60 is relatively unimportant for the human species in terms of survival of the fittest. Survival of the fittest applies to the gradual development of fitter species that increases their proportion of the total gene pool. If our major reproductive period were toward the end of our lives, there would be a much different relationship. But this is a modern phenomenon since more people are alive to retirement, whereas throughout evolution the mean age at death was closer to the reproductive period.

The connection between food supply and survival of species is clear. Animals must be provided with food of the type their species has been consuming and to which they have adapted. There is a wide variation in adaptation, ranging from species that appear to have only one major food supply, like the anteater, to species that can consume a wide variety of plants and animals. This has been recognized by animal nutritionists, especially those in charge of modern zoos, but this recognition has been very slow in coming to human nutritionists. Lack of recognition of the need to match our food supply with our inherited needs underlies the health crises about which we hear so much today. Maladaptation is the major factor and must be corrected if ever we are to halt the inevitable increase in chronic disease and bring it back to levels that a proper match of genetics and food supply would ensure.

Bioindividuality

Every person is unique. Infants know this as soon as they can differentiate their mother from all other mothers. When a child first recognizes a stranger, that child has already mastered the concept that we are all different. In appearance we are not the same. The best test for this is the interest generated when identical twins walk down the street. When quintuplets are identical, public curiosity is enormous, for these phenomena violate the principle of individuality.

The need for individuality has been essential for survival. The outer appearance and behavior of any individual is an expression of that person's physiology and biochemistry. It follows that their biochemistry and nutritional needs must also be individual. Without individuality, there would be no humanity. The individuality of people was necessary for the evolution of our human societies.

We know all about the individuality of fingerprints, how even identical twins do not have identical fingerprints. Blood types also are unique to individuals, as are dental patterns and DNA. Surgeons are not surprised when they try to find the appendix and it is not where it is supposed to be. Sometimes the heart is on the right side. Most organs of the body are not exactly where they are supposed to be, nor are they the same size and shape. Physicians and pharmacologists have known that the optimum doses for drugs can vary enormously between patients, that while there are useful guides for how much to give, many people will need much less and many will need much more. People know that "one man's meat is another man's poison."

However, this principle of bioindividuality has not been applied to the need for developing optimum nutrition for each person. The manufacture and advertising of high-tech food is based upon the principle that we are all alike. They extol the virtues of their product without acknowledging that many people may be allergic or otherwise be made sick by this product and should avoid it. The dairy industry touts its products very highly with support from nutritionists and physicians, but they never mention in their advertisements that many people are made sick by milk.

We are unique as individuals and our needs for nutrients vary, as do other biochemical and physical attributes. There will be a narrow range of variation for some nutrients and a wide range of variation for others. Each nutrient will have its own range. This means that most people will have an optimum range that varies about a mean for the whole group, but there will be a much smaller number of people who will need much less and another group who will need much more.

Recommended Daily Allowances

The optimum amount of nutrients varies for each person, but we do not have the data for each nutrient on large normal populations. The recommended daily allowances (RDAs) generally cover a very narrow range of need. The developers of these recommended doses assumed that vitamins were needed only in very small doses and added what they considered was an ample safety factor by recommending more than they really thought were needed.

These doses apply only to normal and healthy people, however. They exclude people under stress, people who are sick, pregnant women, and nursing women. There are so many exclusions that RDAs have no value for individuals. They have never been of any value for determining what individuals should be taking. Recently, scientists have begun to recognize this, and some have recommended using specific doses for individual diseases. We have done this for many years.

If we constructed a large bell shaped curve showing the range of dosage for any one nutrient along the bottom or the X axis and plotted the area on the curve where each disease properly fell, we would find that healthy people would be in the area from the lowest doses to somewhat above the mean for the whole group. Patients would be in the high dose area, and the sicker they were, the closer they would lie to the extreme right of the diagram. Thus, the average person will get along fairly well with about 3 g per day of ascorbic acid. A person with any infection, such as the common cold, will need perhaps two to three times as much. A person seriously ill with a killing disease, such as cancer, will require doses ranging from 12 to 40 g orally and may need an additional 50 to 100 g given intravenously.

Vitamin C represents the very wide variation of optimum doses. Other nutrients have much narrower ranges. For riboflavin there is little evidence to suggest that we have to give more than 100 or 200 mg per day. The water-soluble vitamins are very safe because they do not build up in the body. They are easily excreted. Fat-soluble vitamins can build up and one has to be more cautious about using high doses. But even here the dangers of these vitamins, such as vitamin D-3 and vitamin A, have been grossly exaggerated.

Orthomolecular Medicine

Dr Linus Pauling, in his fundamental study of "orthomolecular" nutrition and in his celebrated book *Vitamin C and the Common Cold*, has shown how the human body lost its ability during evolution to make certain nutrients. About 60 million years ago man, other primates, the guinea pig, and an Indian fruit-eating bat lost the ability to make vitamin C. The process has not stopped.

> Dr Pauling proposed the word "orthomolecular" to describe the use of optimum (often large) doses of molecules naturally present in the body to treat poor health and to promote optimum health.

Man is going through a process right now where we are losing the ability to make vitamin B-3 from tryptophan, as Dr Pauling and Dr Hoffer have suggested in their book *Healing Cancer* and as Professor Harold D. Foster and Dr Hoffer have documented in their book *Feel Better and Live Longer with Vitamin B-3*. The schizophrenias represent a group of people who have gone far in this direction. As diets have become high-tech, the amount of vitamin B-3 has been lowered, and those people who no longer have the machinery for converting enough tryptophan to the vitamin are becoming sick. We have been convinced for a long time that if we were to add 100 mg of niacinamide to our diet for every person, there would be a major decrease in the incidence of schizophrenia and many other diseases, such as hyperactivity and learning and behavioral disorders in children.

Dr Pauling proposed the word "orthomolecular" to describe the use of optimum (often large) doses of molecules naturally present in the body to treat poor health and to promote optimum health. The new practice of orthomolecular medicine recognizes that most chronic diseases are due to a metabolic fault that is correctable in most patients by good use of nutrition, including the use of vitamin and mineral supplements.

In sharp contrast, drugs are synthetics that are not naturally present in the body and for which the body does not have ready-made mechanisms for their destruction and elimination. They are called xenobiotics – that is, foreign molecules. And unlike conventional medicine, orthomolecular medicine also recognizes the principle of individuality in recommending the optimum diet of nutrients for each of us.

Orthomolecular medicine requires the application of both these basic principles, individuality and the use of optimum doses (large doses if needed).

Whole, Alive, Fresh . . .

Just as we were able to describe the problems of the modern high-tech diet with nine adjectives – artifact, dead, stale, monotonous, toxic, abundant, exogenous, synthetic, complex – so we can describe the naturopathic orthomolecular diet with their opposite attributes – whole, alive, fresh, varied, non-toxic, scarce, endogenous, naturally flavored, and simple. The adequacy of these adjectives can be assessed by anyone who has any familiarity with the way animals eat in the wild and the way they are fed in zoos. Natural food is *whole*. Some fish eat other fish swimming less rapidly and they eat them whole. Lions after the kill eat the whole animal provided they can protect the kill against other predators. A tiger does not cut a steak from its prey and store it either cold or dried or otherwise preserved. Herbivores naturally graze on living vegetable material, although domestic horses and cows are fed grasses that have been cut, dried, and stored.

Whole

Animals that eat their prey will ingest all the available minerals, vitamins, and other food components *whole*. Carnivores often eat the internal organs first and later go after the muscle meats. With plant material, there is a tremendous difference nutritionally between the various fractions of that food. Whole wheat comprises the germ, the bran, and the white endosperm. The outer coating of the wheat berry or the bran is rich in minerals and vitamins and the richest source of nutrients is the germ. In milling white flour, both the bran and the germ are discarded, and by eating the white flour (bread, pastry, pasta), we are depriving ourselves of the most nourishing part of the wheat berry. Nearly 200 years ago it was shown by a French army surgeon that dogs fed on whole-meal bread alone were kept alive and healthy, while similar animals fed on white bread quickly sickened and died. Eating whole grain foods provides all the nutrition available in that plant.

Alive

Natural food is *alive*. Even scavenger animals eat meat that has not been stored very long. The main advantage to eating food that is or has been recently alive is that all the nutrients present in that food are available for use. Fresh food, alive or recently alive, has not had time to deteriorate or to develop infection or infestations with organisms and insects that are harmful. Fresh food that has deteriorated loses substantial amounts of vitamins and enzymes. If live food is not always available, the best means of preserving food value is freezing at very low temperatures, and the next best method is canning. None of the stored and preserved foods, however, can compare in nutritional quality to the original fresh food. Remember that when animals do store foods, it is food like nuts and seeds, which are alive but dormant and which can create new life when given a chance.

Fresh

The third adjective is *fresh*. Fresh and alive are almost the same since alive food is necessarily fresh and fresh food has been recently alive. But there is a difference. Fresh whole-wheat bread will be more nutritious than will be the same bread after it has been stored for a long time. With storage, there is the problem of contamination with organisms, which can destroy the nutrient value of the food and can also cause illness.

Varied

A natural diet is *varied*. Since we are omnivores, we can best ensure getting the nutrients we need by consuming a wide variety of foods. If the foods are varied from meal to meal, from day to day, and from season to season, there is much less danger of developing allergic reactions. If a person is allergic to a food or to several foods, they must be eliminated from the diet, often for a period of time lasting from 6 months to a year. Then it may be possible to follow a rotation diet – to follow a schedule where similar families of food are eaten every fourth day or fifth day. A program of eating is developed that spreads the foods over these days. It may then be possible for the person to eat these foods at these intervals without having the usual reactions they were having before.

Modern diets do not follow this variety principle. Rather, staple foods are consumed daily in large quantities. People will have bread with every meal, meats every day if not in two out of three meals, potatoes every day, and so on. Many individuals eat 50% of their calories as sugar. Early man could not follow these monotonous diets. Their food supply varied from morning to night, from month to month, and from season to season. They had no way of storing their foods so that they could eat the same foods every day for the whole year.

In meats, variety is introduced by eating more than just the muscles. This includes sweetbreads, liver, cartilage, and even softer bones. In fish, it may include whole fish, like sardines. With fruit, one can eat from a large variety depending more on the home-grown types. The same applies to vegetables. One should consume the edible parts, including leaves, seeds, tubers, roots, and stems where feasible from as many kinds of vegetables as are available. The same applies to grains, where one should use all the grains, not just a large number of products made from flour.

Non-toxic

The natural diet is *non-toxic*. It is obvious that our ancestors quickly eliminated those foods that were toxic, probably at first by trial and error. If they ate the food and remained well, this would become part of the diet. They did not have to worry about the addition of chemicals to the food to 'enhance' flavor or to preserve it. The foods they ate were non-toxic, except when they tried to store food and it became contaminated with bacteria and their toxins.

Scarce

The food in a natural diet is *scarce*. In comparison to the abundant food supply available today in high-tech societies, our ancestors had to adapt to fluctuations in food supply by storing fat as a reserve energy source. During periods when food was abundant, their bodies would store more fat, and when food was scarce or when they were starving, their bodies would draw upon this energy reserve. Women had to bear a double burden when they were pregnant, and for this reason they adapted by storing even more fat before pregnancy and during pregnancy, in order to have enough food to provide milk for their babies. They alternated between having enough food and not having enough, but they did not have to contend

> Modern society does not demand as much calorie expenditure of its people, while at the same time providing a huge surplus of attractive artifact foods, which taste good and which can easily be eaten very quickly.

with having poor nutritional quality food. Today, in high-tech societies, there is too much food and there are no periods of starvation or decreased supply. The fat that accumulates when too much is consumed is not taken off by any following period of food reduction or starvation.

Over consumption is less likely with whole meat and fish, fruit and vegetables. It is more of a problem with the grains and nuts and seeds. Sugar is one of the major factors, as are the commercial fats and oils. Natural foods are more bulky, have to be chewed longer, and cannot be eaten as quickly, so it is less easy to overload the system. Prepared foods from ground and refined grains are usually combined with sugar, fat, and other additives. It is very easy to over-eat bakery goods. Many of our patients with eating disorders have told us that they would buy one dozen doughnuts and that they would be gone before they arrived home, or that they would eat a loaf of bread in one evening, or a pound box of candy in a few hours. Primitive societies did not have a surplus of food. They had to work for their food as well. Modern society does not demand as much calorie expenditure of its people, while at the same time providing a huge surplus of attractive artifact foods, which taste good and which can easily be eaten very quickly.

Endogenous

Natural food is *endogenous*. Foods before the dawn of agriculture and for thousands of years afterward were locally grown or harvested. Foods today may come from anywhere on the globe. There are both advantages and disadvantages to this. The advantages arise when the imported food is superior in quality to the home-grown or endogenous foods. The advantage of home-grown food of equal nutritive quality is that there is a better match between the essential fatty acid composition of the foods in local plants and animals and the fatty acids needed by the consumer of those foods.

This is very important in northern and colder climates, where the ratio of essential fatty acids to non-essential fats is important in developing cold tolerance. The colder the climate, the more important is it to both plants and animals to have more essential fatty acids. These are more unsaturated and, therefore, their freezing point is lower. They may be compared to the antifreeze one uses in cars. They are not needed in the tropics but very essential in northern Canada. If a native from Mexico is suddenly transposed to Saskatoon where it is minus 40°F, he will be much more apt to freeze exposed parts of his body – his ears or the rolls of fat around his neck. If the same person moved to Saskatoon in the summer, his body would have time to adjust by laying down more unsaturated fatty acids and he would be much more cold tolerant by the time winter arrived. It is wise to depend as much as possible on endogenous foods and to supplement the diet with exogenous food known to be superior in quality.

Naturally Flavored

Natural food is *naturally flavored*. Ancient foods were not overly processed and no synthetic flavors were known. With more sophistication, our ancestors began to flavor their foods with herbs. This became much more important when food, which had gone bad, had to be consumed. The herbs were used to cover the awful taste of these stale preparations. Fresh food for most people tastes pretty good, even without the addition of salt and sugar. Many people, however, cannot enjoy the taste of food unless it is saturated with salt and sugar because that has been so much a part of their diet for so many years.

Simple

The natural diet is *simple*. Our ancestors did not have our ability or our desire to compound food preparations. Many modern recipes call for over a dozen different ingredients. In the past, the foods were simple, and people eating them could know what it was they were eating. If they knew that rabbit meat made them sick, they did not have to worry that some rabbit meat might be present in other food preparations. Today, we cannot be sure of the ingredients in food unless we make them ourselves. This is why people who know peanuts will kill them (anaphylactic shock) have died eating food they thought was safe because some person had added peanut oil to the preparation. One has to be very careful of all overly processed foods and to distrust even the labels on many prepared foods.

Natural Nutrition Standards

In the perennial dance of the individual and the environment, time does not go backward. We cannot re-establish the world from which we have evolved. We cannot return to the dietary habitat of our prehistoric ancestors, nor do we need to. It is feasible to process our modern foods and to select from these foods the elements we are best adapted to. Eventually, everything that is done to our food from the farm to our kitchens will have to be treated so as to maximize its nutritional quality. One day we may have a public health law that will not permit the sale and distribution of any food preparation unless it is proven to be as safe and as nourishing as the foods from which they were fashioned. This requires no new knowledge – just the will to do so. It would simply force all the food processors to perform animal feeding tests.

Our food should be processed and selected to fit the description of the diets to which we are adapted. We should be able to describe our foods as almost whole, alive, and fresh and distinguish them from the artifacts that are dead and stale. Visualize a scale or line ranging from whole at one end (or alive or fresh) to artifact at the other end (or dead or stale). The objective is to move toward the healthy end of the scale as far as possible, knowing that this is an ideal most people won't reach. Nevertheless, it is healthier to be close to the healthy end than it is to be close to the disease end where we are today. Perhaps each item could be rated with a quality item or number starting with 100 and decreasing in value to the pathological end at zero. At the zero end, life would be barely sustainable with maximum disease, while at the healthy end of the scale, life would be sustainable with optimum good health. A quick look at our traditional food groups will reveal how close they come to meeting this natural nutrition standard.

Food Groups

All animal products – meat, fish, eggs, and dairy products – must be as fresh as possible or properly preserved or stored (freeze dried, frozen, or heat dried, which is the less desirable). These foods will have to be cooked unless one is absolutely certain they are free of bacterial or parasitic infection. The only dairy product that can be considered whole is milk. All the other products are derivative of this. Milk should be fresh and not heat treated if one could be certain it was free of bacterial contamination. Pasteurized milk for most is essential. Cheeses are deliberately contaminated, seeded with organisms that ferment or ripen them. Cheeses cannot be fresh or whole and thus cannot be ideal foods because of the way they are made and stored. Only cottage cheese can meet the fresh criterion; all other cheeses are artifact, dead, and stale, as is ice cream and many other products made from dairy products.

Fresh fruit is alive and almost whole (the seeds are often not consumed). Fruit that has to be stored and shipped is alive and whole to a degree. In storage, the fruit will lose a fair amount of its nutritive value, especially the vitamins. This loss is accelerated if the fruit is cut and exposed to air and to light. Frozen fruit is next best to fresh fruit, followed by dried and then by preserved fruit. A can of pears is an artifact. The least desirable are the jellies and jams that are mostly sugar flavored by the fruit. Most juices are not wholly healthy foods because they do not meet this criterion.

Fresh vegetables are alive and whole (edible parts only). The quality decreases with processing in factory or in the kitchen in the following order: fast frozen, freeze-dried, cooked, and preserved. All edible parts can be used, including roots, tubers, leaves, and stems. In storage, vegetables lose vitamins, and when cooked they lose more vitamins and water-soluble minerals. They also can become contaminated with bacteria and fungi. Processed fractions from vegetables, such as potato flour, do not meet the criteria since they are artifact, dead, and stale.

Most plant material cannot be digested by people. If consumed, it will be toxic by virtue of this fact and the bulk. Cellulose is indigestible for us, but not for fungi and some insects. Straw is indigestible for humans, but can be digested by ruminants that have special digestive apparatus for dealing with this. Over the years, we have learned which foods are edible. Once we have a tradition about foods, it becomes very difficult to change it. For many years tomatoes were considered toxic in the U.S.A. but not in Europe. Americans began to eat tomatoes after a public demonstration in front of a courthouse, where one person ate tomatoes. Natural food excludes all the plant and animal material that is inherently toxic or indigestible. The toxic properties of the edible foods arises from the addition of chemicals, which have not been proven to be non-toxic in chronic toxicity trials in animals in combination with other additives, or which have not been used by people long enough to have demonstrated its safety.

Whole grains meet the natural standard before they are processed, milled, or ground. They are alive because they can grow. When given the right conditions, they will sprout and produce a whole new plant. They can be consumed whole or may be ground and eaten very soon after that. But once ground, they quickly go stale, especially flax, which turns rancid very quickly. Bread made from wheat is pretty healthy, even though it is now dead. The nutritive quality for many is enhanced by the cooking, which makes them easier to chew and to digest. The quality decreases quickly with increased refinement in processing.

Balanced Diet

The term 'balanced diet' has been corrupted by dietitians and food processors, who use it as a justification for allowing the many degradations in the food they make. For many years, apologists for white bread maintained that since no one lived on bread alone, it did not matter if it was deficient in some nutrients; the rest of the nutrients needed to balance the diet would be provided by other food groups.

> A diet consisting of natural foods is inherently balanced, provided enough variety is introduced.

This is not true. If 90% of the diet were good, it would not matter too much if 10% were corrupted. But where 75% of the diet is corrupted, it really does matter. Ideally, each food should contain its full share of nutrients required by the person. Whole foods are balanced already by nature. A diet consisting of natural foods is inherently balanced, provided enough variety is introduced. In the animal world, monotonous foods are well balanced. An anteater eats a diet of live ants only and the koala bear eats only leaves from a few species of the eucalyptus tree. The term 'balanced' should apply only to combinations of natural foods – only to the naturopathic orthomolecular diet.

(7) | OPTIMUM ABSORPTION

Not only good food but also a healthy digestive system is essential for optimal health. Our digestive system needs to be working efficiently if we are to absorb nutrients so that they can get into the blood and tissues of the body and if we are to fend off environmental toxins and bacteria.

The digestive tract is a tube-like structure, approximately 30 feet long, running from the mouth to the anus and including the pharynx (throat), esophagus, stomach, small intestine, and large intestine (colon). Our digestive system is one of the only systems in the body that is in direct contact with the outside world (environment) in terms of the foods we eat, the fluids we drink, and the incidental products (bacteria and dirt, for example) that we accidentally ingest.

However, many individuals do not absorb the maximum nutrients available in their diet or derive the maximum protective effects of these nutrients because of low stomach acid. They might be on the best nutritional plan, but only when their acid problems are corrected, do they reap the healthy benefits of their food.

Most nutritionally oriented healthcare practitioners know the value of proper digestion and begin their investigations with the stomach. Numerous treatments are available that can replace the stomach acid that is no longer being produced. Treatments might also be used to stimulate the specialized cells of the stomach to increase their production of acid. Regardless of the types of treatments employed, the goal is to optimize the functioning of the stomach, improve nutrient absorption, and resolve troublesome clinical signs and symptoms.

Stomach Functions

The stomach is one of the most important parts of a good digestive system. It is a J-shaped, saclike reservoir located between the esophagus and the small intestine. The stomach itself is divided into three sections – fundus, body, and antrum. When fasted the stomach's volume is around 50 ml, one-fifth of a regular 250 ml glass of water. The stomach expands greatly when a meal is consumed, potentially reaching a volume of 1 liter.

> Not only good food but also a healthy digestive system is essential for optimal health.

The primary functions of the stomach are to store food temporarily, digest protein, and provide an adequate acid environment for the absorption of nutrients. Food is stored in the stomach until the small intestine is ready to receive it. It takes hours to digest and absorb a meal that might have taken only minutes to be consumed. The stomach must empty into the small intestine at a rate that does not overwhelm the capacities of the small intestine and at a rate that is appropriate for optimal digestion and health.

Stomach Acid (HCl)

For the digestion of protein the stomach must secrete a sufficient amount of stomach acid, also known as hydrochloric acid (HCl). Stomach acid is the most important substance secreted by the stomach. The acid directly influences the acid-base (pH) balance of the fluids and food within stomach. When a meal is consumed, the pH becomes more acidic due to the release of additional stomach acid. The range in terms of pH when a meal is consumed is somewhere between 1-3. When a meal is not consumed, the stomach pH is much higher (greater than 3) and thus is more basic or alkaline.

> **Without adequate stomach acid, the nutrient composition does not favorably change and absorption from the small intestine becomes significantly impaired.**

With the additional stomach acid present, many enzymes systems are activated, helping to break down proteins from the ingested meal. Stomach acid stimulates other organs to function optimally by facilitating the flow of bile from the liver and encouraging the production of pancreatic enzymes. Bile helps with the absorption of fats and oils and is involved with the regulation cholesterol. Pancreatic enzymes, released from the pancreas into the small intestine, digest protein, fat, and carbohydrate.

The additional stomach acid allows for the proper absorption of a variety of nutrients, such as calcium, iron, folic acid, vitamin B-6, vitamin B-12, vitamin A, vitamin E, and other B vitamins. The stomach acid changes the nutrient composition so that they can eventually be absorbed from the small intestine. Without adequate stomach acid, the nutrient composition does not favorably change and absorption from the small intestine becomes significantly impaired. This acidic environment also prevents infections from developing because it sterilizes and safeguards against the growth of bacteria and other harmful pathogens within the stomach and the small intestine.

Acid Deficiency Symptoms

There are many people who do not secrete sufficient amounts of stomach acid even when a meal is consumed. This can lead to numerous digestive symptoms, the most common being chronic gas and bloating. Many symptoms of low (deficient) or absent stomach acid are similar to the symptoms of too much stomach acid, also known as heartburn or gastroesophageal reflux disease (GERD). Thousands of people are medicated for GERD or heartburn before an underlying deficiency or absence of stomach acid is adequately explored.

> ### Common Signs and Symptoms of Deficient Stomach Acid
>
> A sense of fullness after eating
> Abnormal intestinal flora
> Acne
> Bloating, belching, burning, and gas immediately after meals
> Chronic Candida albicans infections
> Chronic intestinal parasites
> Dilated blood vessels in the cheeks and nose
> Hair loss in women
> Indigestion, diarrhea or constipation
> Iron deficiency
> Itching around the rectum
> Multiple food allergies
> Nausea after taking supplements
> Poor tolerance to dentures
> Progressive loss of bone from the jaw
> Soreness, burning and dryness of the mouth
> Swollen tongue
> Undigested food in the stool
> Upper digestive tract gassiness
> Weak, peeling and cracked fingernails

Many of the signs and symptoms of low or absent stomach acid can be found through a simple (routine) physical examination. For example, gassiness in the upper abdomen, hair loss and cracked nails are associated with stomach acid problems. Other findings include a reddened face with scattered medium-to-large acne-like bumps on the forehead and cheeks. Dilated capillaries in the cheeks and at the edges of the nose are also physical exam findings of low stomach acid.

Low Stomach Acid Questionnaire

Symptom Rating Scale:

0 = Never
1 = Occasionally
2 = Frequently
3 = Almost Always

___ Gas

___ Bloating

___ Heartburn

___ Upper abdominal heaviness after eating

___ Nausea after eating

___ Nausea when taking supplements

___ Diarrhea

___ Constipation

___ Acne

___ Hair loss

___ Food allergies

___ Swollen tongue

___ Soreness, burning and/or dryness of the mouth

___ Week, peeling and/or cracked fingernails

___ Itching around the rectum

Scores in the range of 30 and over possibly indicate severe low stomach acid

Scores in the range of 20-29 possibly indicates moderate low stomach acid

Scores in the range of 10-19 possibly indicates mild low stomach acid

Scores under 10 are normal

Diagnosing Low Stomach Acid

Baking Soda Test

This crude test is not the most reliable method of diagnosing low stomach acid. When baking soda (a base) is added to a solution of vinegar (an acid), the result is foaming and bubbling due to the release of carbon dioxide (a gas). The same holds true when a solution of baking soda is swallowed. Upon entering the stomach, the reaction between the baking soda and stomach acid should cause a release of carbon dioxide. Instead of visible foaming, burping will occur.

To do this test, it is necessary to fast for at least 8 hours. It is easiest to begin the fast after dinner so that you will do the majority of fasting while sleeping. Upon waking up, add 1 tablespoon of baking soda to 1 cup (240 ml) of water and drink the solution. If burping occurs within 2 to 3 minutes, low stomach acid is not likely. If burping does not occur by 5 minutes, it is necessary to do more extensive testing for low stomach acid.

Hair Analysis

In this method of assessment, a sample of hair from the nape of the neck is taken and sent to a specialized lab for analysis. If the hair analysis comes back and shows that five or more minerals are low, excluding sodium and potassium, then an investigation into low stomach acid should be performed. Once the stomach acid problems are corrected, follow-up hair analysis often shows a trend toward normal or the complete normalization of the previously deficient minerals.

Stool Analysis for Meat Fibers

In this method of assessment, a stool sample is sent to a lab and analyzed. It is normal to have no undigested meat fibers in a stool sample. If, however, the test result demonstrates numerous undigested meat fibers, the cause is typically low stomach acid. After a period of treatment, the undigested meat fibers do not show up on a repeat stool analysis.

Urine (Indican) Test

This test in an indirect method for the assessment of low stomach acid. Since it is a urine test, it is simple, noninvasive, and quick. When too much bacteria is present in the small intestine, a compound known as indole is converted to indican, which eventually gets excreted in the urine. Remember that stomach acid sterilizes unwanted organisms in the stomach and intestine. If there is a deficiency of stomach acid, it is likely that 'bad' bacteria will build up in the intestines. Therefore, if a high amount of indican is present in the urine, it is likely due to low stomach acid. After instituting the appropriate treatments, it is typical for the indican test to normalize.

Causes of Low Stomach Acid

The causes of low stomach acid have not been determined, but most cases are of the type B gastritis variety. Low stomach acid is associated with gastric atrophy or atrophic gastritis (a condition where there is loss and damage to the acid-producing cells of the stomach). It has been reported to occur in some 28% of an adult Caucasian population. Although there are different types of atrophic gastritis (Types A and B), both are characterized by impairments in the secretion of stomach acid and are differentiated on the basis of clinical and histological findings.

Type A gastritis is also called autoimmune gastritis, characterized by a severe impairment in gastric acid secretion. Pernicious anemia almost exclusively develops from Type A gastritis, which is also associated with greater incidences of other diseases, such as hypo- or hyperthyroidism, Hashimoto's thyroiditis, insulin dependent diabetes mellitus, and vitiligo. Type B gastritis, which is about four times more common in the general population than type A, is characterized by moderate-to-severe impairment of gastric acid secretion. Type B gastritis has no relationship to autoimmunity, but appears to result from environmental factors that irritate the gastric mucosa. The incidence of gastric carcinoma (stomach cancer) is greater in type B gastritis.

Food Allergies

Some research points to the possibility that food allergies might cause low stomach acid. When common allergic foods (for example, corn, dairy, eggs, milk, and wheat) are consumed, they might stimulate specialized immune cells, known as mast cells, to release histamine. Histamine is made from the amino acid histidine and stored in mast cells located in the stomach and many other locations throughout the body. Histamine and other inflammatory mediators cause many of the common symptoms of food allergies, such as hives, itchy eyes, runny nose, and skin rashes. The histamine contained within the stomach is one of the most important stimulators of stomach acid. When allergic foods are consumed, the histamine stores in the body become depleted, and, therefore, less histamine is available in the stomach for the proper release of stomach acid. Over time, this chronic depletion of histamine stores might lead to a deficiency or absence of stomach acid.

Stress

A second possible cause of low stomach acid is stress. Although stress is a fundamental part of life, when it becomes overwhelming, it can bring about adverse changes in the stomach. Dr Hans Selye, in his book *The Stress of Life*, described ulcers in the lining of the stomach as a response to extreme or prolonged stress. It is possible that prior to the development of stomach ulcers, stress could suppress stomach acid secretion. Part of the control of stomach acid is mediated by the relaxing system in the body, known as the parasympathetic nervous system (PNS). With chronic stress, the PNS might function less efficiently and the secretion of stomach acid would be impaired.

> The fact that the incidence of low stomach acid appears to increase with age means that many people are suffering from low stomach acid and are probably not receiving appropriate treatment.

Helicobacter pylori (H. pylori)

A third possible cause of low stomach acid is infection by a specific bacterium, known as *Helicobacter pylori (H. pylori)*. *H. pylori* is the prime cause of stomach and small intestinal ulcers. Infection from this bacterium requires specific treatments to eliminate it. Research has further demonstrated that infection from *H. pylori* might cause low stomach acid because this bacterium increases the stomach pH and induces changes in the lining of the stomach that impairs the secretion of acid. Antibodies to *H. pylori*, indicating infection, have been found in 80% of people in the United States by the age of 75 years.

Environmental Irritants

The final factors involved in the production of type B gastritis include environmental irritants, such as alcohol, aspirin use, and non-steroidal anti-inflammatory drugs. All of these substances, especially when used long-term, will damage the lining of the stomach, cause inflammation, and create problems with the ability to secrete stomach acid.

At Risk

Based on the above facts, it is not surprising that the population group having the highest incidence of low stomach acid is the elderly. Studies have shown that 11% to 50% of the elderly population has lost the ability to make stomach acid because of degenerative changes in the stomach. This fact is made worse when one considers how common it is for elderly people to take antacids for heartburn or for an 'acid' stomach. Compared to the elderly, the incidence of low stomach acid among adults is significantly lower. Low stomach acid affects approximately 14% of the younger population group (mean age, 30 years). The fact that the incidence of low stomach acid appears to increase with age means that many people are suffering from low stomach acid and are probably not receiving appropriate treatment.

Associated Clinical Conditions and Diseases

Many common medical conditions and diseases are associated with low stomach acid. Many people suffering from these diseases likely have low stomach acid, but are not receiving treatment for it.

Clinical Conditions and Diseases Associated with Low Stomach Acid

Addison's Disease	Gastric polyps
Alcoholism	Gastritis
Anemia/Pernicious Anemia	Hepatitis
Arthritis/Rheumatoid Arthritis	Hyperthyroidism (Grave's disease)
Carcinoma of the stomach	Hypothyroidism
Celiac Disease	Lupus erythematosus
Childhood asthma	Myasthenia gravis
Chronic autoimmune disorders	Osteoporosis
Depression	Psoriasis
Dermatitis herpetiformis	Rosacea
Diabetes mellitus	Sjögren's disease
Diabetic neuropathies	Thyrotoxicosis
Eczema	Ulcerative colitis
Flatulent dyspepsia (maldigestion)	Urticaria (hives)
Gallbladder disease	Vitiligo

Food Allergies

A possible consequence of low stomach acid is food allergies. When proteins are not broken down through the combined actions of stomach acid and other enzymes to individual amino acids, these larger protein structures might pass through the small intestine into the bloodstream. These larger protein molecules might cause the body's immune system to attack itself, consequently causing allergic symptoms (for example, itchy eyes, runny nose, and skin rashes).

Stomach Emptying Problems

Food stored in the stomach temporarily is eventually emptied into the small intestine at a certain rate. In the low acid stomach, there is a delay in the passage of food from the stomach to the small intestine. This has health consequences because the delay changes the way nutrients from foods are absorbed. The delay can adversely affect blood and urine tests as well.

Intrinsic Factor Secretion

The cells that line the stomach to produce acid also produce a compound known as intrinsic factor (IF). The function of intrinsic factor is to bind to vitamin B-12 and ensure its absorption once it reaches the part of the small intestine known as the ileum. In the low acid stomach, intrinsic factor secretion is deficient and vitamin B-12 absorption often is impaired.

Pathogenic Overgrowth in the Small Intestine

Normally, the acid secreted by the healthy stomach sterilizes most of the ingested or swallowed pathogens from foods or liquids, such as bacteria, parasites, and fungi. When the stomach pH is less than 3, most of these pathogens are destroyed. The stomach acid also enters the small intestine through waves of acidity, killing off unwanted fecal organisms. Thus, the acid secreted by the stomach is an important defense against unwanted organisms from foodstuffs or liquids. In a low stomach acid environment, these unwanted organisms breed in the small intestine and become markedly elevated. It has been demonstrated that bacterial concentrations in the small intestine are increased in 50% to 100% in individuals with low stomach acid. The health consequences are impaired nutrient absorption due to binding and inactivation of nutrients by bacteria. The overgrowth of bacteria in the small intestine also affects health by altering the ways nutrients are metabolized in the body.

Altered Small Intestinal pH

The pH of the stomach in a low acid environment is above 3. When this occurs, the elevated stomach pH causes the pH of the small intestine to be increased as well. Many nutrients depend on a normal small intestinal pH so that they can be effectively separated from the foods they are combined with. When the small intestinal pH exceeds its normal value, nutrient absorption is greatly impaired since the nutrients cannot be released from their food complexes. Instead, they pass from the small intestine to the large intestine and end up in the stool, having not been adequately absorbed.

Drug Absorption Problems

A sufficient amount of stomach acid enables a number of prescription drugs to dissolve properly in the stomach and to be absorbed from the small intestine. In the low acid stomach, medications are rendered less effective due to the deficiency or absence of stomach acid. The consequences of this might mean more side effects since more of the prescription drug is necessary to overcome the acid deficit. If the stomach acid problem were to be corrected, then the drugs would likely work better at smaller dosages and have less potential side effects.

Nutrient Consequences of Low Stomach Acid

Low stomach acid can lead to various nutrient deficiencies, but these deficiencies can be treated by eating nutrient-rich food. For a guide to these foods, see the section in this book on the Nutrient Content of Common Foods. If an adequate level of nutrients cannot be obtained from your diet, you may need to take supplements. A guide to taking supplements for low stomach acid is provided at the end of this chapter.

Amino Acid Deficiency

Protein digestion occurs in the stomach due to the beneficial actions of enzymes and stomach acid. The process of protein digestion is called hydrolysis, which simply means the breaking down of large protein structures into smaller protein units, referred to as amino acids. Proteins need to be broken down to individual amino acids because every physiological system in the body depends on them for optimal health.

Amino acids maintain muscle mass, nourish the organs and tissues, optimize immune function, and preserve brain function. In a low stomach acid environment, the proteins do not adequately breakdown, and many critical amino acids do not get absorbed. For example, the amino acids L-tryptophan and L-tyrosine are involved in feelings of well-being and mood regulation. It is hypothesized that low stomach acid might create or even precipitate depression by leading to a reduction in the blood levels of these amino acids.

Low stomach acid can lead to various nutrient deficiencies, but these deficiencies can be treated by eating nutrient-rich food.

Another example worth considering is the relationship between amino acids and antibodies. Antibodies are specific cells of the immune system that bind to foreign substances and render them inactive. When amino acid absorption is impaired, the production of these important immune cells might be compromised. The net result would be increases in both the incidence and frequency of infections. In fact, a study does show that patients with a confirmed antibody deficiency syndrome have an increased incidence of low stomach acid.

Calcium Deficiency

Calcium plays many roles in the body, most of which are to provide strength and stability to bones and teeth. Calcium also helps with blood clotting, muscle contraction, and nerve transmission. When calcium is deficient, osteoporosis develops, tooth enamel weakens, muscles cramp and spasm, nerve cells do not function optimally, and blood does not clot well. Calcium also prevents colon cancer and lowers blood pressure.

For calcium to be absorbed from the stomach, there needs to be a sufficient amount of stomach acid to separate it from food complexes so that the calcium can be absorbed from the small intestine. That is why supplemental calcium is often necessary.

The absorption of the most common type of calcium in supplement form (calcium carbonate) appears to be significantly impaired in a stomach that is low in acid. Another type of calcium (calcium citrate) is very well absorbed even in a stomach that is low in stomach acid. Since low stomach acid appears to be a factor in calcium malabsorption, it might lead to deficiency of this extremely critical mineral.

Food Sources: Most people do not consume enough calcium in order to meet their daily requirements. The absorption in a healthy stomach of calcium from milk products and calcium supplements is approximately 25% to 35%. Other food sources with good amounts of calcium include Swiss cheese, cheddar cheese, broccoli, collard leaves, almonds, salmon, and yogurt.

Iron Deficiency

Iron is vital to our survival. It functions to transport oxygen from the lungs to the tissues of the body. Iron is stored in muscle cells and provides energy to our muscular system during any type of physical activity. Iron is involved in cellular energy production and is an essential facilitator of numerous enzymes in the body. For example, iron facilitates a system of liver enzymes that helps to detoxify chemicals and toxins in the body. Iron also stimulates enzymes to produce brain chemicals (neurotransmitters) and thyroid hormones.

However, iron deficiency is the most common nutrient deficiency, occurring frequently in children and women. Iron-poor diets are usually responsible for this deficiency among infants and children. In women, the most frequent cause is heavy menstrual bleeding. Some of the common signs and symptoms of iron deficiency are anemia, brittle hair, dry skin, fatigue, increased susceptibility to infection, learning difficulties, loss of appetite, pallor, muscle cramping, and up-turned nails. Many women continue to have iron deficiency despite having taken high-dose iron supplementation for years. When tested, many of these women have low stomach acid. Only when their stomach acid problems are corrected does their iron status return to normal and their iron deficiency resolve.

Like calcium, the absorption of iron is impaired in a low stomach acid environment. Stomach acid frees the iron bound to food and converts it to the well-absorbed ferrous form of iron. Without adequate acid, iron remains in its poorly absorbed ferric form and cannot be adequately absorbed. Only in the presence of adequate amounts of acid will the ferric form of iron convert to the well-absorbed ferrous form of iron.

Food Sources: In other words, most food sources of iron do depend upon stomach acid for proper absorption. Some of these foods include soy flour, lentils, white beans, oatmeal, figs, dried dates, and carrots. The only exception is that the iron contained in meat products (heme iron), such as liver, beef, veal, pork and chicken, absorbs very well even in the presence of low stomach acid.

Zinc Deficiency

Zinc is critical for antioxidant function, cellular protection, immune function, proper enzyme function, and protein structure and function. Zinc has been successfully used therapeutically to treat several conditions, including impaired growth in children, infertility, rheumatic disease, and skin diseases.

When stomach acidity is compromised, so too is the absorption of zinc. In studies using acid-blocking medications to create a low stomach acid state, zinc absorption was significantly impaired. However, when a very good supplement of zinc is used, such as zinc acetate, the absorption is adequate, even in a low stomach acid environment. Although low stomach acid might significantly affect zinc absorption, the available evidence indicates that the absorption defect can be overcome by utilizing certain forms of zinc supplements. Zinc supplementation appears to be warranted since chronic, marginal deficiency is common, even among healthy adults.

Mild-to-severe zinc deficiency might arise as a consequence of poor intake and/or low stomach acid. Zinc deficiency is common, especially among children, adolescents, pregnant and lactating women, and the elderly.

Food Sources: Excellent food sources of zinc include oysters, lamb chops, pecans, pumpkin seeds, green peas, white beans, wheat bran, and eggs. Zinc deficiency is characterized by skin changes (dermatitis), impaired taste, infertility, inflammatory acne, poor wound healing, reduced sense of smell, weakened immune function, and white spots on the nails.

Folic Acid Deficiency

Deficiency of folic acid is one of the most common vitamin deficiency disorders, characterized by anemia, birth defects, depression, fatigue, hostility, impaired cell growth within the digestive tract, impaired fetal growth and development, paranoid behavior, shortness of breath, and weakness. Folic acid is of prime importance to cell growth, protein metabolism, and fetal growth and development. It is used in supplement form to guard against heart disease, improve immune function, prevent birth defects, and reduce the risk of certain cancers, including cervical, colon, and lung cancers.

When the stomach pH is in the low acid range, it causes the pH of the small intestine to be more basic than it normally is. As a result, the ability of the small intestine to absorb folic acid is impaired and a deficiency of this vitamin will develop. Other research has demonstrated that bacterial overgrowth occurring in the small intestine as a consequence of low stomach acid might be able to synthesize enough folic acid so as to prevent against deficiency.

Food Sources: Good food sources of folic acid include wheat germ, kidney beans, spinach, broccoli, calf liver, eggs, soybeans, and beets.

Vitamins B-1, B-2, and B-3 Deficiency

People with low stomach acid are at risk for deficiencies of critical B vitamins. Vitamins B-1 (thiamin), B-2 (riboflavin), and B-3 (niacin or nicotinic acid) are involved in antioxidant protection, carbohydrate metabolism, energy production, fat metabolism, liver detoxification, and the functioning of the nervous system. Deficiencies of these B vitamins have overlapping features and include anxiety, cardiovascular problems, cracks at the corners of the mouth, diarrhea, depression, dermatitis, dementia, fatigue, nervousness, insomnia, psychosis, and swollen tongue.

There is experimental evidence demonstrating that an adequate intake of B vitamins is needed to maintain proper stomach acid function. When animals were fed a diet deficient in B vitamins, the secretion of stomach acid was impaired. Upon providing adequate B vitamin intake, the impairment reverted to normal. There are also some documented case reports of patients who developed deficiencies of these B vitamins as a consequence of low stomach acid.

Among the B vitamins, the most critical one in terms of optimal stomach functioning is likely niacin. A severe niacin deficiency is known as pellagra. Some of the symptoms of classical pellagra overlap with those of low stomach acid. For example, in pellagra, the changes in the gastrointestinal tract are manifested as diarrhea and diminished secretion of stomach acid. Three published reports have demonstrated dramatic improvements in symptoms of low stomach acid in three patients supplementing with optimal doses of niacin.

Food Sources: It is extremely important to ensure an adequate intake of B vitamins from food sources. Foods that contain high amounts of these B vitamins are brewer's yeast, wheat bran, sunflower seeds, soybeans, wild rice, turkey, and chicken.

Vitamin B-6 Deficiency

Vitamin B-6 functions in the body to facilitate protein synthesis, to maintain normal blood sugar levels, to aid fat metabolism, to preserve red blood cell function, and to help with the production of brain neurotransmitters.

There is conflicting evidence about the effect of low stomach acid upon the absorption of vitamin B-6. It is known that when stomach acid is insufficient, the intestinal absorption of vitamin B-6 (in its active form of pyridoxal-5-phosphate) from food sources is impaired. It is also believed, however, that in a low stomach acid environment, the increased amount of bacteria in the small intestine might be able to synthesize enough vitamin B-6 to prevent deficiency.

Even though debate exists, low stomach acid might lead to a vitamin B-6 deficiency. As a result, numerous signs and symptoms of deficiency can develop. Some of the well known clinical manifestations of a vitamin B-6 deficiency include anemia; anxiety; burning and tingling of the hands and feet; cracks and fissures at the angle of the mouth; depression; increased risk of calcium-oxalate kidney stones; increased risk of heart disease; purplish and painful tongue; and walking difficulties.

Food Sources: Good food sources of vitamin B-6 include liver, potatoes, banana, lentils, brewer's yeast, trout, and spinach.

Vitamin B-12 Deficiency

The body needs vitamin B-12 in order for optimal metabolism of folic acid, amino acids, and fat to occur. Vitamin B-12 is also important for maintaining antioxidant protection and for the adequate functioning of the nervous system.

The vitamin B-12 found in foods needs the appropriate amounts of stomach acid and other enzymes to be liberated from food proteins. Once liberated, the vitamin B-12 from food combines with a compound known as intrinsic factor. The vitamin B-12-intrinsic factor complex then travels to the farthest part of the small intestine, where it is absorbed. In a low stomach acid environment, vitamin B-12 cannot dissociate from food proteins and bind to intrinsic factor, and, therefore, cannot be absorbed. Another feature of a low stomach acid state is increased overgrowth of bacteria in the small intestine. This overgrowth causes vitamin B-12 to be bound to the bacteria, which also impairs absorption.

Vitamin B-12 deficiency is characterized by anemia, confusion, constipation, fatigue, impaired immune function, insomnia, poor memory, shortness of breath, sore tongue, and weight loss.

Food Sources: The best food sources of vitamin B-12 are liver, mussels, salmon, beef, eggs, hard cheese, and milk.

Vitamins A and E Deficiency

Vitamins A and E are part of the fat-soluble vitamin family, which also includes vitamins D and K. Fats are required in order for these vitamins to be absorbed. Vitamin A is involved in hormone synthesis, vision, reproduction, and resistance to infection. Some of the functions of vitamin E include protection against free radicals and the thinning of blood.

An absence or deficiency of stomach acid might adversely affect the absorption of vitamins A and E. Deficiency of vitamin A can lead to brittle hair, brittle nails, dry skin, fatigue, increased risk of infections, infertility, and loss of smell and taste. Vitamin E deficiency causes cardiomyopathy, degeneration of nerve cells, red blood cell destruction, infertility and muscle atrophy.

Food Sources: Good food sources of vitamin A include liver, cod liver oil, dandelion greens, carrots, eggs, cheddar cheese, sweet potato, butter and milk.

Some good food sources of vitamin E are sunflower seeds, wheat germ, sweet potatoes, safflower oil, shrimp, salmon and eggs.

Treating Low Stomach Acid

In the first half of the 20th century, there was considerable medical interest in stomach acid. The consensus among interested medical authorities was that low stomach acid is a real medical condition that necessitates appropriate medical treatment. Numerous studies were undertaken and the results were startling. In a 1935 study, low stomach acid was found among 26% of female arthritic patients. In a 1937 study, almost 100% of all alcoholics evaluated had low stomach acid. In 1945, the incidence of low stomach acid among patients with various skin conditions was studied.

Skin Conditions and Low Stomach Acid

Skin Condition	Number of Patients	Percentage who had absent or low (deficient) acid production	Percentage who had normal stomach acid production
Acne Rosacea	30	87	13
Alopecia (Hair Loss)	19	95	5
Avitaminosis	37	79	21
Eczema	106	74	26
Lupus	9	100	0
Psoriasis	9	89	11
Seborrheic Dermatitis	68	87	13
Staphylococcus Infection	12	75	25
Urticaria (Hives)	77	85	15
Vitiligo	29	90	10

In this case, treatment with stomach acid and a B-complex vitamin (as brewer's yeast) improved the skin conditions in all cases. The patients with more mild cases of stomach acid deficiency responded the fastest to treatment.

Other conditions associated with low stomach acid were childhood asthma, gallbladder disease, and rheumatoid arthritis.

Maldigestion

Clinical interest in low stomach acid has subsequently waned, with a more comprehensive evaluation of digestive complaints being favored. The clinical focus has shifted toward the evaluation and management of indigestion (maldigestion). Symptoms of indigestion include chronic or recurrent discomfort concentrated at the upper abdomen, associated with belching, bloating, heartburn, nausea, or vomiting. Common conditions, such as hyperacidity and heartburn, are often considered when a doctor evaluates a patient for indigestion. People afflicted with indigestion certainly require medical attention, but the problem is that the majority of doctors are no longer investigating the possibility that low stomach acid is responsible for their digestive symptoms.

> Assuming that low stomach acid is a factor in the symptoms of functional indigestion, the potential savings in terms of healthcare dollars could be in the billions if low stomach acid were to be properly investigated and treated.

Indigestion affects approximately 25% of the population each year; however, most affected persons do not seek medical care for it. Approximately 50% to 60% of patients with indigestion are considered to have a functional problem because no specific cause can be identified. Up to 40% of indigestion is caused by peptic ulcer disease and reflux esophagitis, with less than 2% of cases being the result of gastric or esophageal cancer. The common symptoms associated with low stomach acid are strikingly similar to those symptoms associated with functional indigestion.

An estimated 40% of adults in the Western world have repeated episodes of indigestion. In the United States (and likely Canada), 2% to 5% of visits to primary care providers are for this condition. More than $1.3 billion is spent annually on prescription drugs for dyspepsia in the United States, not including the cost of over-the-counter (OTC) medications, which are presumed to be at least equal to the annual prescription costs for this condition. Assuming that low stomach acid is a factor in the symptoms of functional indigestion, the potential savings in terms of healthcare dollars could be in the billions if low stomach acid were to be properly investigated and treated.

HCl Supplements

To re-acidify the stomach, it is best to supplement with stomach acid. The best acid supplement is known as betaine hydrochloride (HCl). Each betaine HCl capsule should be at least 500 to 650 mg (equivalent to 10 grains). It is best to find a betaine HCl supplement that also has pepsin in it because pepsin helps with digestion. Betaine HCl supplements must always be taken with a meal and never on an empty stomach.

Dosage

The best way to supplement with betaine HCl is to swallow 1 capsule of betaine HCl with every large meal. The next day, 2 betaine HCl capsules are taken with every large meal. Do this until you are taking 6 capsules with every large meal, or stop at the dose that causes you to experience some warmth or slight burning in your stomach. The slight burning or warmth indicates that stomach tolerance has been achieved. At this point, if your stomach feels too irritated, you can swallow 1 teaspoon of baking soda dissolved in a glass of water for immediate relief.

By following the instructions outlined above, your therapeutic dose can easily be figured out. If, for example, your stomach tolerance occurred at 4 betaine HCl capsules with every large meal, your therapeutic dose would be 3 betaine HCl capsules with every large meal and 1 to 2 capsules with smaller meals. It is important to reduce your dose of betaine HCl by half when eating smaller meals. As your stomach regains its ability to make more HCl, you might reach stomach tolerance at doses that initially did not cause any slight burning or warmth.

It takes about 3 to 12 months for normal stomach acid production to come back. In some cases, especially in persons 45 and older, daily use of HCl capsules is required for life in order to continue to feel healthy and be free of symptoms.

The betaine HCl capsules should never be opened or sprinkled on food because the HCl will be very corrosive to the teeth when administered this way. This therapy cannot be administered to patients who have been identified as hypersecretors of HCl or are suspected as having a condition where there might be too much stomach acid present. Please do not try this treatment if you have been on long-term aspirin therapy or other non-steroidal anti-inflammatory therapy, or if you are currently taking prednisone.

Liver Extract

Liver extract is a potent source of vitamins and minerals and other important physiological factors. Liver extract provides the most absorbable form of iron, known as heme iron. Heme iron is effectively absorbed, even in a stomach that has low stomach acid. In other words, the lack of acid does not interfere with the utilization of the heme iron from the liver extract. Liver extract also contains crucial B vitamins, such as folic acid, vitamin B-2, and vitamin B-12.

We often recommend liver extract for various reasons. First, patients with iron-deficiency anemia do better when they take this form of iron. Second, patients often respond better to betaine HCl supplementation when combined with liver extract. Third, liver extract improves the overall functioning of the liver and helps other digestive functions in the body.

Specifically, the liver has three main functions: vascular, secretory, and metabolic. It filters approximately 1450 ml per minute and removes harmful blood products, such as bacteria, endotoxins, and immune complexes, from the circulation. The liver's main secretory function is in synthesizing and secreting bile. Bile is useful in absorbing fat-soluble vitamins and helps to bind many toxic substances and eliminate them from the body. The liver's metabolic functions include carbohydrate, fat, and protein metabolism; the storage of vitamins and minerals; the formation of vital physiologic factors; and the detoxification of foreign or endogenous chemical compounds.

Dosage

The best type of liver extract are hydrolyzed (water is added to it) and are known as "liquid liver extracts." Make sure that at least 3 to 4 mg of heme iron is provided per capsule of the liver extract. The typical of dose iron prescribed is 1 to 2 capsules, three times daily with meals. The only contraindication is that this natural medicine cannot be given to people having an iron-overload disorder, such as hemochromatosis.

Niacin or Inositol Hexaniacinate

Niacin or its flush-free form, inositol hexaniacinate (IHN), are potent stimulators of HCl production. These forms of vitamin B-3 supply the mitochondria with fuel, and in doing so, help to facilitate the release of HCl into the stomach. In the stomach, parietal cells secrete HCl when stimulated through the actions of consuming a meal or by the actions of other known stimulators. Within the parietal cells are a group of structures called mitochondria, which are known as the "powerhouse" of all cells. The parietal cells of the stomach contain the highest amounts of mitochondria compared to all other metabolic tissues within the body. Vitamin B-3 feeds the mitochondria with cellular energy and makes the parietal cells release of HCl more effectively when stimulated to do so.

When taking niacin, you feel healthier, have more energy, and low stomach acid improves. Even though niacin is easy to find, it is not a nutrient that any person should simply purchase over-the-counter. A healthcare provider should prescribe it. The best form of niacin is the "pure" form that is not in a time-released capsule or tablet. Another excellent form of niacin is the "non-flush" form. If you take the pure form, a flush occurs due to the release of histamine and prostaglandins.

Dosage

For our patients less than 45 years of age, we often try niacin or IHN to remedy the low stomach acid. For patients who are 45 years of age and older, we use betaine HCl since it is necessary to directly replace the deficient stomach acid. The dose of niacin or IHN that we start with is 500 mg, three times daily with meals. After 3 days, we increase the dose to 1000 mg, three times daily. The therapeutic response is usually excellent and patients tolerate it very well.

Herbal Bitters

There is a long history regarding the use of herbal bitters to stimulate HCl production. Many herbal medicines are very effective for mild cases of low stomach acid. We prefer betaine HCl or niacin for the more moderate-to-severe cases. The best herbal stimulator is *Gentiana lutea* (gentian). It has been shown to stimulate certain receptors in the taste buds, referred to as gustatory receptors. By stimulating the gustatory receptors, there is a reflex increase in saliva and HCl production. Other herbal bitters, such as *Zingiber officinale* (ginger) or *Centaurium minus* (common or red centuary), might work equally as well.

The preferred form is an herbal medicine in tincture form, which is simply an alcohol-based preparation. The alcohol helps to dissolve all the necessary ingredients in the herbal, and, at the same time, acts as a preservative. The dose, regardless of the concentration, is 5 to 15 drops 15 to 20 minutes before meals, three times daily. There are no side effects to herbal bitters. Any healthcare provider can prescribe these herbal medicines or they might be available at your local health food store.

If you are unable to locate herbal bitters, lemon juice or apple cider vinegar is an option. Try 1 teaspoon of lemon juice or apple cider vinegar 15 to 20 minutes before meals, three times each day.

Enteric-Coated Peppermint Oil (ECPO)

Supplementing with enteric-coated peppermint oil (ECPO) can be extremely helpful, especially in cases where there is overgrowth of bacteria in the small intestine. A positive indican test is associated with an overgrowth of bacteria and low stomach acid. The aromatic oils in ECPO both inhibit the growth of and destroy bacteria. ECPO has also been shown to help with certain digestive symptoms, such as abdominal pain, bloating, gas, and indigestion.

Dosage

The best dose to use is 90 mg, twice daily, away from food. Side effects are extremely rare, but can include skin rash, heartburn, slowing of the heart rate, and muscle tremor.

Nutritional Supplementation

When normalizing stomach acidity, it is equally important to maintain an optimal nutritional intake. The chart below summarizes the main nutrients that need to be supplemented in low stomach acid, with suggested doses. For specific information about proper dosing and whether or not some of the nutrients should be taken with or without meals, see a qualified healthcare professional.

Nutritional Supplements for Low Stomach Acid

Nutrient	Recommended Daily Dose
Calcium	1000-1500 mg
Vitamin D-3	1000 IU
Iron (only when a diagnosed iron deficiency anemia is present)	150-200 mg
Zinc	25-50 mg
Folic Acid	1 mg (1000 mcg)
B-Complex 50 or 100	1-2 capsules or tablets
Vitamin B-3	1500-3000 mg
Vitamin B-6	50-200 mg
Vitamin B-12	1000-2000 mcg
Vitamin A (if pregnant do not exceed 5000 IU per day)	5000-10000 IU
Vitamin E (mixed tocopherols)	400-800 IU

8 | NATUROPATHIC HEALTHCARE

A fascinating side effect of using naturopathic nutrition to prevent and treat health conditions is the relatively low cost of doing so when compared to drug therapy and surgery. In addition, naturopathic nutrition can complement traditional practices of medicine, thus improving therapeutic outcomes. For the sake of everyone's health, it makes sense to integrate these healthcare practices.

Reducing Healthcare Costs

Healthcare expenses include the cost of professional services (physician, surgeon, nurse, social worker, physiotherapist, psychologist), the cost of drugs, and the cost of operating clinics and hospitals. Naturopathic nutrition and orthomolecular medicine are much more economical than standard healthcare for several reasons. They lead to recoveries in a shorter period of time and, therefore, require fewer visits to the doctor. There is nothing more economical than getting the patient healthy quickly.

Each year for the past 25 years, Dr Hoffer has examined his pattern of practice (a profile provided by the medicare program) and compared it against the average of all the psychiatrists practicing in Saskatchewan and, since 1976, in British Columbia. Each year, he has seen nearly twice as many patients as the mean for all other psychiatrists, and his billings to the governments have been about 10% higher than for the average billing. He does not work particularly hard and, for the past 10 years, has been seeing patients only 4 days each week. If every psychiatrist practiced this efficiently using naturopathic nutrition and orthomolecular psychiatry, we would need 50% fewer psychiatrists for the same population in North America.

> To reduce the costs of healthcare, the medical profession will need to adopt the principles and practices of naturopathic nutrition and orthomolecular medicine.

This practice of medicine also reduces the costs of drugs. Most nutrients prescribed by naturopathic doctors and orthomolecular physicians are available over the counter at a remarkably reasonable price when compared to prescribed drugs. They also carry little potential for the kind of side effects characteristic of drugs, which perpetuate illness, treating one symptom while creating another.

With less reliance on professional healthcare services and drug treatments, there is also less demand for clinics and hospitals to house these services and patients. These facilities are at their breaking point in most states and provinces in North America, overwhelmed by patients with chronic diseases resulting from our modern high-tech diet. Paying for professional services, drug plans, and medical institutions is also overwhelming the individual taxpayer.

To reduce the costs of healthcare, the medical profession will need to adopt the principles and practices of naturopathic nutrition and orthomolecular medicine. This can be achieved in two main ways. (1) Increase the amount of information on the value of good nutrition and nutrient supplements for the public and for the profession. The public is already getting more and more information since the major media have lost their fear of so-called alternative health practices, and the profession is also beginning to get more in the form of reports, articles in the medical journals, and papers delivered at medical meetings. (2) Make it possible for physicians to practice nutritional medicine. The medical establishment must remove the fear that physicians will lose their medical license if they begin to work with vitamins and minerals.

Integrative Healthcare

The pressure on physicians to avoid nutritional therapy has been immense; many physicians have lost their license because they would not give up their practice of nutritional medicine. However, opinion is changing.

In 1990, a legislative bill was passed in Washington State stating that the medical board may not base a finding of professional incompetence solely on the basis that a licensee's practice is unconventional or experimental in the absence of demonstrable physical harm to the patient.

In 1992, Alaska Governor Walter J. Hickel appointed Dr R. Rowento to the medical board, who stated, against the protests of many fellow physicians, that "there is as much room for divergent opinions in medicine as there are for divergent beliefs in God. I have stated it is time for medicine to be responsible to the people rather than to the needs of the profession. Organized medicine must take an honest look at itself, acknowledge that it does not have all the answers and reach out to embrace other avenues to healing as both orthodox and complementary medicine have much to offer. Each can fill in some of the gaps left by the other." We could not have stated our own position better. Embracing this belief in the value of nutritional healthcare, we can look forward to a new age of optimum health for all in the 21st century.

NUTRITIONAL THERAPY

9 | NUTRIENT DEFICIENCIES

Optimum adaptation is not perfect adaptation. Perfect adaptation would exist if every cell in the body, every tissue, every organ, and every system were provided with the amount of each nutrient required for optimum growth and function. At the same time, all waste products of metabolism would be removed so as not to interfere with the operation of these cells and tissues. Obviously, this is impossible.

Optimum adaptation exists when the organism, plant or animal, is in balance with the environment, especially the biochemical environment, so that it can grow, function, and reproduce to perpetuate the species. It does not necessarily mean long life, although long life will accompany optimum adaptation.

Since perfect adaptation may not be possible, each cell and each tissue must, therefore, learn to function adequately with less than optimum provision of nutrients, and to respond quickly to more optimum conditions. The chief means of providing optimum conditions is through the use of nutrient supplements – vitamins, minerals, amino acids, and essential fatty acids.

Vitamins as Medicine

The history of the use of food and vitamins for medicinal purposes has been divided into five ages by Dr L.J. Machlin. The first period ranges from about 1500 B.C. to 1900 A.D. Foods were used empirically to heal certain diseases. The second period ranges from 1880 to 1900. During this period, deficiency diseases were produced in animals and the vitamin hypothesis was developed. The third period ranges from 1900 to 1930. During this phase the vitamins were discovered, isolated, their structure determined,

> Since perfect adaptation may not be possible, each cell and each tissue must, therefore, learn to function adequately with less than optimum provision of nutrients, and to respond quickly to more optimum conditions. The chief means of providing optimum conditions is through the use of nutrient supplements – vitamins, minerals, amino acids, and essential fatty acids.

and their synthesis established. The fourth period begins about 1930 when biochemical functions of the body were studied, dietary requirements were introduced, and commercial production of vitamins became prominent. We are now into the fifth period, which began in 1955 and is characterized by the recognition of therapeutic health effects beyond prevention of deficiency disease.

Vitamins as Prevention

From 1880 to 1955, vitamins were limited in their application to the prevention of deficiency diseases, such as scurvy, beri beri, and pellagra. During this vitamin-as-prevention era, it was believed that the only role of vitamins was to prevent vitamin deficiency diseases – and that they were needed in small amounts. This made sense since vitamins are catalysts of reactions in the body, and catalysts are known to be needed only in small amounts because they are used over and over.

Any dose above these small preventive doses was considered bad medical practice. In fact, physicians have lost their medical license because of allegations that they were prescribing large doses of vitamins that harmed their patients. Some hospitals still do not permit the use of intravenous ascorbic acid. These 'principles' make up the preventative vitamin or vitamin deficiency paradigm. They are still adhered to very vigorously by many dietitians, nutritionists, and physicians.

> A nutrient deficiency is present when the diet is so bad that even the small preventive doses are not provided. A nutrient dependency is present when the needs of the body are so great that even the best diet cannot provide the right amount.

The vitamin deficiency paradigm led to the creation of recommended daily allowances (RDAs) for *healthy* people, but have little application to individuals who are not average – not of value to 50% of the total population. Recently, Professor David Mark Hegsted, appointed to Harvard's New England Regional Primate Research Center in Southborough, Massachusetts, recommended the RDAs be abolished, arguing that the system is unworkable because it was based on estimates using healthy young males – the group least likely in the population to have nutritional deficiencies. Dr J. Blumberg, Professor of Nutrition at Tufts University, argues that "the RDA committee is locked into the old paradigm of nutrition – how much is needed to prevent deficiency disease. It has not shifted gears to where medicine is today."

In the middle 1930s, just after it was recognized that niacin cured pellagra, pellagra specialists found that the small doses of vitamin B-3 that prevented pellagra and that cured early (acute) pellagra did not help patients who had chronic pellagra. Chronic patients required 600 to 3000 mg per day, a huge quantity compared to the tiny dose of less than 20 mg needed to prevent pellagra. Chronic pellagra changed body chemistry (in humans and dogs) so that the small doses effective as a preventive measure were no longer adequate. Much larger amounts were needed, for they had developed a dependency on vitamin B-3.

A nutrient deficiency is present when the diet is so bad that even the small preventive doses are not provided. A nutrient dependency is present when the needs of the body are so great that even the best diet cannot provide the right amount.

Despite its application to deficiency diseases, the preventive vitamin paradigm has impeded nutritional research, inhibiting the investigations of the *therapeutic* use of vitamins for nutrient dependencies and general health.

Vitamins as Therapy

The original impetus to use vitamins therapeutically started in 1955 when we published a research paper showing that niacin (vitamin B-3) lowered cholesterol levels in people. L.J. Machlin, in the *Annals of the New York Academy of Sciences* (1992), credits this report as having started a new age in the medical use of vitamins with our "recognition of health effects beyond prevention of deficiency diseases."

For the 30 years following our report, there was a slow accumulation of papers in the medical literature confirming our findings and expanding them. However, most physicians at the time were swayed by pharmaceutical companies promoting their own products for lowering cholesterol. Niacin cannot be patented and, therefore, it was never promoted by any major drug companies.

There was little interest until the final report of the Coronary Drug Study was published in 1986, showing that of all the compounds tested, only niacin decreased the death rate (by 11%) and increased longevity (by 2 years). The other compounds decreased mortality a little from cardiovascular disease, but there was a compensating increase in deaths from accidents, suicides, and homicides. This did not occur with niacin. The use of niacin as therapy for lowering cholesterol is rapidly expanding worldwide. Niacin is now recognized as one of the safest and most effective compounds for lowering LDL cholesterol and increasing HDL cholesterol.

We also showed that vitamin B-3 was therapeutic for schizophrenics in our initial studies in the 1950s, a discovery chronicled in the book *Vitamin B-3 and Schizophrenia: Discovery, Recovery, Controversy*. Despite many subsequent clinical studies proving the efficacy of niacin in treating schizophrenia, the psychiatric establishment has not yet wholly embraced this low-cost therapy.

Interest also spread to the therapeutic use of other vitamins, particularly the antioxidant vitamins, such as vitamin E, vitamin C, and beta carotene, and to the antioxidant minerals, such as selenium, in treating cancer, AIDS, mental disease, cardiovascular disease, and senility.

Our research published in 1955 proposed the therapeutic use of vitamins in large doses. The therapeutic vitamin paradigm is based on the following four observations.

- We are each different and have different nutrient requirements.
- Optimum amounts of vitamins are needed, which range from smaller doses necessary to prevent deficiency disease to much larger doses to treat vitamin dependent conditions – conditions like elevated cholesterol levels and too low levels of high density lipoprotein (HDL) cholesterol.
- The following variables determine the optimum need: age, sex, physical stress (including pregnancy), psychological stress, lactation, diseases (whether acute or chronic), use of xenobiotic drugs.
- Thus, there can never be one useful Optimal Daily Dose (ODD) schedule for everyone. There must be an Optimal Recommended Dose (ORD) specific for each condition and for each disease.
- Vitamins can be taken safely for a lifetime.

The therapeutic vitamin paradigm opens up the use of vitamins for optimum health to everyone. In sharp contrast to drugs, which are very toxic and must be carefully controlled by trained professionals, vitamins can be experimented with by any person secure in the knowledge that they are as safe as any of the over-the-counter medications readily available today. People can become their own therapists. Experimentation will not do them any harm, provided they have taken a little time to examine the vitamin literature. With drugs, too little is much safer than too much, but with vitamins, a little more is much safer than too little if one wishes to obtain optimum health. If more than needed is taken, there is no harm because the extra amount is not stored and is readily eliminated. There are very few exceptions.

Thus, you can try to find the optimum dose by taking increasing doses until it is reached. And if that dose is exceeded, the body can readily deal with it. If too little is taken, the desired therapeutic effect will not be obtained. The difference between optimum and less effective doses can be narrow. We have seen schizophrenic patients who did not respond to 3 g per day of niacin, but when this was doubled, they began to improve very quickly. The same principle does not apply to minerals and may not apply to amino acids, even though they also have a wide tolerance range.

Paradigm Shift

The year 1992 was a watershed year in public attitudes toward vitamin therapy, marking a great change in medical interest in the use of vitamins for therapy, using doses much larger than ever before recommended or accepted. It was inevitable but pleasant at last to see. The lay press, which had for years been toeing the party line about nutrients and the RDAs, suddenly began to publish reports about the remarkable new therapeutic properties of the vitamins. Since the media feel free, at last, to publish this information, it is clear they are no longer afraid of the censure of the old medical establishment and that the profession has become interested enough that it no longer objects as vigorously as it did in the past. There are a few fossilized physicians who are still living in the early 20th century, but they are rapidly fading from the scene.

One of the first signs of this new age of vitamin therapy was an article published in *The New York Times*, March 10, 1992, under the headline "Vitamins Win Support as Potent Agents of Health." *Time Magazine*, April 6, 1992, was next with their cover story "The Real Power of Vitamins," subtitled "New Research Shows They May Help Fight Cancer, Heart Disease and the Ravages of Aging."

While the U.S. Food and Drug Administration (FDA) disputed nutrient health claims, Dr Walter Willett of the Harvard School of Health said, "at this time I say don't take megadoses, but I'm not ruling out that in two or three years we might change our mind." The *Time* report concluded: "But stay tuned. Vitamins promise to continue to unfold as one of the great and hopeful health stories of our day." *The Medical Post*, April 23, 1992, reported that vitamin C may lower heart disease risk, and on May 8, 1992 the *New York Times* reported, "Vitamin C Linked to Heart Benefit: It May Also Help Prevent an Early Death from Other Disease."

Newsweek finally joined ranks on May 8, 1992, with their story "Live Longer With Vitamin C." *The Harvard Health Letter*, *Johns Hopkins Medical Letter*, and the *Diet-Heart Newsletter* have reported with similar stories. Finally, the U.S. National Institutes of Health has created a new Office of Alternative Medicine, which will explore various alternative practices. We hope the study of vitamins will be included in their mandate – unless they now consider megavitamin therapy as mainstream medicine.

The medical profession has been alerted to this new age by the *New England Journal of Medicine* in a 1993 article reporting that in 1990 more

Americans consulted alternative practitioners than all U.S. primary care physicians, 425 million visits versus 388 million. The social demographic group who consulted these alternative practitioners were non-black, ranging in age from 25 to 49 years, with relatively more education and higher incomes. They consulted them for chronic conditions. Of this group, 12% sought megavitamin therapy – 51 million visits were devoted to megavitamin therapy. The authors advised the profession should ascertain from their patients information about their use of alternative therapies. We do not think this will be much help since most patients who have consulted us are not willing to discuss it with their practitioners because of the negative reactions they have had in the past. The article concluded that "medical schools should include information about unconventional therapies and the clinical social sciences (anthropology and sociology) in their curriculums. The newly established National Institutes of Health Office for the Study of Unconventional Medical Practices should help promote scholarly research and education in this area."

British and Canadian doctors are also facing growing pressure from alternative medicine, as C. Gray in the *Canadian Medical Association Journal* writes: "It is impossible to ignore the growing acceptance of alternative medicine in today's Britain." She predicts that in Canada the future promises a "similar change. Alternative medicine is beginning to find a ready and healthy market. And our doctors as a group are feeling unloved and unrewarded." Nutrient therapy, using large doses of supplements when needed, is well on the way to becoming established medical practice.

10 | NUTRIENT DEPENDENCIES

We have seen many patients whose nutrition was excellent, but who still were sick and needed one or more vitamin supplements. A recent example was a man in good health except that for the past 5 years he had suffered from severe peripheral neuropathy of his feet. Five physicians skillfully diagnosed him, but no one offered him any hope. His diet was good. When we prescribed niacin 1 gram, three times daily after meals, he was well on the way to recovery in 1 month.

We are convinced there are some common diseases that are dependent on one or more nutrients. A dependency is present when the amount of any nutrient, which would be enough for the vast majority of people, is not adequate for a smaller proportion of the population due to a large number of genetic and other factors. For every nutrient, there are individuals who are dependent upon it, and if it is not provided, they will suffer a disease or a syndrome. Dr Heaney describes these nutrient dependencies as a "long-latency deficiency disease," but we prefer to call them nutrient dependency diseases. Dr Bruce Ames suggests that only about 10% of the possible dependency diseases are known. Most schizophrenics, for example, are dependent upon niacin; without receiving optimum amounts of this nutrient, the susceptible person will develop schizophrenia and general health will deteriorate.

Such dependency diseases will not be adequately treated until the nutrient dependency is discovered and the nutrient is given in optimum quantities. There are fewer individuals who are dependent upon two nutrients (we think Huntington's Disease is a double dependency on vitamin E and vitamin B-3), and even fewer who are dependent upon three or more. The greater the number of dependencies, the less likely that individual will survive beyond infancy.

Optimum Dosage

The need for a specific nutrient is determined by the general nutritional state of the person. There are many people whose diets are relatively good, but they still need extra nutrients due to biochemical individuality and many other factors, such as genetics or chronic deficiency.

Individual nutrients will not replace a grossly inadequate diet. Because vitamin deficiencies are usually multiple, we assume that most of our patients have several deficiencies, and even if they need only one, say niacin, we will still add others, such as vitamin C and the B complex vitamins. As Dr Linus Pauling pointed out so many years ago, they will do no harm and they may be very helpful.

The only rational way of treating with nutrients is to ensure first that the diet is optimal and then to use optimal amounts of the nutrients that are needed for individual patients. Standard nutritionists recommend the

> There are many people whose diets are relatively good, but they still need extra nutrients due to biochemical individuality and many other factors, such as genetics or chronic deficiency.

usual small vitamins doses, while orthomolecular and naturopathic therapists use optimum doses, which may be small or large. The important characteristic of the dose is not its size, but its efficacy – whether it is doing the job it is supposed to do to make the patient well.

After restoring our food as closely as possible to the nutritional state we have are adapted to, it is then necessary to determine whether supplements are needed. One day this will be done by careful laboratory tests, but these are still in the experimental stages and are not readily available. Furthermore they are expensive.

The easiest and most accurate way is to use yourself as the test organism, proceeding by trial and error. The trials are simple and the errors are minimal. There is no better method.

The starting dose must be enough to produce the desired effect. A dose too small would not be helpful. Once it has been found that the nutrient has had an appreciable effect, you could then increase the dose to determine if more would improve health even more. The dose range will be indicated for each nutrient. Side effects should be recorded. With an increase in dose, these side effects would be more pronounced. You would have to be sure that the side effects are coming from the active nutrient and not from some other ingredient in the composition. For example, many people are allergic to yeast, and if the nutrient is yeast based, there will be side effects from the yeast, wrongfully ascribed to the nutrient.

If you wanted to be even more precise, you could have your pharmacist make up the vitamin to be tested and a matching set of pills that are identical in everything except they would contain an inert substance. They could be coded so that you would not know which was which. Then one set of pills would be taken, say for 2 months, and after that the other. Notes would be kept of any changes in health to determine which is the superior product. If this could not be determined, it would mean that this particular vitamin or nutrient is not needed. This would be a so-called double-blind controlled experiment with a series of one.

NUTRIENT SUPPLEMENTS

11 | VITAMINS

Most nutrients can be obtained from the natural diet. Supplements, no matter how valuable, do not replace food. You cannot compensate for a poor diet by taking huge quantities of supplements. They are to be taken after the diet has been made as good as possible and if thereafter the state of health desired has not been reached. Before launching into a nutrient supplement regimen, be sure to read the chapter on "The Nutrient Content of Common Foods" later in this book. You may find that your needs can be met by increasing your consumption of nutrient-rich foods, that is, if you do not have a nutrient dependency. In the case of a health condition, you may need to supplement your diet with nutrients to derive therapeutic value from them.

Some people may be reluctant to change their cooking and eating habits. If a natural diet cannot be wholly restored, supplements can provide some of the nutrients that are missing from the diet. For some, it may be simpler to swallow pills than to change their diet. If this is the only concession some people will make to change, then at least they should increase their intake of all the water-soluble vitamins.

You will have to find out for yourself which vitamin and other nutrients you should take as a supplement and how much from the information we supply for each nutrient. The nutrients we do not describe have not been used therapeutically, but it is likely that, in time, every nutrient will be found to be essential in large amounts for some disease.

We start with vitamin C, followed by the B complex group, and then the remaining vitamins in order of their popularity and common usage. Even though more emphasis will be placed on vitamin C and the B complex vitamins, all of the vitamins discussed are essential for preventing diseases, treating specific clinical conditions, and ensuring optimum health.

Vitamin C

Vitamin C is the best known and most popular vitamin supplement, partly due to its historical role in preventing scurvy and partly due to the so-called vitamin C controversy. Besides preventing scurvy, vitamin C is our chief antioxidant, effective in treating arteriosclerosis, low stomach acid, various cancers, and aging conditions when taken in optimum doses.

Scurvy

Scurvy is a vitamin C (ascorbic acid) deficiency disease. When we do not get enough vitamin C in our food, we all become scorbutic. Every human suffers from subclinical scurvy, what Dr Irving Stone calls hypoascorbemia, because we cannot make vitamin C in our bodies, and the amount present in even the best possible diet will not provide more than 100 mg per day. This amount is totally inadequate for optimum health. Since we lost the capability of making vitamin C about 20 million years ago, our bodies have had to adapt to chronic deficiency after we moved away from a natural diet to a food supply that did not provide adequate amounts. We are still paying the price of this dietary change.

Although the connection between vitamin C and scurvy was first scientifically established by Nobel Laureate Dr A. Szent-Gyorgyi in the early 20th century, the importance of eating vitamin-C rich fruits and vegetables in preventing illness was known in some parts of our globe many centuries before. Historians believe that as early as the 15th century, the Chinese were cultivating fruit and vegetable gardens on board their large 'junk' ships during voyages of discovery that may have taken them as far afloat as Africa and North America. During this period, Admiral Zheng led a series of voyages, involving more than 300 ships and nearly 30,000 men. Largely because of their diet, these sailors did not suffer from the symptoms of scurvy that plagued the European crews on board the ships led by Ferdinand Magellan and Sir Francis Drake during their voyages of discovery.

In the 18th century, Dr James Lind in England conducted a controlled nutritional trial showing that sailors suffering from scurvy symptoms recovered in a few days after eating citrus fruit, most notably lemons and limes (thus the reference to English sailors as "limeys"), whereas control patients not given this treatment got no better. By the time of the Battle of Trafalgar in the early 19th century, Lord Nelson's sailors were receiving a regular 'dose' of fresh fruit and juice, whereas Napolean's sailors were not. Some historians speculate that this dietary regime may have saved England

> You cannot compensate for a poor diet by taking huge quantities of supplements. They are to be taken after the diet has been made as good as possible and if thereafter the state of health desired has not been reached.

from defeat. Napolean's sailors could not stand out to sea more than a few weeks, while the English sailors could stay out for months, if necessary. Interestingly, the British naval custom at the time of the Battle of Trafalgar was for officers to stand on board exposing themselves to fire "as an act of honor and as a sign of their status as gentlemen officers," one historian notes. "Captains would coolly fold loose sails or munch grapes as shots fell around them." While munching grapes on deck may have exposed these officers to physical danger, this sign of courage was protecting them from scurvy.

Because of our modern high-tech diet, the symptoms of scurvy are still alive and well. Several doctors have documented cases in the United States among men ranging in age from 35 to 61 who suffered painful edema on the legs, red spots on their arms, abdomen, and legs, as well as large purple discolorations on the lower limbs. They ate frequently in restaurants, avoided fruits and vegetables. Given ascorbic acid, they responded in a few days.

Vitamin C Controversy

Despite Dr Szent-Gyorgyi's discovery of the therapeutic value of vitamin C in treating scurvy, very few people knew about vitamin C until Professor

Linus Pauling published his book on *Vitamin C and the Common Cold* in 1970. There was a marked increase in sales of vitamin C as a result — and a marked increase in debate over the therapeutic value of nutrient supplements, especially when taken in optimum or megadoses.

Dr Pauling's conclusion that vitamin C was preventive *and* therapeutic for the common cold and for other conditions was so disturbing to some members of the medical community that they began a major effort to discredit him. The main complaint was that Dr Pauling, awarded two Nobel Prizes, one for Biochemistry and one for Peace, was not a medical doctor and, therefore, should not be commenting on medical matters. On the one hand, they argued that large doses of vitamin C, beyond RDA levels, were useless; on the other hand, they argued that so-called megadoses of vitamin C were dangerous.

Megadoses

Dr Pauling introduced the orthomolecular theory that the optimum therapeutic dose of vitamin C is much higher than the RDA preventive dose. This has been amply confirmed by the patients who have been taking the vitamin in higher doses and who report that the frequency of their colds has been greatly decreased, compared to the number of colds their close relatives are still getting.

Opponents of the use of vitamin C claim that taking more than a few milligrams a day is useless because the extra vitamin C is simply excreted into the urine, creating nutrient-rich urine. However, this argument fails to recognize how vitamin C is absorbed in the body. With vitamin C, research has shown that the more that is taken into the body, the greater is the amount retained and used by the body. In our early studies, we found we could inject chronic schizophrenics with 90 g of vitamin C and still find none in the urine. If the dose is 1 g, a fraction of that will be retained. If the dose is 10 g, many grams will be excreted but many grams will also be retained. To increase the retention, the dose must be increased.

For any substance to be therapeutic, in most cases, enough of the compound must be given before it can be therapeutic. This sometimes means allowing a major part to appear in the urine until the optimum dose is determined. If a person is given 50 g per day of penicillin to save his life, most of that also appears in the urine.

Safety

The medical establishment has tried to link vitamin C to every possible toxicity imaginable. The news media features so many stories of the dangers of vitamin C that you would think there are bodies laying all over the country who have died from this hugely popular vitamin. The chief claims are that large doses of vitamin C cause kidney stones, DNA damage, and cancer.

With vitamin C, research has shown that the more that is taken into the body, the greater is the amount retained and used by the body.

Early in this controversy, one physician in Australia tried to link the increased use of vitamin C following the publication of *Vitamin C and the Common Cold* to an equally dramatic rise in the incidence of kidney stones. However, he did not mention that the increase in kidney stones had begun long before Dr Pauling's book appeared and that after it appeared, the incidence did not rise further. Since then there has been a massive effort on the part of many doctors, dietitians, professors of biochemistry, and others to educate people against taking vitamin C supplements.

The potential danger from ascorbic acid to produce kidney stones is grossly exaggerated. There is a known frequency of kidney stone episodes among the general population; it is much less than expected among ascorbic acid users. Dr Roger Cathcart, who has more experience with more patients using ascorbic acid than any other physician, told us that, in his practice, he saw very few cases. The main factor in kidney stones formation appears instead to be a magnesium deficiency, not a vitamin C excess.

Two large studies have put the kidney stone controversy to rest. In a study published in 1996, 45,251 men (aged 40 to 75 years), with no history of kidney stones, were followed to determine if there was any relationship between vitamins C and B-6 and kidney stones. During the 6 years of follow-up, there were 751 cases of kidney stones; however, vitamin C and B-6 intakes were not significantly associated with the risk of stone formation. In fact, the results were so promising that the investigators concluded that the data does not support an association between a high daily intake of these vitamins and the risk of kidney stone formation.

Another study published in 1999 evaluated the intakes of both vitamin C and B-6 on the risk of symptomatic kidney stones in a cohort of 85,557 women with no history of kidney stones. The risk of kidney stones among women taking greater than or equal to 1500 mg per day of vitamin C was the same as women taking less than 250 mg per day. In either group, the intake of vitamin C was not associated with an increased risk of kidney stone formation. The investigators of this study concluded that routine restriction of vitamin C to prevent kidney stone formation is unwarranted.

Another unfortunate myth about vitamin C came from a report published in 2001 that linked vitamin C with DNA damage and cancer. In that report, an in vitro (test-tube) experiment did show that vitamin C could transform a fatty molecule into something that could damage DNA. However, no cause-and-effect association between vitamin C and cancer was actually identified in this study. Antioxidants like vitamin C are often given together for their therapeutic effects, and not separately, as this study reported.

Many oncologists believe that vitamin C, because of its antioxidant properties, decreases the efficacy of chemotherapy and radiation. Vitamin C decreases the toxicity of these treatments and thus prevents them from being fully effective. However, this belief is not based on published biochemical or clinical studies. In the *Journal of Orthomolecular Medicine* (Special Issue, Fourth Quarter, 2004), J.A. Stoute reviewed every available published paper dealing with these issues and concluded: "All but one of the studies and reviews presented in this bibliography support the use of vitamin C with chemotherapy. It confirmed the conclusions of key workers in this area that antioxidants, including vitamin C, do not protect cancer cells against free radical and growth-inhibitory effects of standard therapy. On the contrary, they enhance its growth-inhibitory effects on tumor cells, but protect normal cells against its adverse effects."

This brings us to the final vitamin C myth – that sudden cessation or stoppage of large doses causes rebound scurvy. Early reports demonstrating rebound scurvy after stopping supplemental vitamin C were uncontrolled and unsubstantiated. Moreover, studies in guinea pigs (mammals that do not synthesize vitamin C like humans) found no link between an increased break down of vitamin C following withdrawal from large doses.

Benefits vs. Risks

Every time an organism interacts with the environment two possibilities have to be evaluated. Is the interaction beneficial or is it harmful? Given an answer to these questions, then we need to ask, how can we determine the risk involved? How do we balance the potential benefit against the potential harm? There is always a risk-benefit ratio, even in crossing the street.

Activities may be risk free and enormously beneficial – for example, eating good food to which we have been adapted. The potential benefit also may be minimal and the risk enormous – for example, in smoking and drinking alcohol or imbibing other poisons. The same applies to all medicines – and to all nutrients.

In pharmacology, each drug is assessed for its therapeutic effect and for its toxicity. This is mandatory. The drug will not be released for general patient use unless government agencies are convinced that the drugs are effective and relatively safe. These studies are conducted by feeding the drugs to a variety of animals for a long enough period of time to receive clear results. Since animals used in the laboratory are short lived, they are on the drugs for a substantial proportion of their life span. The animals are examined for any pathological changes in their organs, for the effect the drugs have on growth rate and their ability to reproduce, and, of course, for their LD_{50}. This is a measure of the ability of drugs to kill. If, given over a certain amount of time, a dose kills 50% of an animal population (for example, rats or mice), this dose is called the LD_{50}. In a survey of the literature on the toxicity of vitamin C and other vitamins, Dr Andrew Saul found that there has not been a single death from vitamin use, compared to over 100,000 deaths annually in the United States from prescription drugs.

Despite some claims to the contrary, vitamin C has passed these tests. As Dr John Marks, Fellow, Tutor, and Director of Medical Studies, Girton College, Cambridge, concludes: "This is a vitamin that has been consistently administered in high dosages for very prolonged periods. Quantities in excess of 1 gram are being ingested by many people as a prophylactic against the common cold, in various cancers, in the detoxification of drug addicts, in schizophrenias, for wound healing and for the prevention of the formation of nitrosamines in the stomach. Some critics of high-dose vitamin C administration have alleged that the substance causes kidney stones through the increased excretion of oxalate; interference with vitamin B-12 metabolism; rebound scurvy upon sudden cessation of therapy; excessive iron absorption and a mutagenic effect. An extensive and very thorough analysis of the data during the past years has disproved all the serious allegations. Some patients, particularly in the early days of high-dose administration, do experience a laxative effect. Even this mild and harmless adverse effect is not found consistently."

The case for the safety and efficacy of vitamin C has been supported in many recent medical journals and monographs, including *Ascorbate: The Science of Vitamin C* and *Injectable Vitamin C and the Treatment of Viral and Other Diseases*, which is an excellent compilation of the impressive early clinical reports establishing this vitamin as valuable in preventing and treating various disease conditions.

The public also has its own way of dealing with medical ideas. It goes by how it feels. When patients find that they get fewer colds after taking vitamin C, no amount of rhetoric will persuade them that their own convictions are unscientific. Vitamin C is the most popular nutrient supplement on the market. Despite early intense opposition, Linus Pauling's conclusion that vitamin C is helpful in decreasing the frequency and improving the symptoms of the common cold has won the day. Many scientific studies have shown that vitamin C consistently decreases the duration of cold episodes and the severity of symptoms.

"Since I began writing in this field," Dr Pauling once remarked, "I've had the support of scientists. They say that I've been right so often that I'm probably right here too. It's the medical community that has been blind. Rene Dubois, who discovered the first antibiotics, said that he was always working in the mainstream of science, but I was 20 years ahead of everyone else. I myself don't consider myself a maverick in science. I'm just ahead of it."

As Dr Pauling recognized, vitamin C is not only effective for preventing and treating scurvy and the common cold, but also for other common health conditions, including coronary disease and cancer, largely because of its antioxidant activity.

Therapeutic Uses

Antioxidant Activity: Vitamin C is needed by everyone, not only to prevent diseases, such as scurvy, but also to insure optimum health of the whole body. In the presence of any pathology or stress, the amount needed increases very rapidly. It has been found that the more serious the condition, the more vitamin C is needed.

==Vitamin C is indeed our chief antioxidant.== We live in an atmosphere that contains about 20% oxygen. This is used in respiration to create energy. But excessive oxidation will be very harmful. Free radicals are formed, which are very active and can damage cells and tissues. A free radical can pull another electron from another molecule and convert that into another free radical. This chain reaction will continue until the electron reacts with another electron or is deactivated by an antioxidant, a scavenger, or an enzyme. The body has developed a system of antioxidants to protect itself against excessive oxidation. A potato will turn brown once it is peeled if not protected from oxidation by being immersed in water. The brown pigment formed is the result of excessive oxidation in a tissue not protected by antioxidants. Free radicals are involved in a large number of processes in the body, including cancer, aging, Parkinson's disease, cardiovascular disease, cataracts, arthritis, and diabetes. By controlling these reactions, antioxidants have a therapeutic role in all these conditions.

Vitamin C is the main water-soluble antioxidant, but the body's defense system also includes other nutrients that work in conjunction with vitamin C, including antioxidant enzymes, superoxide dismutase (sod), catalase, glutathione peroxidase, vitamin E, beta carotene, non-enzymatic scavengers, uric acid, glutathione, and thiols in proteins. These substances work together both within the cell and in the fluids outside the cells. They also reinforce each other's activity: for example, vitamin E spares vitamin C. Vitamin C works mainly in the water medium, while vitamin E works primarily in the fat medium and on cell membranes.

Anti-Aging Activity: In his book *How To Live Longer and Feel Better*, Linus Pauling concluded that people taking ascorbic acid would live longer. All the information we have about ascorbic acid supports this conclusion.

Normally, less than 5% of the total vitamin C in the body is in the oxidized state (dehydroascorbic acid), so that the ratio of ascorbic acid to dehydroascorbic acid is greater than 20:1. However, when the individual is close to death, almost all the vitamin C is in the oxidized dehydroascorbic acid state. To supplement with ascorbic acid to improve this ratio would seem to make sense.

But the final test is the practical one – does it work? In fact, it does. Dr James Enstrom, School of Public Health, University of California at Los

Angeles, analyzed a 10-year study of 11,348 people, aged 25 to 74. Men who consumed at least 300 mg of ascorbic acid suffered 41% fewer deaths during that period than men who took only 50 mg in their food. They lived on the average 6 years longer. Had they used gram doses daily, we think the results would have been more striking.

Stress Reduction: Modern society is filled with stresses from work, family life, and even daily driving on highways. Sometimes stress leads to depression, anger, and even violence. Vitamin C can reduce the deleterious effects of stress and help us to withstand the inevitable stresses that we encounter each day. A randomized double-blind, placebo-controlled trial involving 120 healthy young adults assessed the ability of vitamin C to moderate stress. The trial lasted 14 days, with one group of 60 healthy adults given sustained-release vitamin C (1000 mg, three times daily), and with another group of 60 adults given an identical looking placebo, three times daily. The study evaluated blood pressure, cortisol (a stress hormone), and the subjects' subjective responses to acute psychological stress. The results of this study demonstrated that vitamin C palliates blood pressure, cortisol, and subjective response to acute psychological stress. In other words, vitamin C helped the subjects to handle stress more efficiently, and even reduced physiological parameters commonly increased in response to stressful events or stimuli.

Arteriosclerosis: Dr Linus Pauling and Dr Rath have shown that the body increases its production of lipoprotein cholesterol (a) in an attempt to overcome some of the symptoms of scurvy. A major problem with scurvy is that the blood vessels can no longer retain their integrity and fluid leaks from them, into the skin, into the tissues. The lipoprotein (a) present in the blood plugs small leaks, which develop and decreases the leakage of fluid from the vessels. But if too much is made – and this could be a *too* successful attempt to prevent fluid loss – the extra lipoprotein(a) is deposited in the vessel wall and initiates arteriosclerosis. This is one of the main factors responsible for cardiovascular disease, including strokes and coronary disease. There are probably other mechanisms, which have developed over the past 20 million years to try and overcome the problems generated by the lack of ascorbic acid.

Stomach Acid Supplement: Vitamin C is a weak organic acid, comparable to lemon juice. Compared to the strong acid present in the stomach, the addition of any amount of ascorbic acid makes a minor contribution to the stomach fluid acidity.

Laxative Effect: Vitamin C is a very good laxative. Since at least one third of the population over 65 is constipated, it would seem to us to be wise for all elderly people to control this problem not only by consuming enough fiber but also by taking enough vitamin C. This is done by starting with doses of 3 to 6 g each day and gradually increasing it until the sublaxative dose is reached. Then the dose is decreased to just below this level. If the laxative level is 20 g, the optimum oral level will be around 18 g.

Idiopathic Thrombocytopenic Purpura (ITP): Dr A.G. Brox and his colleagues at McGill University in Montreal found that ascorbic acid, given 2 g daily, successfully treated 7 out of 11 patients with idiopathic thrombocytopenic purpura (ITP). They had all been sick more than 2 months and had not responded to adrenocorticosteroids. Three had had splenectomies. Four had failed additional treatment, including the current usual treatments. We have one patient now with ITP on ascorbic acid, who has been well over 5 years, but only as long as she remains on her ascorbic acid. If she discontinues, her platelet count begins to sink within a few weeks.

Cancer Prevention and Treatment: In 1990, the National Cancer Institute cosponsored a meeting on Ascorbic Acid and Cancer. Thirty-three presenters, including Linus Pauling, outlined the current state of research connecting vitamin C and cancer. Based upon these abstracts, it is clear ascorbic acid must be considered a major component in the treatment of cancer for the following reasons.

Vitamin C protects plasma lipids against peroxidation. Higher vitamin C levels in the blood provide the most protection. Since both chemotherapy and radiation increase peroxidation, vitamin C decreases the toxicity of these treatments for normal tissue. In vitro ascorbic acid protects cells against transformation by methyl cholanthrene and against Rous sarcoma virus. In hairless mice, it decreases the incidence and delays the onset of malignant lesions when exposed to ultraviolet light. It also decreases incidence of spontaneous mammary tumors in mice. Other workers reported similar protective effects of ascorbic acid on animals. A review of the literature showed that in 33 out of 46 studies, vitamin C was protective, decreasing incidence and mortality. Individuals in the top one-quarter vitamin levels had only a 50% risk of cancer compared to those in the lowest quarter. The final conclusion was that ascorbic acid was an important part of any cancer treatment.

> Ascorbic acid must be considered a major component in the treatment of cancer.

Ewan Cameron and Linus Pauling's conclusion in their book *Cancer and Vitamin C* that ascorbic acid increased the survival of patients with terminal cancer first aroused our interest. Subsequently, we began to give cancer patients a comprehensive orthomolecular program, which included ascorbic acid, 12 g or more daily, plus a large number of other nutrients, including vitamin B-3, beta carotene, selenium, and, in some cases, vitamin E. Our patients were also concerned, anxious, or depressed, and were given psychiatric treatment, including medication for this, if required. Our treatment program proved to be very successful, to the point where many doctors began referring their cancer patients in substantial number.

The first case was a woman with cancer of the pancreas, after a by-pass operation. On this vitamin program, she recovered and was still well 15 years later. She began to tell all her friends and others about her own recovery and gradually the number of referrals began to increase. When we had seen 134 patients, we reviewed their state and sent the information to Dr Pauling for analysis. He had just developed a new, elegant way for examining the outcome of cohort studies. We first published the results in the *Journal of Orthomolecular Medicine*; an expanded study appears in the 1993 edition of Cameron and Pauling's *Cancer and Vitamin C*; our final work is published in two books, *Vitamin C and Cancer: Discovery, Recovery, Controversy* and *Healing Cancer: Complementary Vitamin and Drug Treatments*.

Of the 134 cases studied, there were 33 patients who did not follow the treatment regimen and 101 similar patients who did. To analyze the results of the vitamin treatment, we used the Hardin Jones biostatistical analyses of mortality for cohorts or groups of cancer patients, developed by Dr Pauling.

This method applies to the problem of evaluating mean survival time for a cohort with a few survivors at the termination of the study, and for a cohort with many survivors at the termination of the study. There were three cohorts. (1) The pseudo control group of 33 who did not follow the treatment protocol; they survived 5.7 months. This group included all the cancer cases. (2) The cohort of 40 patients with cancer of the breast, ovary, uterus, cervix, and fallopian tubes. There were 22 survivors. Mean survival time was estimated to be 99 months. (3) The remaining cohort of 61 patients with the other cancers. There were 29 survivors; mean estimated survival time was 67 months.

We concluded that 80% of the patients who followed our orthomolecular nutritional regimen had a probable survival time 21 times that of the controls for cohort 2, and 13 times that of the controls for cohort 3 – or, for all patients, 16 times that of the controls. The mean survival of patients from each group who did not survive was about 10 months or about twice as high as it was for those who did not follow the program. The mean survival of the controls, 5.7 months, is about what is observed for ambulatory patients who have reached or are close to the terminal stage of cancer, with 85% having received potentially curative or palliative conventional therapy.

We concluded that "the much longer mean survival time of 81 of the similar patients who followed the regimen, 92 months, must surely be attributed to this regimen." We also said that "on the basis of these results and of those reported by Cameron and his collaborators we strongly recommended that patients with cancer follow the regimen described in this paper, as an adjunct to appropriate conventional therapy." We also joined Ewan Cameron in recommending that physicians consider administering large amounts of sodium ascorbate by intravenous infusion to patients with advanced cancer. Cameron himself gave intravenous ascorbate, usually 10 g per day for about 10 days, as well as oral ascorbate continued indefinitely, to each of his patients, and other physicians have reported the successful use of intravenous ascorbate.

Patients started on treatment soon after they have been diagnosed appear to have a better prognosis compared to those who are started several years after they have been diagnosed. This may mean that the treatment they have already had has decreased their ability to respond as well to orthomolecular treatment.

We have examined the relationship between the interval between first symptoms and when patients first consulted me. From this group of 40 female patients, those who started on therapy about the same time as they were started on xenobiotic therapy (chemotherapy and radiation therapy) had a 10-month advantage over those who were started after an average of 9 months. We have also completed a further evaluation of a larger group, not included in the 134 group. Their follow-up period is less, but comparing the outcome over the 3 years of follow-up, it is apparent that their outcome will be very similar to the outcome of the previous group.

Skin Disorders: Another remarkable benefit of vitamin C is that it can reduce common symptoms and signs associated with skin disorders. Skin cancer is becoming more prevalent, resulting in the need for better sunscreens. These must protect us against ultraviolet damage.

Apparently, the ultraviolet light, after penetrating the skin, increases the formation of free radicals. It makes sense to increase the protection against free radicals by using nature's antioxidants, vitamin C, vitamin E, beta carotene, and selenium. The frequent, recurring reports in the media about the dangers inherent in excessive exposure to sunlight continually frighten some people about the possibility of getting skin cancer. However, these reports do not discuss the connection between the nutritional health of the population and their susceptibility to cancer of the skin. Since ultraviolet irradiation increases the formation of free radicals, it would not be surprising that increasing the availability of antioxidants would prevent some of the toxic reactions to ultraviolet radiation.

Dr John Murray, Professor of Dermatology at Duke University, found that vitamin C decreased the intensity of the reaction to ultraviolet light. Subjects were pre-treated with a vitamin C solution or with placebo. The protective effect was immediate. The vitamin C was not a sunscreen, but it decreased the effect of ultra violet light by its antioxidant properties – that is, it wiped out some of the free radicals that were formed.

The fat-soluble antioxidant vitamin E should also have protective properties. Many years ago, Dr Evan Shute reported that vitamin E in ointment or oral form protected against radiation burns. For many years, we have been advising friends and family to apply vitamin E cream or to use the contents of the vitamin E capsules to protect themselves against sunburns.

Even after they have burned, application of this vitamin has quickly removed the pain and has prevented serious burns. It, too, acts as an antioxidant.

> We would, therefore, suggest that the three best known natural antioxidants – ascorbic acid, vitamin E, and selenium – be used to protect people against the toxic effect of excessive ultraviolet irradiation.

Selenium is also a preventive nutrient. Selenium given to hairless pigmented mice protected them against damage from ultraviolet irradiation. Both a lotion containing 0.02% L-selenomethionine and oral administration of water containing 1.2 p.p.m. were protective. These dosages did not cause any toxic reactions. This study concluded that "SeMet is effective in protecting against skin cancer induced by UV irradiation, both by retarding the onset and reducing the number of lesions." They were also "effective in reducing the acute damage induced by UV irradiation-inflammation (sunburn), blistering, and pigmentation (tanning)." Selenium is a good antioxidant. It is synergistic with vitamin E, the body's best known fat-soluble antioxidant. The daily recommended dose is 200 mcg. We have given 600 mcg and more to certain patients for many years and have seen no toxic side effects.

We would, therefore, suggest that the three best known natural antioxidants – ascorbic acid, vitamin E, and selenium – be used to protect people against the toxic effect of excessive ultraviolet irradiation. It would be prudent to use optimum amounts of vitamins C and E and selenium and to apply a sunscreen containing all these antioxidants – vitamin C, vitamin E, and selenium. The dose would be 200 mcg selenium, 800 IU of vitamin E, and 3 g or more per day of ascorbic acid. It should not take too much time to test these antioxidants in controlled studies. Because the danger from ultraviolet-induced skin cancer and melanoma is potentially so great, it would appear to us to be prudent to take these simple nutrients as a precaution. They would, of course, have other advantages as well.

Vaccinations and Inoculations: One of the most interesting benefits of vitamin C is that it can protect against side effects from vaccinations/inoculations. C.A.B. Clemetson, Department of Obstetrics and Gynecology,

Tulane University School of Medicine, in a 2004 article described how the level of histamine in the blood could rise following a vaccination. Symptoms of an increase in blood histamine can be severe and include retinal petechiae (small hemorrhages in the retina), and subdural hemorrhage (bleeding within the brain).

According to Dr Clemetson, the high blood histamine and low vitamin C levels following a vaccination in an infant might be the cause of some cases of shaken baby syndrome. To remedy this, he suggests that every infant should receive 500 mg of vitamin C (in crystals or powder form) in fruit juice prior to receiving a vaccination. Because vitamin C helps to clear histamine from the blood, it will mitigate the rise in blood histamine following a vaccination, reducing any potential side effects from the elevated levels of histamine in the blood.

Optimum Dosage

There is no need to ask the question, do I need any vitamin C? The only question is, how much do I need? But how much do we need and in what form?

Nature offers some clues to determining an optimum dose. Of these clues, the best is the amount of vitamin C animals make in their body normally and under severe stress. They are able to convert glucose into vitamin C because they have the enzyme, L-gulonlactoneoxidase, which human beings lack. They make much more than we take in from our food. A goat, weighing about as much as a man, will make 14 g of vitamin C per day. Apparently, all animals that make vitamin C produce about the same amount per kilogram of body weight. Every person should take ample quantities to replace what nature took away from us.

To derive this amount of vitamin C from our diet would require eating huge quantities of fruits and vegetables – more than 100 oranges each day, for example. Rather than overeat, we can supplement our diet with synthetic ascorbic acid, which is readily available and very inexpensive.

The maximum recommended oral dose of vitamin C is 75 g each day, but very few can tolerate this extremely high dose because it exceeds the laxative dose. While the majority of people take under 12 g per day, it is best to think in terms of the optimum tolerable dose. You can determine this for yourself.

When more vitamin C is taken than that individual can absorb from the gastrointestinal tract, it causes increased formation of gas and the bowel contents become very fluid. If the dose greatly exceeds this level, diarrhea will develop. The ideal dose has optimum functions in the body without causing any effect on the bowel except to help regulate it.

Dr Roger Cathcart discovered that the more the body needs the vitamin, the more it can tolerate. We have observed the same, as have almost all orthomolecular physicians. Our personal optimum dose has ranged between 30 and 3 g daily, depending on our state of health. If a lot more is needed, it is possible to train the body to accept more. Some AIDS patients in Australia have been trained to take 200 g daily. If the higher doses cannot be reached, it may be necessary to take intravenous vitamin C. When given in intravenous drip, up to 200 g can be given over several hours without any gastrointestinal effect.

Ascorbates

A number of people do not like the sour taste of ascorbic acid in tablet or water-soluble powder form This problem can be solved with the use of ascorbic acid salts, such as sodium ascorbate, potassium ascorbate, and calcium ascorbate. A few preparations on the market, called mineral ascorbates, contain a variety of these salts of vitamin C. They do represent an improvement over the straight ascorbic acid, which is never present in nature as the pure acid, as it is in tablets, but is associated with other nutrients. One such preparation we have been using for several years is Supergram Plus, non-acidic vitamin C. It contains calcium, magnesium, zinc, manganese, molybdenum, and chromium ascorbates, but most of the vitamin C contained there is sodium ascorbate. Mineral ascorbates are more tolerable for many and are equivalent to taking the pure vitamin C (hydrogen ascorbate).

A very small number of people, fewer than 20 seen over the past 30 years, cannot tolerate any amount of vitamin C. They have developed an allergy or idiosyncrasy to either the synthetic vitamin C or to some of the other ingredients of the preparations. They might try preparations made from other sugar sources. The common vitamin C is made from corn syrup. It is preferable to take the vitamin several times per day to decrease the amount lost in the urine.

Vitamin B Complex

Vitamin B complex preparations are available and labeled B-complex 25s, B-complex 50s, B-complex 75s, or even B-complex 100s. The first one contains 25 mg per tablet of thiamin, riboflavin, nicotinamide, and pyridoxine, plus small amounts of the other B vitamins. Similar preparations are called anti-stress vitamins. These are useful preparations made by many drug and vitamin companies. Very few people have any problem with them, though some may be worried about the yellow urine caused by the riboflavin in the preparations. It is a useful marker whether or not the tablet gets absorbed into the body.

> **Thiamin is essential for the metabolism of carbohydrates. When deficient, the disease beri beri results.**

These complexes are very useful in ensuring that all the B-vitamins will be provided. They are also very helpful in determining whether vitamins in general are needed. For those who are allergic to yeast, the preferred ones are yeast free.

Vitamin B-1 (Thiamin)

The early scientists recognized only two kinds of vitamins, fat-soluble vitamin A and the water-soluble ones. Thiamin was the first water-soluble vitamin to be identified. When more water-soluble vitamins were found, they were named in order of discovery as B-1, B-2, and later B-3. After their structure was determined, they were given their chemical names – thiamin, riboflavin, and nicotinic acid with its amide.

Thiamin is essential for the metabolism of carbohydrates. When deficient, the disease beri beri results. Ironically, thiamin would never have been discovered if it had not been first removed from staple foods. In the Far East, white rice became fashionable in this century. White rice is made by polishing off the outer layers of the whole original or brown rice, thereby removing the bran, germ, and adjacent layers. In cereal grains, such as rice or wheat, this is where the major part of the thiamin is located.

Therapeutic Uses

Beri beri: People living mostly on white rice suffer a thiamin deficiency or beri beri. The Japanese navy wanted to solve the problem of so many of their sailors having beri beri. This led to the studies showing that a food factor had been removed, later identified as thiamin. Adding this to the food prevented the disease beri beri. More recently, brown rice has been heat treated to drive the thiamin further in so that polishing the rice does not remove as much of the thiamin. Thiamin is one of the vitamins added to white flour in North America. Beri beri is very rare now that thiamin has been restored to processed grains. The amount available in food due to fortification of white flour will ensure that very few will get beri beri.

Wernicke-Korsakoff Syndrome: There are only a few indications for using large doses of thiamin. Most people will need less than 50 mg daily, the amount that is found in the vitamin B-complex preparations called B Complex-50. The exceptions are people who consume large quantities of carbohydrates. They usually are on a diet too rich in refined carbohydrates and fats, which provides minimal amounts of all the vitamins and increases the need for thiamin. The best example is alcoholism.

Some alcoholics develop a very serious killer disease called Wernicke-Korsakoff syndrome. The recommended treatment for this is to give large amounts of thiamin, parenterally at first and later by mouth. Up to 500 mg per day are recommended. We also add vitamin B-3 in large doses to our patients. They respond much better to the combination. This syndrome may be an example of a double dependency, vitamin B-1 and vitamin B-3. After the syndrome has been controlled, smaller amounts of thiamin will keep them well if they stop drinking. We think people who are obese because of their heavy sugar intake would also be helped by extra thiamin. It has been used for some patients with depression.

In one study, 8 out of 39 patients (23%) with AIDS had evidence of the same type of clinical features associated with the Wernicke-Korsakoff syndrome of alcoholism. None of the deficient patients had any history of alcoholism or neurological symptoms. AIDS patients on mainstream treatments (for example, AZT) for their illness would benefit from taking supplemental thiamin each day to prevent deficiency.

Congestive Heart Failure: Some of the most notable features of thiamin deficiency include cardiomyopathy, irregular heartbeat, and shortness of breath — clinical signs that mimic congestive heart failure. In fact, a pilot study did find thiamin deficiency among many congestive heart failure patients on long-term therapy with the drug furosemide. Based on this evidence, it is a wise idea for all patients with congestive heart failure on diuretic medication to take replacement doses of thiamin each day.

Psychiatric Disorders: Psychiatric patients are another group in which supplementation with thiamin might be beneficial. Up to 30% of all patients entering a psychiatric ward were found to be deficient in thiamin. Another study found that chronic borderline thiamine deficiency was associated with a heightened experience of anxiety among healthy male adults who were not normally anxious individuals.

Other Conditions: Other clinical indications for supplementing with thiamin include AIDS, congestive heart failure, and psychiatric disorders.

Optimum Dose

The therapeutic dose ranges from 50 to 3000 mg daily, but the highest doses are very seldom used. Most doses are less than 100 mg daily, except for alcoholics when it will have to go as high as 500 mg. We have given 3 g per day with no difficulty and no side effects. It may be given by injection as well.

Safety

As Dr John Marks notes, "The only reaction found in humans is of the hypersensitivity type. In the vast majority of cases these have occurred after injection of thiamin, and a skin-test dose is advised before undertaking parenteral administration of thiamin in patients with a history of allergic reactions. For parenteral administration the dose that has produced these reactions varies from 5 to 100 mg, although the majority of the reactions occur in the higher part of this range. Since the RDA is 1.4 mg, this means the margin of safety is still high. Very rare cases of transient hypersensitivity reactions have also been reported after oral high doses usually in the range of 5 to 10 g (but with one case report at 17 mg). Hence for oral administration the safety factor is at least 100 times the RDA."

A few patients find that on high doses of thiamin there is a thiamin odor on their skin, which they find offensive. Others have told us it was also offensive to mosquitoes.

Vitamin B-2 (Riboflavin)

Riboflavin has not been studied very intensively. This vitamin is water soluble, easily destroyed by light and heat. It is yellow with a beautiful fluorescence when exposed to ultra violet light. It is also added to white flour. Very few people are deficient in riboflavin.

Therapeutic Uses

Migraine Headaches: One of the most recent indications for riboflavin is in the prevention of migraine headaches. Migraines headaches impose a significant burden upon our society and its working force. According to the National Headache Foundation, some 45 million Americans suffer from chronic, recurring headaches and 28 million from this total suffer from migraine headaches annually. Furthermore, the work force loses approximately 50 billion dollars per year due to absenteeism and medical expenses caused by headache, with more than 157 million workdays lost each year to migraine sufferers. One of the leading theories of migraine headaches is that there is some degree of mitochondrial dysfunction. This leads to impaired energy metabolism, and causes biochemical shifts that activate the trigeminovascular system, resulting in migraine attacks.

> One of the most recent indications for riboflavin is in the prevention of migraine headaches.

Riboflavin improves energy metabolism within most cells of the body through its ability to optimize the functioning of cellular components called mitochondria. Several randomized controlled clinical trials have shown that 400 mg per day of riboflavin is effective at reducing the frequency and pain of migraine headaches in as little as 3 months.

Other Conditions: Riboflavin is helpful in preventing cataracts in elderly patients if the treatment is started very early. This vitamin is also effective against carpal tunnel syndrome. There is a report that phenothiazine tranquilizers will increase the need for riboflavin.

Optimum Dose

The more common dose ranges for riboflavin are 50 mg to several hundred daily. The majority of people will not need more than 50 mg. There are no side effects with these doses.

Vitamin B-3 (Niacin and Niacinamide)

The third water-soluble vitamin to be discovered was the anti-pellagra vitamin, now known as niacin. As Dr Hoffer recalls, he first heard about vitamins in his second year at the university in 1935 in a class called Biochemistry 1. The professor was Roger Manning, a biochemist. He systematically covered all the known vitamins, beginning with vitamin B-1, then vitamin B-2, and later vitamin B-3. But the use of the number B-3 did not stay in the literature very long, replaced by nicotinic acid and its amide (also known medically as niacin and niacinamide). The name was changed to remove the similarity to nicotine, a poison. We once had a chronic paranoid patient who refused to take nicotinic acid because he thought it was nicotine, but he did not object to taking niacin.

The term vitamin B-3 was reintroduced by our friend, Mr. Bill W. (Bill Wilson), co-founder of Alcoholics Anonymous. We met in New York in 1960, where we introduced him to the concept of megavitamin therapy. We described the results we had seen with our schizophrenic patients, some of whom were also alcoholic. We also told him about its many other properties. It was therapeutic for arthritis, for some cases of senility, and it lowered cholesterol levels.

Bill was very curious about it and began to take niacin, 3 g daily. Within a few weeks, fatigue and depression, which had plagued him for years, were gone. He gave it to 30 of his close friends in AA and persuaded them to try it. Within 6 months, he was convinced that it would be very helpful to alcoholics. Of the 30 friends, 10 were free of anxiety, tension, and depression in one month. Another 10 were well in 2 months. He decided that the chemical or medical terms for this vitamin were not appropriate.

He wanted to persuade members of AA, especially the doctors in AA, that this would be a useful addition to treatment and he needed a term that could be more readily popularized. Bill asked what the names had been used. Dr Hoffer then recalled Professor Manning's lectures and told Bill it was originally known as vitamin B-3. This was the term Bill wanted. In his first report to physicians in AA, he called it "The Vitamin B-3 Therapy." Thousands of copies of this extraordinary pamphlet were distributed. Eventually, the name came back and today even the most conservative medical journals are using the term vitamin B-3.

Bill soon became unpopular with the members of the board of AA International. The medical members who had been appointed by Bill felt that he had no business messing about with treatment using vitamins. They also believed vitamin B-3 could not be as therapeutic as Bill had found it to be. For this reason, Bill provided information to the medical members of AA outside of the National Board, publishing and distributing three more pamphlets, which are still in demand.

Professor Harold Foster and Dr Hoffer have concluded that at least half of our population suffers from some form of vitamin B-3 deficiency or dependency. The clinical evidence shows that these people feel better, become healthier, and live longer if they take vitamin B-3 supplements.

Vitamin B-3 exists as the amide in nature, in nicotinamide adenine dinucleotide (NAD). Pure nicotinamide and niacin are synthetics. Niacin was known as a chemical for about 100 years before it was recognized to be vitamin B-3. It is made from nicotine, a poison produced in the tobacco plant to protect itself against its predators, but in the wonderful economy of nature, which does not waste any structures, when the nicotine is simplified by cracking open one of the rings, it becomes the immensely valuable vitamin B-3.

Vitamin B-3 is made in the body from the amino acid tryptophan. On the average, 1 mg of vitamin B-3 is made from 60 mg of tryptophan, a 1.5% conversion rate. Since it is made in the body, it does not meet the strict definition of a vitamin, which is defined as a substance that cannot be made by the body. It should have been classified with the amino acids, but long usage of the term vitamin has given it permanent status as a vitamin. We suspect that one day in the far distant future none of the tryptophan will be converted into vitamin B-3 and it then will truly be a vitamin.

The 1.5% conversion rate is a compromise based upon the conversion of tryptophan to N-methyl nicotinamide and its metabolites in human subjects. According to M.K. Horwitt, the amount converted is not inflexible, but varies with patients and conditions. For example, women pregnant in their last 3 months convert tryptophan to niacin metabolites three times as efficiently as in non-pregnant females. Also there is evidence that contraceptive steroids or estrogens stimulate tryptophan oxygenase, the enzyme that converts the tryptophan into niacin.

This observation raises some interesting speculations. Women, on average, live longer then men. It has been shown in men that giving them niacin increases their longevity. Is the increased longevity in women the result of greater conversion of tryptophan into niacin under the stimulus of their increase in estrogen production? Does the same phenomenon explain the lower incidence of coronary disease in women? Elsewhere, we have suggested that in schizophrenics there is a decrease in the production of niacin from tryptophan, and that this is part of a slow evolutionary change that will one day totally remove this source of niacin, and we will have to depend entirely on external sources. It was observed a long time ago that pregnant women were to a degree less prone to develop schizophrenia, and when it did occur, it often took the form of a post partum psychosis.

In their book, *Feel Better and Live Longer with Vitamin B-3*, Professor Harold Foster and Dr Hoffer have concluded that at least half of our population suffers from some form of vitamin B-3 deficiency or dependency. The clinical evidence shows that these people feel better, become healthier, and live longer if they take vitamin B-3 supplements.

Humanity has virtually lost the ability to synthesize niacin. This probably had relatively little negative consequence when diets were high in this vitamin. Unfortunately, mineral deficient fertilizers and food processing are depleting diets of a wide range of essential nutrients, including vitamin B-3. As a consequence the numerous niacin deficiency diseases, which include arthritis, heart diseases, and schizophrenia, are becoming much more common.

There have, however, also been advantages associated with this loss of the ability to synthesize niacin. This vitamin is an antagonist of adrenochrome and its derivatives, which appear to promote intelligence and creativity and reduce susceptibility to cancer. There seems, therefore, to be a balanced polymorphism at work, which ensures that genetically the benefits and costs of a decreased ability to metabolize niacin are offset against those associated with high levels of adrenochrome and its associated derivatives.

Ideally, then, we should attempt to obtain the benefits of both niacin and adrenochrome without the disadvantages of either. On the one hand, niacin deficiency can be easily overcome by supplementation, usually combined with high dose vitamin C. Elevated adrenochrome is a double-edged sword. It appears to promote both intelligence and psychosis, while protecting against cancer. As seen in the treatment of schizophrenics, where excessively elevated levels of adrenochrome cause psychosis, levels must be lowered by natural methyl acceptors, such as niacin and coenzyme Q10. However, the successful treatment of cancer may require deliberately stimulating adrenochrome levels to the point at which they cause temporary psychosis. As a species, we need to be smart enough to manipulate the body levels of niacin and adrenochrome and its derivatives so that we can gain their benefits without paying the health costs of shortages of either.

There are now 16 clinical indications, and probably many more, that can be improved or even reversed by supplementing with vitamin B-3. How can one nutrient be so useful for so many apparent different conditions? Pellagrins suffer from serious skin lesions, from gastrointestinal disease, from a schizophrenic type of dementia and they die. A tiny dose of B-3, one nutrient only, will cure all these major apparently different diseases. That is how nutrients work. A deficiency of any one is expressed by a multiplicity of signs and symptoms, and when these deficiencies are corrected, the many diverse diseases vanish. This is a common property of nutrients, never of drugs.

Therapeutic Uses

Pellagra: The best known vitamin B-3 deficiency disease is pellagra. More accurately, it is a tryptophan deficiency disease because tryptophan alone can cure the early stages. Pellagra was endemic in the Southern United States until the beginning of the last world war. It can be described by the four Ds – dermatitis, diarrhea, dementia, and death. The dementia is a late stage phenomenon. In the early stages, it resembles much more the schizophrenias and can only with difficulty be distinguished from it. We consider it one of the schizophrenic syndromes.

Blood Lipids (Cholesterol): We have been involved in establishing two of the major uses for vitamin B-3, apart from its role in preventing and treating pellagra. These are its action in lowering high cholesterol levels while elevating high density lipoprotein (HDL) cholesterol levels; and its therapeutic role in the schizophrenias and other psychiatric conditions.

Of the two major findings made by our research group in Saskatchewan, the nicotinic acid cholesterol connection is well known. Nicotinic acid is now used worldwide as an economical, effective, and safe compound for lowering cholesterol and elevating high density lipoprotein cholesterol.

However, its therapeutic value in treating schizophrenia has been almost totally ignored by psychiatry, in spite of the four double-blind controlled experiments we did in the early 1950s and in spite of over 50 papers published in the medical literature by our colleagues dealing with various aspects of this treatment. This suggests to us that psychiatry is at least 20 years behind general medicine in adopting new paradigms. We suspect that it will take another 20 years before every schizophrenic is given the benefit of orthomolecular treatment, which includes mainly vitamin B-3 and vitamin B-6, for treating even chronic patients who do not respond in a few months, but may need many years of treatment in an overall comprehensive program that includes diet, nutrients, and drugs in an optimum combination. In two books, *Vitamin B-3 and Schizophrenia: Discovery, Recovery, Controversy* and *Healing Schizophrenia: Complementary Vitamin and Drug Treatments,* we have told the story of this discovery in full.

Schizophrenia: In 1951, we developed a unified hypothesis of schizophrenia that united biochemical and psychosocial factors. We suggested that in schizophrenia there was an abnormal production of adrenochrome, which then acted on the brain much as does the hallucinogen d-lysergic acid diethylamide (LSD). Adrenochrome is one of the more reactive derivatives of adrenaline. Noradrenochrome is the derivative from noradrenalin.

Over the next 10 years, our research group in Saskatchewan established that adrenochrome is an hallucinogen, that the biochemical conditions necessary for its formation in the body were all present, and that using a compound that blocked its activity on the brain was therapeutic for schizophrenia. That compound was vitamin B-3, either nicotinic acid or nicotinamide. Recently, it was shown that adrenochrome is made in the body and then rapidly converts into adrenolutin, a reduced derivative. Both have hallucinogenic properties.

As we developed our research program, we met some opposition from the Canadian professors of psychiatry who did not like our hypothesis and tried to block us from getting research grants. However, with the help of Dr Nolan D.C. Lewis, then Director of the Psychiatric Institute in New York, we were awarded our first Government of Canada grant in 1952. Dr Hoffer was appointed Director of Psychiatric Research for the Province of Saskatchewan. Later, we were given a large grant from the Rockefeller Foundation, which made it possible to enlarge our research group substantially over the next 6 years.

We then discovered that this vitamin given in gram doses per day lowered cholesterol levels. Since then it has been found that vitamin B-3 also elevates high density lipoprotein cholesterol, thus bringing the ratio of total cholesterol over HDL to below 5. This was a very fortunate finding because it led to the approval by the FDA for using this vitamin in megadoses for cholesterol problems and opened up the use of this vitamin in large doses for other conditions as well. This occurred at a time when the FDA was doing its best not to recognize the value of megavitamin therapy.

By 1957, our research group had published a large number of papers dealing with various aspects of psychiatric disease and we were recognized as one of the better research groups in North America. Apart from skepticism about our adrenochrome hypothesis, we did not run into much opposition. This changed, though, after we published our first report that vitamin B-3 was useful for the treatment of acute schizophrenia. Suddenly, psychiatry found its basic concepts of schizophrenia challenged as no other finding ever had before. Tranquilizers were being introduced at the time, but they were accepted as better sedatives, which simply made psychotherapy more effective. This did not run counter to psychodynamic theories, which had swept into psychiatry after the last world war.

The four double-blind controlled studies we did between 1952 and 1958 showed that adding one vitamin, vitamin B-3, to the current treatment doubled the 2-year recovery rate from 35% to about 75%. Since then, a large number of studies from our group and from many other practitioners have shown that these results were improved by the addition of other nutrients and by more attention to the use of the optimum diets for these patients.

Still, our earlier studies were not promising for the chronic patients. Vitamin B-3 therapy, as the single vitamin, did not appear to help chronic patients. Later, we found that if the treatment was combined with other treatment and maintained for several years, the results were more promising.

> We were surprised by the extent and intensity of the opposition, but accepted it as the inevitable result of promoting new ideas in medicine. New ideas historically have had to run the gauntlet of opposition for up to 40 years before they are incorporated into the body of medicine.

Recently, we examined the outcome of treatment of 27 chronic patients who remained under our care for 10 years and more. They were ill on the average 7 years before they came under our treatment program. This is only a relatively small portion of the large number of chronic patients we are treating. The average age of this group was 40 years when they started the program, they had failed to respond to all previous treatments, and they were still following the program. This consisted of a good diet, the correct vitamin and mineral supplements, and medication, such as tranquilizers and antidepressants, as required. A survey showed that today 11 are working, two are married and looking after their families, two are single mothers caring for their children with no difficulty, three are managing their own business. One patient received his BSc from the local university, one was awarded her MA, another got a certificate from the community college. From this total group, 18 are well today, three are much improved, five are improved. None are worse.

Using the best xenobiotic drug therapy, it is clear that from a similar group of chronic patients one would expect almost no cases of recovery, while at best a few might have reached an improved state. As reported in *The British Journal of Psychiatry*, E.C. Johnston and his colleagues studied 532 schizophrenic patients treated over a 10-year period beginning in 1975 for their recovery rates. It was found that only two patients were now in the best occupational levels (this means that they were well) and 25 were found in the next best occupational level. That is, only 5% of this large group had shown any significant recovery. They found that close contact between patients and their treating doctors did not improve the results any – closer supervision was not helpful. They even questioned whether there was any benefit to closer monitoring of these patients. This group must have included a large number of acute and chronic patients. Only their most chronic patients would be comparable to the 26 described in our report.

In the 1970s, we treated the sick daughter of a prominent New York resident, who had been diagnosed as having schizophrenia. She became ill after graduating from a women's college. She began to experience hallucinations and became obsessive. She was admitted to hospital, treated with electro shock therapy (ECT) and tranquilizers. At the end, after having spent $250,000 vintage 1975 dollars, she was catatonic. Over the next 5 years, she was treated in seven hospitals by a number of top specialists. The parents consulted us and we advised them to start her on our vitamin B-3 program. In discussing what we thought was the most correct diagnosis for this condition, we pointed out that it closely resembled the psychosis of pellagra and that in our opinion was a variant of it – it was a vitamin B-3 dependency. This appealed to the parents' good sense, and they began to look upon it as a form of pellagra. After a discussion with the family, they discovered that just before she graduated she had gone onto a crash diet supported by medically prescribed amphetamines, losing 12 pounds weekly. After she was started on the orthomolecular program we recommended to them, she began to recover and remains well.

Our finding that this vitamin helped schizophrenics, but only when used in large doses, also challenged the nutritional establishment, which was still preoccupied with the idea that the average balanced diet was so good it did not need to be supplemented, and that taking any quantity of vitamin above these small doses would be ineffective because the extra amounts would be excreted in the urine. Their view of vitamins was very primitive. Thus, our report stirred up a massive amount of criticism based almost entirely upon theoretical ideas and not upon clinical research.

We were surprised by the extent and intensity of the opposition, but accepted it as the inevitable result of promoting new ideas in medicine. New ideas historically have had to run the gauntlet of opposition for up to 40 years before they are incorporated into the body of medicine.

There were two attempts by official medical bodies to prevent us from doing our work. The College of Physicians and Surgeons of Saskatchewan, a body that controlled licensure of all physicians in Saskatchewan, tried to censure us. Behind that attempt at censure was the psychiatric dislike of our view that vitamins could be helpful in treating schizophrenia and perhaps antagonism toward the Saskatchewan Schizophrenia Association, which was promoting the view that vitamins were helpful.

The American Psychiatric Association attempted to suppress our work several years later. We had published a paper in 1967 describing the results of treatment on five California patients. The patients had failed to respond to the best treatment they could get in California, including psychoanalysis, family therapy, medication, and so on. One of them came to us for treatment, and the rest were treated in California by other orthomolecular physicians. They all recovered. One of this group is now a research psychiatrist.

Following this publication, a few California psychiatrists complained to the American Psychiatric Association that we were promulgating treatments not acceptable to the profession. We received a letter from the APA advising us that this kind of behavior was unacceptable. At the end of a rather heated hearing, the APA announced they would let us have their decision in a few days. We had protested vigorously their right to even investigate us, pointing out that we were engaged in a scientific debate, and we had not been unethical in promulgating views, for which we had ample evidence.

We have still not heard from the APA. They concluded they had no case, but neglected to let us know this, or else they were fearful that we would announce that we had been investigated by them and that they had not found us to be unethical.

The onus is now on orthodox psychiatry to demonstrate by research of their own that there is a major fault in our conclusions. It is not good enough to assume that this is all due to a series of unproved assumptions, such as a placebo effect, faith, or even some monstrous conspiracy to show something works when in fact it does not. Or will the profession adopt the stance of a California psychiatrist who recently testified for 15 minutes before a judge that one of the patients was psychotic since she believed that vitamins had been helpful to her? World psychiatry experienced similar types of reasoning and conclusions from Russian psychiatrists who labeled dissidents psychotic simply because they were dissidents.

Our major problem today is the slow pace of recognition of new therapeutic ideas in medicine and, especially, in psychiatry. This is very costly in terms of lives. The British Navy began to issue limes to their sailors 40 years *after* Dr James Lind proved that citrus fruits cured and prevented scurvy. During those 40 years, the Navy lost 100,000 seamen from scurvy. How many schizophrenics today are being condemned to permanent and debilitating disease for the rest of their lives because of this slow pace in accepting new treatments? We must develop a mechanism by which new discoveries are promptly used in all of medicine. This should not be beyond the wit of humanity. It could be done very economically and with scientific precision – if only there was the will to do so.

Hypochlorhydria (Low Stomach Acid): When stomach acid is deficient, numerous gastrointestinal symptoms develop, including frequent gas and bloating, heartburn, nausea from taking supplements, a sense of fullness, thinning or loss of hair, brittle nails, and unexplained iron deficiency anemia. Unfortunately, many sufferers of these common gastrointestinal

> Vitamin B-3 plays an integral role in the proper functioning of the stomach and a healthy digestive system.

complaints are given acid blocking medications and other drugs for conditions mainstream medicine has termed dyspepsia (poor digestion) and heartburn. Dr William Kaufman's book on aniacinamidosis (a term that denotes a lack of vitamin B-3) describes patients afflicted with aniacinamidosis as having digestive upsets, an occasional sense of fullness when only small amounts of food are eaten, heartburn, frequent belching, indigestion, abdominal discomfort or pain, loose stools up to three times per day or constipation, glossitis, and general malaise. While sifting through Dr Kaufman's detailed clinical observations, it became apparent to us that many signs and symptoms of the aniacinamidosis disease were strongly suggestive of hypochlorhydria. Moreover, the symptoms of patients lacking optimal amounts of vitamin B-3 mimicked those commonly associated with mainstream diagnoses of dyspepsia and heartburn.

When looking at the mechanism of vitamin B-3 and the physiology of gastric (stomach) acid secretion, it is appears that vitamin B-3 plays an integral role in the proper functioning of the stomach and a healthy digestive system. Niacin increases the production of histamine. When eating a meal, a set of signals occur, one of which causes histamine to be released, which then triggers the production of stomach acid. The release of histamine in the stomach facilitates proper digestion. Vitamin B-3 also interacts with cellular components called mitochondria. Numerous mitochondria live in cells of the stomach (parietal cells). When the mitochondria are functioning adequately, they generate cellular energy in the form of adenosine triphosphate (ATP), which drives the production of stomach acid. Vitamin B-3 is a required substrate for the mitochondria, ensures the proper production of ATP, and, therefore, the adequate release of stomach acid when digesting a meal.

Migraine and Tension-type Headaches: A systematic review of previous research and published anecdotal reports has demonstrated that intravenous and oral supplementation of niacin is effective at aborting acute migraine headaches and alleviating tension headaches. It is probably an effective prophylactic agent for the prevention of migraine headaches as well. When taken intravenously or orally, niacin causes cutaneous flushing that might abort the acute symptoms of migraine by vasodilating the intracranial vessels, thus preventing the subsequent vasoconstriction of the extracranial vessels. Chronic tension-type headaches are also associated with cerebrospinal pressure or intracranial venous pressure (or both). In fact, tension-type headaches are more similar to migraine headaches than they are dissimilar, in that they seem to progress into migraine headaches due to an escalating pathophysiological process. Thus, niacin might mitigate the acute phase of tension-type headaches through the same mechanism of action that occurs with migraine headaches.

Anxiety Disorders: The form of vitamin B-3 that is the most effective for the treatment of anxiety disorders is niacinamide. Niacinamide might pass through the blood-brain-barrier more efficiently than niacin. Although this point is debatable, niacinamide likely has a better ability to influence the central nervous system and reduce the debilitating symptoms of anxiety. Dr Prousky has documented this therapeutic use of vitamin B-3 in his book *Anxiety: Orthomolecular Diagnosis and Treatment,* while Dr Prousky and Dr Hoffer have discussed this therapy in their DVD *Anxiety Disorders: Grand Rounds.*

The anti-anxiety properties of niacinamide are mostly achieved by the correction of an underlying vitamin B-3 dependency. One the key features of a vitamin B-3 dependency is mental/emotional symptoms. Niacinamide also has benzodiazepine-like effects, which accounts for some of its anti-anxiety properties. Benzodiazepines are a class of drugs

> **Dr M.F. Murray of Harvard University has done extensive research on niacinamide as a potential AIDS preventive factor.**

that have a significant ability to reduce anxiety, but they also cause significant amount of dependency, side effects, and addiction. It appears that niacinamide has therapeutic effects comparable to the benzodiazepines. Both the benzodiazepines and niacinamide exerts similar anxiolytic effects through the modulation of neurotransmitters (serotonin, norepinephrine, dopamine, and GABA) commonly unbalanced in anxiety. Niacinamide, however, has none of the negative side effects associated with benzodiazepines.

Niacinamide also has the ability to increase the production of serotonin, which is commonly deficient among anxiety sufferers. Niacinamide has the ability to modify the metabolism of blood lactate (lactic acid). Lactate sensitivity or an increased responsiveness to lactate might provoke anxiety symptoms. Niacinamide supplementation appears to increase the conversion of lactate to pyruvate, reducing lactate levels in the blood, which would reduce many anxiety symptoms (especially panic).

HIV Infection: Dr M.F. Murray of Harvard University has done extensive research on niacinamide as a potential AIDS preventive factor. He has found a marked similarity between pellagra and AIDS. In his research, he described a pentad reflective of pellagra in HIV-infected patients that is characterized by plasma tryptophan depletion; intracellular NAD depletion; idiopathic dermatitis; idiopathic diarrhea; and idiopathic dementia. His studies indicate that niacinamide and antiretroviral drugs can increase plasma tryptophan levels and favorably impact the secondary effects of tryptophan depletion. He has also shown that niacinamide is an oral antimicrobial agent with activity against both *Mycobacterium tuberculosis* and HIV. Considering the deaths due to HIV and *M. tuberculosis* were estimated to be 1 million in 1999, safe and cost-effective treatments like niacinamide might prove extremely valuable in the fight against these deadly diseases.

Detoxification: Detoxification simply means enhanced excretion of chemicals and their metabolites in urine and feces, and the facilitation of excretion through the sweat or sebum (a fatty secretion of the sebaceous glands of the skin). There are numerous published reports that have shown niacin to be an extremely valuable agent for the mobilization of stored xenobiotics (foreign toxins) from fatty tissues in the body. Many individuals exposed to environmental chemicals, pesticides, and polychlorinated biphenyls and their byproducts have benefited from a detoxification program that used niacin to encourage detoxification.

Other Conditions: Niacin has been found helpful for many other diseases or conditions, including learning and behavioral disorders among children, alcoholism and drug addiction, some of the senile states, absorption problems, and Huntington's disease. It is also a good antidote against d-lysergic acid diethylamide (LSD) intoxication. Niacin has anticancer properties and decreases risk of leukemia after the original cancer is cured.

It is useful in improving healing, inhibiting development of Alzheimer's disease, decreasing onset of dementia and increasing longevity, preventing juvenile diabetes, treating the arthritides, and preventing cardiovascular disease. It has been used to treat kidney disease with success.

Optimum Dose

The optimum dose range for vitamin B-3 is not as wide as it is for ascorbic acid, but it is wide enough to require different recommendations for different classes of diseases. As is always the case with nutrients, individuals must determine their own optimum level.

With nicotinic acid, this is done by increasing the doses until the flush (vasodilatation) is gone or is so slight it is not a problem. One can start with as low a dose as 100 mg, taken three times each day after meals, and gradually increase it. We usually start with 500 mg each dose and often will start with 1 g per dose, especially for cases of arthritis, for schizophrenics, for alcoholics, and for a few elderly patients. However, with elderly patients it is better to start small and work it up slowly.

Very few can take more than 6 g per day of the nicotinamide. With nicotinic acid it is possible to go much higher. Many schizophrenics have taken up to 30 g per day with no difficulty. The dose will alter over time, and if on a dose where there were no problems, they may develop in time. Usually, this indicates that the patient is getting better and does not need as much.

For people who are well or nearly well and have no obvious disease, who are interested in maintaining their good health or in improving it, or who may be under increased stress, the optimum dose of nicotinic acid varies between 1 and 3 g daily. The same doses apply to nicotinamide. For everyone under physiological stress, such as pregnancy and lactation, or suffering from acute illness, such as the common cold or flu or other diseases that do not threaten immediate death, the dose range is 1 to 10 g daily for nicotinic acid, 1.5 g to 6 g for nicotinamide. All the psychiatric syndromes are included in this group, including the schizophrenias and the senile states. It also includes the very large group of people with high blood cholesterol levels or low HDL when it is desired to restore these blood values to normal.

Side Effects

Patients should not be given nicotinic acid without explaining to them that they will have a flush, which will vary in intensity from none to very severe. If this is explained carefully and if they are told that in time the flush will not be a problem, they will not mind. The flush may remain too intense for a few patients, and the nicotinic acid may have to be replaced by a slow release preparation or by some of the esters, for example, inositol niacinate. Inositol niacinate is a very good preparation with very little flush, and most find it very acceptable even when they were not able to accept the nicotinic acid itself. It is rather expensive, but with quantity production, the price will come down.

The flush starts in the forehead with a warning tingle. Then it intensifies. From the forehead and face the flush travels down the rest of the body, usually stopping somewhere in the chest but may extend to the toes. The rate of the development of the flush depends upon so many factors it is impossible to predict what course it will follow. The following factors decrease the intensity of the flush: a cold meal, taking it after a meal, taking aspirin before, and using an antihistamine in advance. The following factors make the flush more intense: a hot meal, a hot drink, an empty stomach, chewing the tablets, and the rate at which the tablets break down in liquid.

With continued use the flush gradually recedes and eventually may be only a tingling sensation in the forehead. If the person stops taking the vitamin for a day or more, the sequence of flushing will be re-experienced. Some people never do flush, and a few only begin to flush after several years of taking the vitamin. With nicotinamide, there should be no flushing, but we have found that about 2% of people will flush. This may be due to rapid conversion of the nicotinamide to nicotinic acid in the body.

When the dose is too high for both forms of the vitamin, the patients will suffer from nausea at first, and if the dose is not reduced, from vomiting. These side effects may be used to determine what is the optimum dose. When they do occur, the dose is reduced until it is just below the nausea level. With children, the first indication may be loss of appetite. If this does occur, the vitamin must be stopped for a few days and then may resumed at a lower level.

Safety

The safety of taking vitamin B-3 in niacin or nicotinic form has been described by Dr John Marks as follows. "Doses of 200 mg to 10 g daily of the acid have been used therapeutically to lower blood cholesterol levels under medical control for periods of up to 10 years or more and though some reactions have occurred at these very high dosages, they have rapidly responded to cessation of therapy, and have often cleared even when therapy has been continued.

"In isolated cases, transient liver disorders, rashes, dry skin and excessive pigmentation have been seen. The tolerance to glucose has been reduced in diabetics and patients with peptic ulcers have experienced increased pain. No serious reactions have been reported, however, even in these high doses. The available evidence suggests that 100 times the RDA is safe (about 100 mg)."

Dr Marks is cautious about recommending that doses over 100 mg are safe. In our opinion, based upon 40 years of experience with this vitamin, the dose ranges we have recommended are safe. However, with the higher doses, medical supervision is necessary. As well, you should avoid using slow-release preparations, which may cause hepatitis or jaundice and even more serious problems.

Jaundice is very rare. Fewer that 10 cases have been reported in the medical literature, and we have seen none in 10 years. When jaundice does occur, it is usually an obstructive type that clears when the vitamin is discontinued. We have been able to get schizophrenic patients back on nicotinic acid after the jaundice cleared and it did not recur. Since jaundice in people who have not been taking nicotinic acid is fairly common, it is possible this is a random association. The liver function tests may indicate there is a problem when in fact there is not. Nicotinic acid should be stopped for 5 days before the liver function tests are given. There have been three cases of severe liver damage attributed to slow-release preparations, though, and of these three, one patient died and another needed a liver transplant. One patient who had no problem with nicotinic acid for lowering cholesterol switched to the slow-release preparations and became ill. When he resumed the original nicotinic acid, he was well again with no further evidence of liver dysfunction. We have not seen any cases reported anywhere else.

Vitamin B-6 (Pyridoxine)

Vitamin B-6 is the second major vitamin of the water-soluble B series to be studied extensively by orthomolecular physicians. A major impetus was given to this study by Dr Carl C. Pfeiffer, when he discovered that in the absence of enough pyridoxine and zinc, there was in many patients an increase in the excretion of a substance in the urine called kryptopyrrole (KP). He described the syndrome under the term pyrroluria. Kryptopyrrole is a member of the pyrrole family and may be correctly referred to as urinary pyrrole. Dr Pfeiffer showed that this syndrome produced a double deficiency of pyridoxine and zinc. Patients with this condition had clear signs, such as white areas in their fingernails, stria, pain in their knees, changes in their skin, and PMS.

Our research group was first found this substance in the urine of schizophrenic patients. In looking for a unique compound that might be present in the urine of schizophrenics, we tested the urine of a non-schizophrenic alcoholic who was given LSD. After he took the LSD, he began to excrete large amounts of a substance that turned pink on a paper chromatogram when it was developed with the correct chemicals. Later, we found that this compound, which we called the mauve factor, was present in the majority of early schizophrenic patients, and that when they become well, it was no longer present. Dr Pfeiffer found that when it was present, there was also a double deficiency of zinc and pyridoxine. When these nutrients were given in adequate doses, the kryptopyrrole disappeared. Today, this compound is being studied by many investigators, including Dr Woody McGinnis.

> There are several good reasons for using vitamin B-6 (pyridoxine) therapeutically, both for psychiatric patients and for patients with physical disease.

KP is a measure of oxidative stress, found in approximately 75% of schizophrenic patients, depending upon the duration of their sickness and their treatment. While seldom present in healthy people, KP is seen in about one third of all non-psychotic patients, no matter what their diagnosis. About half of the children with infantile autism test positive. It is also produced is a small number of alcoholics given LSD as a psychedelic treatment for their alcoholism. We use its presence in urine as an indication to use vitamin B-3 therapy.

The urine test for KP is relatively simple, and any modern laboratory can learn to do it with little difficulty. The double deficiency of vitamin B-6 and zinc produces symptoms in the skin, including stretch marks on the body and white spots in the fingernails. These are not calcium spots. When the two nutrients are provided, they clear.

There are several good reasons for using vitamin B-6 (pyridoxine) therapeutically, both for psychiatric patients and for patients with physical disease.

Therapeutic Uses

Autism: Dr Bernard Rimland has shown in a double-blind prospective controlled experiment that pyridoxine is therapeutic for autistic children, who often excrete large amounts of KP. Subsequent studies have confirmed this finding, as he notes: "There are now 17 published studies – all positive – showing that high dosages of vitamin B-6 and magnesium are a safe and often helpful treatment for autism. Thousands of parents are using B-6 and magnesium to help their children. Almost 50% show worthwhile improvement and the vitamins are immeasurably safer than any drug."

Carpal Tunnel Syndrome: Dr John Marion Ellis and Dr Karl Folkers concluded that vitamin B-6, 50 to 200 mg, taken daily for 12 weeks, cured the less affected hand in patients suffering from carpal tunnel syndrome who were selected for surgery on the more crippled hand. The vitamin B-6 treatment halted atrophy of the thenar muscle. They suggested it is a cofactor for normal cortisone activity in tendons and synovium. They also reported one case where riboflavin alone was very effective in treating carpal tunnel syndrome, but when both vitamin B-2 and B-6 were given together, the results were even better. They concluded that this syndrome was the result of a double vitamin deficiency.

Arteriosclerosis, Heart Disease, and Stroke: Pyridoxine is receiving increasing attention as a nutrient involved in protection against arteriosclerosis, heart disease, and strokes. It is one of the nutrients essential in the conversion of homocysteine to the non-toxic cystathionine. Dr Moses M. Suzman has theorized that arteriosclerosis is a vitamin deficiency disease, primarily vitamin B-6. In his study, he administered to patients pyridoxine 200 mg, folic acid 5 mg, and vitamin E 100 to 600 IU, all daily. He also used other nutrients in smaller amounts. Of 62 typical heart patients followed for an average of 52 months, there were four reinfarcts (two were fatal). Dr J.M. Ellis, who had been using pyridoxine for a long time to treat carpal tunnel syndrome with great success, observed that few of his patients on this vitamin had heart attacks.

Other Conditions: Other clinical uses of vitamin B-6 include the prevention of diabetic complications, asthma attacks, monosodium glutamate (MSG) reactions, and nausea and vomiting of pregnancy. Vitamin B-6 can also be used as a treatment for a variety of conditions, such as seborrheic dermatitis (dandruff), pyridoxine-dependent epilepsy, lupus (improves general well being), and sickle cell disease (prevents sickling of red blood cells and reduces the number of acute crises). Premenstrual syndrome also responds well to vitamin B-6 and zinc.

Optimum Dose

For people who are well or nearly well and who wish to ensure they will have enough vitamin B-6, we recommend 50 to 100 mg daily. For specific indications of deficiency or disease, we recommend between 100 and 500 mg daily. Larger doses have been used, but they are seldom needed. In children, it may be necessary to also use magnesium to prevent the pyridoxine from activating hyperactive behavior in the child.

Side Effects

There are very few side effects, and these are minor and transient. Some patients can experience an acneiform eruption (a worsening of acne vulgaris) when supplementing with this vitamin. Once the vitamin is discontinued, the skin lesions fade away.

Safety

Much has been made of a study of a few patients collected from several medical schools who took between 2000 and 6000 mg per day. These patients developed a peripheral neuropathy, which cleared after a year, but based on this report the idea became current that vitamin B-6 was toxic. Dr John Marks has proven otherwise: "It has been claimed that high doses of pyridoxine can lead to liver damage, interference with the normal functions of riboflavin, and a dependency state. With the possible exception of the dependency states, these suggestions are not substantiated by scientific data. The dependency states were very transient."

Pantothenic Acid (Vitamin B-5)

Pantothenic acid, once known as vitamin B-5, is very safe with no known side effects. A deficiency of this vitamin can cause fatigue, in addition to listlessness, insomnia, sullenness, and depression.

Therapeutic Uses

Adrenal Dysfunction (Burn Out): One of the principal roles of pantothenic acid is its positive effect upon the adrenal glands. There are four adrenal glands in the body; each pair sits atop of the kidneys. When an individual is stressed in any way, the adrenal glands go into action and prepare the individual to meet the demands of the stressful stimulation. One of the ways in which the adrenal glands operate is to release hormones and chemicals, such as cortisol and norepinephrine, which improve tolerance to stress. Over time, however, continual stress depletes the adrenal glands reserve and reduces an individual's capacity to handle stress. In several studies, pantothenic acid has been shown to prevent the adrenal glands from under-functioning or "burning out."

Acne, Obesity, Lupus: Some very important clinical uses of pantothenic acid have been the subject of some excellent research papers by D. Lit-Hung Leung linking a deficiency of pantothenic acid with the pathogenesis of acne, obesity, and even lupus. He has shown that liberal doses of pantothenic acid (10 g or more per day) are effective for treating obesity and acne, as well as controlling lupus by putting the disease into remission. He feels that these high doses are necessary as a means to overcome the long-standing vitamin deficiency.

Swinging Gait: One of the most interesting features of a pantothenic acid deficiency is a swinging gait while running. Dr C. Hemingway has found that supplemental pantothenic acid with a B-complex tablet improved running gait and strength in three young women. He hypothesized that a deficiency of this vitamin can cause an awkward, swinging running gait, and that it probably has some relationship to metabolism and female hormone production. Up to 10 to 12 g per day have been given with only occasional diarrhea and water retention.

Other Conditions: Pantothenic acid also has a role to play in keeping the immune system healthy. In animals, it has been shown to extend life. It has been used to help control food allergies and as a mild anti-anxiety or anti-tension substance.

Optimum Dose

Even though the optimum doses have not been determined, it does appear that doses up to 10 g per day are very safe, and doses of 20 g per day can safely be used without any toxicity. Pantothenic acid deserves to be studied in more detail.

Folic Acid
(Folinic Acid, Folacin, Pteroglutaminic Acid)

Folic acid is another safe water-soluble vitamin, basic to the methylation cycle in the body. The exchange of methyl groups is one of the basic reactions in the body.

Folic acid is essential for the metabolism of methionine, which, in turn, is converted into homocysteine. Homocysteine is converted back into methionine, which needs folic acid and vitamin B-12, and can even be catabolized to cysteine. The amino acid cysteine is essential for the synthesis of glutathione, one of the most important natural antioxidants. High bloods levels of homocysteine are correlated with disease and with low folic acid blood levels. Homocysteine is needed for the synthesis of adenine and thymine.

About one quarter of the population is low in folic acid, which may be an underestimate since it is based upon RDA standards. A large number of conditions, such as arthritis, alcoholism, depression, pregnancy, poor diet, smoking, diabetes, aging, and cancer are influenced by folic acid. Use of certain drugs, such as methotrexate and Dilantin, also lowers folic acid levels. Genetic factors that impair homocysteine metabolism are also involved. The importance of these genetic polymorphisms has been recently re-emphasized by Bruce Ames in a remarkable series of recent publications.

Therapeutic Uses

Neural Tube Defects: It has been proven that women will give birth to babies with spina bifida and similar neural tube defects (NTDs) much less frequently if they take supplemental folic acid, 1 mg. We generally recommend 5 mg daily.

Dr Smithells in 1981 showed that giving pregnant women extra folic acid decreased the incidence of NTDs. Before that he had measured the red cell folate and white cell vitamin C levels of mothers who had babies with NTDs and found they were lower in both. This finding created tremendous interest in using orthomolecular doses of folic acid.

However, the initial reaction was one of strong disbelief and hostility;

the establishment refused to advise women to take folic acid until the requisite number of double-blind experiments were done. Almost a decade later, the *Journal of the American Medical Association* published a report proving that folic acid provided protection for most causes of the defect. Even in women with a family history of NTD, where the frequency of babies with the defects was more than five times greater than normal (18 per 1000 against 3.5 per 1000), this treatment was effective.

The U.S. Public Health Service has issued the following advisory: "In order to reduce the frequency of NTDs and their resulting disability, the United States Public Health Service recommends that: All women of childbearing age capable of becoming pregnant should consume 0.4 mg of folic acid per day for the purpose of reducing their risk of having a pregnancy affected with spina bifida or other NTDs." This amount will not be provided by most diets and requires supplementation. The U.S. Public Health Service now fortifies bread with folic acid. Folic acid is destroyed by heat but some will survive.

Folic acid can decrease neural tube defects by 75%. If all the other vitamins were used, we are certain that figure would be closer to 100%. We cannot recall in the past 40 years a single female patient of ours on vitamins giving birth to any child with a congenital defect.

Health and Welfare Canada has likewise recommended that "as early as possible when planning a pregnancy women should consult their physician about folic acid supplements. Women with a previous NTD affected pregnancy are at higher risk of having another affected pregnancy. These women should consult their physician about folic acid supplements. All women of child-bearing potential should follow *Canada's Food Guide to Healthy Eating* and take care to choose more foods higher in folate. For protection against occurrence, 0.4 mg folic acid alone is likely to be beneficial and not toxic."

The truth is that 0.4 mg is probably not the best dose to reduce NTDs in women of childbearing age. It is known that about 5% to 15% of the population has a defect in the enzyme, 5,10-methylenetetrahydrofolate reductase (MTHFR), which cannot be overcome by 0.4 mg per day. This defect does increase homocysteine levels and the chance of having a baby with a NTD. At present, the best recommendation for preventing NTDs is for all women of childbearing age to supplement with at least 1 mg of folic acid per day.

Folic acid can decrease neural tube defects by 75%. If all the other vitamins were used, we are certain that figure would be closer to 100%. We cannot recall in the past 40 years a single female patient of ours on vitamins giving birth to any child with a congenital defect. We have been able to advise them all that not only would they not harm their developing baby by taking vitamins, but that their chances of giving birth to a defective child would be greatly diminished. However, some of our patients have been told by their doctors that they must stop all their vitamins while pregnant. They still look upon vitamins as toxic drugs.

Arteriosclerosis: Folic acid is also one of the nutrients involved in the prevention of arteriosclerosis. Arteriosclerosis is a complicated phenomenon, with a large number of factors involved, including ascorbic acid, nicotinic acid, pyridoxine, and choline. Jack Challem in his *The Nutrition Reporter* reviewed the recent literature suggesting that the common factor is homocysteine, which is quickly changed to cystathionine in the body. High levels of homocysteine are now recognized as a risk factor in heart disease.

Dr M. Stampfer analyzed blood from 14,916 male physicians, all of whom had not had a heart attack. Five years later, 271 had suffered heart attacks. Of these, 31 had extremely high blood levels of homocysteine. A study at Oregon Health Sciences Center showed that 40% of patients who had a stroke had high homocysteine levels. In a normal population, it is elevated in 5%. There was an inverse correlation between homocysteine and intake of vitamins. Folic acid is one of the vitamins needed for the rapid conversion of homocysteine to the non-toxic cystathionine. A dose of 1 to 5 mg of folic acid should be taken daily. This is enough to decrease elevated homocysteine levels in blood.

Cancer: Folic acid has been found to decrease the odds of getting lung cancer. It has also been shown to reverse changes found in the cervix as measured by the Pap smear; patients with low folate levels are more likely to develop cervical dysplasia. We use it for these reasons.

Anti-Aging: Folate supplements can enhance memory and slow the decline seen with aging. Eight hundred and eighteen people with normal brain function, aged 50 to 75 years old, were given either a placebo or 800 mcg of folate for 3 years. Those on folic acid had better memory scores. Some high-potency multivitamin formulas contain 800 mcg of folate. Doses of 5 to 20 mg of folate may be needed to have additional benefits. It is interesting to note that as we age, we have a reduced capacity to absorb the form of folic acid present in foods, known as folylpolyglutamates. This is another reason why optimal supplementation with folic acid each day is warranted, especially as we age.

Another indication we have found is in elderly patients who develop a hand tremor, which makes it difficult for them to write. Giving them folic acid 5 to 10 mg daily will often remove this problem in a week or so.

Recently, we have seen what folic acid can do for an elderly male who had been a little more unsteady and who had to be more careful in walking because of this. He had also infrequent episodes of tachycardia, which responded in a few minutes to changes in body position, and at other times his pulse rate was too slow and too unresponsive to the demands of exercise. He had been on niacin for many years. The addition of 15 mg of folic acid, twice daily, changed this dramatically. The unsteadiness was gone within one hour, and the tachycardia no longer occurred. The low pulse rate has been slowly improving and is no longer a problem on most days.

Psychiatric Disorders: A deficiency of folic acid is also clearly related to psychopathology. Folic acid deficiency is high in patients with depression, senility, and schizophrenia, as well as in epileptic patients on Dilantin. Medical patients with folic acid deficiency suffer more from psychiatric symptoms. The addition of folic acid to the diet of these patients produces substantial improvement. Patients with acute psychiatric disorders show a significant response if they are given high dose supplements (15 mg) of folate. We use 25 mg daily for our depressed patients and have gone higher. We consider it a very good antidepressant and free of side effects. Dr Carl Pfeifer recommended 1 to 2 mg daily for psychotic patients who have too low blood histamine levels, called histapenia.

Depression: Folate can prevent and treat depression. People with low folate levels are more apt to be depressed, and depressed patients have lower blood levels of folic acid. Dr Paul Godfrey, Institute of Psychiatry, London, has reported that folic acid speeds recovery from depression. One third of their depressed patients were folate deficient. The overall outcome of folic acid therapy was impressive. Every one improved to some extent. The best results were obtained at 3 to 6 months. Patients given 10 mg daily responded in 2 to 3 months, but gastrointestinal and neurological symptoms were improved in 5 months on 10 mg weekly. Patients treated with Prozac respond sooner, and they are less likely to have relapses if they have adequate folate levels.

Optimum Dose

A recent study showed that half of the American population does not get enough folic acid. For most diseases, the therapeutic daily dose should be 5 mg or less. For other conditions, much more may be needed – for example, for the treatment of depression, doses up to 50 mg per day or more have been helpful.

Although at one time in Canada, folic acid was available in 25 mg tablets over the counter, a prescription is now needed for the 5 mg tablets. In the United States, 30 mg tablets can be obtained by mail order.

There can be no one ideal dose for everyone. The ideal dose depends upon too many other factors. Our rule of thumb for vitamins is that slightly too much is better than too little, whereas with drugs, our rule is that too little is better than too much.

Safety

Only 1 mg tablets are available over the counter based upon the false idea that folic acid in larger amounts may cover the symptoms of pernicious anemia. There is a very remote danger (discussed earlier) that giving folic acid will mask a vitamin B-12 deficiency (pernicious anemia), but a vitamin B-12 blood level will show whether this is a problem. The fear that it will mask pernicious anemia is unjustified but pervasive. Giving patients any of the current B complex preparations will provide enough vitamin B-12 to assure anyone that pernicious anemia will not be covered up.

Vitamin B-12 (Cobalamin)

Vitamin B-12 is involved in numerous biochemical reactions as a cofactor and coenzyme. Its main functions involve DNA synthesis, methionine synthesis from homocysteine, and conversion of propionyl into succinyl coenzyme A from methylmalonate. The psychiatric manifestations of a vitamin B-12 deficiency include agitation or restlessness, dementia, depression, fatigue, irritability, panic and phobic disorders, personality change, psychosis, mild memory impairment, and negativism. Patients most likely to develop vitamin B-12 deficiency have clinical conditions, such as atrophic gastritis, bacterial overgrowth of the small intestine, or pernicious anemia, but there are many other conditions that benefit from vitamin B-12, even though they do not present with classical deficiency signs.

Vitamin B-12 is absorbed from the intestine, except in patients with pernicious anemia, who cannot do so. It is usually given by injection, but recent evidence shows that giving tablets or sublingual lozenges will be as effective. Up to 100 mg per day have been given with no side effects.

Therapeutic Uses

Breast Cancer: One of the most interesting developments of recent years is the association between vitamin B-12 deficiency and breast cancer. In a 1999 article published in the journal *Nutrition Reviews*, it was postulated that a deficiency of the vitamin might cause DNA strand breaks and alteration of DNA methylation. Both factors could promote the development of breast cancer. In a 2002 article published in the same journal, a new mechanism was found to be associated with a vitamin B-12 deficiency. Professor J. Miller or the University of California, Davis, Medical Center, reviewed research demonstrating that vitamin B-12 deficiency can cause increased levels of tumor necrosis factor-α and decreased levels of epidermal growth factor in both rats and humans. This may be a new factor in certain clinical disorders, such as Alzheimer's disease, rheumatoid arthritis, multiple sclerosis, and AIDS.

Chronic Fatigue Syndrome: Vitamin B-12 has been used in megadoses by many physicians for many years for their patients with chronic fatigue, even though their blood levels are normal. There is no doubt that these patients have benefited. Injecting 1000 mcg per day provides 1000 times the recommended daily dose. Dr Simpson has found that many chronic conditions, such as chronic fatigue syndrome (CFS) and multiple sclerosis (MS), benefited from optimal doses of vitamin B-12. Patients with MS had a large proportion of their erythrocytes (red blood cells or RBCs) that were too large and could not traverse the capillaries. Thus, much of the body tissues would be deficient in oxygen. He found that injections of hydroxocobalamine in large doses was very effective in treating these conditions. He also used essential fatty acids (EFAs) to make the RBC membrane more elastic.

Patients most likely to develop vitamin B-12 deficiency have clinical conditions, such as atrophic gastritis, bacterial overgrowth of the small intestine, or pernicious anemia.

In our practice, we have added niacin to the hydroxocobalamine and EFAs to prevent adhesion of RBCs to each other (sludging). We have found that this triple attack on these chronic disorders, especially CFS, has been very effective. We start patients on 1 mg subcutaneous hydroxycobaline injections, three times per week, and as they recover, we reduce the frequency to a maintenance dose of once per month. Since vitamin B-12 deficiency is clearly correlated with larger than normal RBCs (called macrocytosis) and is characteristic of pernicious anemia, these disorders may be a form of subclinical pernicious anemia.

Psychiatric Disorders: Vitamin B-12 is involved in the synthesis of serotonin, and serotonin dysfunction is associated with many psychiatric disorders. Another conceivable benefit from supplementing with vitamin B12 is the resulting increase in the amount of vitamin B-12 that would gain entrance into the central nervous system (CNS). In a study involving 13 patients (29-50 years of age) with neurasthenia (characterized by profound fatigue, depression, and anxiety), the vitamin B-12 levels were assessed in both the serum and cerebrospinal fluid (CSF). All 13 patients had normal serum levels of vitamin B-12 (range, 280-750 pg/ml), but 11 of them had deficient CSF levels (<5 pg/ml). The other 2 patients had CSF levels of 10 pg/ml and 15 pg/ml, respectively. By not performing routine

CSF analysis, the majority of these patients would not have been found to have a vitamin B-12 deficiency. The authors concluded their report by stating that all patients displaying organic mental symptoms should have their CSF levels of vitamin B-12 assessed.

In a similar study involving 49 patients with organic mental disorders, deficient CSF levels of vitamin B-12 (<5 pg/ml) were found in 30 patients. When the serum levels of vitamin B-12 were tested, normal values (200 to 800 pg/ml) were found in 45 of them, indicating a marked difference between both compartments. A group of 10 patients were also given injectable hydroxocobalamine at a dose of 1000 mcg twice weekly for 6 weeks. The injectable group was also instructed to take a capsule containing 50 mg zinc DL-aspartate and 250 mg of taurine, three times daily. This group was compared against a group of 2 patients given 0.1 mg of oral cyanocobalamin in a capsule with 50 mg zinc DL-aspartate and 250 mg taurine, prescribed three times daily for 6 weeks. The group given the injections achieved a much greater increase in their CSF levels of vitamin B-12.

Given that serum levels of vitamin B-12 can be normal yet deficient in the CSF, patients responding to regular injections of hydroxocobalamine might have an improvement in their mental condition due to marked (supraphysiological) increases in their CSF vitamin B-12 levels, or from the correction of deficient CSF levels of vitamin B-12. The best way to achieve high CSF levels of vitamin B-12 is probably by the administration of regular injections.

The major transport protein that shuttles vitamin B-12 into the CNS is transcobalamin II. High serum levels of vitamin B-12 might also increase CSF levels by circumventing defects in the ability of this transport protein. The use of injectable hyrdoxocobalamine presumably optimizes the functioning of transcobalamin II and enables more of vitamin B-12 to shuttle into the brain. These reasons support the idea that many patients suffering from psychiatric and neurological conditions have an increased need for or a dependency upon vitamin B-12, which cannot be satisfied through diet alone.

Other Conditions: Clinically, there are a number of additional clinical indications for the use of vitamin B-12, especially when provided in the methylcobalamine form. These are Bell's palsy, cancer, diabetic neuropathy, eye function, heart rate variability, HIV, male impotence, and sleep disturbances (regulates melatonin secretion, augments light sensitivity, and normalizes circadian and sleep-wake rhythms).

Optimum Dose

The frequency and amount of supplemental or injectable vitamin B-12 is dependent upon the serum level desired. Studies have shown that the psychological benefits of vitamin B-12 are best achieved when serum levels range from 1000 to 2000 pg/ml. However, this serum range might not be optimal because extremely high serum levels (average 465,173 pg/ml) have relatively no side effects and appear to be necessary when improving patients' psychological health. To get serum levels in this range (1000 to 2000 pg/ml), the amount of vitamin B-12 is at least 1000 mcg given by injection every 2 weeks, or at least 5 mg (5000 mcg) of B-12 taken orally each day. To bring serum levels to the higher range, the amount of vitamin B-12 required is 3000 mcg given by injection 4 times each week, or 9000 mcg by injection daily. The most preferred form of oral vitamin B-12 is the methylcobalamine form because it has greater tissue retention than cyanocobalamine and appears to produce good clinical results irrespective of the method of administration.

Patients getting the best therapeutic response from vitamin B-12 are those presenting with a psychiatric and/or neurological disorder with some degree of fatigue. Such patients typically require 1000 to 5000 mcg of injectable vitamin B-12 once or twice each week until their symptoms improve. The serum level of vitamin B-12 usually needs to be greater than or equal to 1000 pg/ml to have the best therapeutic benefits. The form of injectable vitamin B-12 most recommended is hydroxocobalamine.

Side Effects

The only rare side effect from supplemental vitamin B-12 is an acneiform exanthema, particularly in women. These lesions have only been reported to occur from oral supplementation, but they can occur (albeit, rarely) from hydroxocobalamine injections as well. The lesions consist of loosely disseminated small papules or papulopustules on the face, the upper parts of the back, and chest that can spread to the upper arm. They will go away within a week once vitamin B-12 is discontinued.

Inositol

Inositol is one of the B complex vitamins, a precursor of the phosphatidylinositol cycle. It plays a role in the metabolism of cholinergic, noradrenergic, and serotoninergic systems. These systems are considered most important in regulating mood and other disorders of the brain.

Therapeutic Uses

Professor C. Belmaker, Hoffer-Vickar Chair in Psychiatry, Unit for Orthomolecular Clinical Research, Ben Gurion University, has reported that high doses of inositol, about 200 mg per kilogram, was therapeutic for mood disorders, including anxiety and depression. In their first trial of 11 depressed patients, given 6 g daily for three weeks, nine improved. The mean Hamilton Depression score was decreased by 50%. A subsequent double-blind study yielded similar results. It also had value in treating obsessive-compulsive behavior and bulimia nervosa. Inositol niacinate (known as 'no flush niacin') is also effective in treating the schizophrenic disorders.

Optimum Dose

The optimal dose of inositol is 6 to 18 g daily in divided doses with some fruit juice. Patients can have significant gastrointestinal bloating and indigestion when taking these high daily doses. To reduce gastrointestinal symptoms, the dose should be increased gradually over several weeks until the desired dose is reached.

Vitamin E (The Tocopherols)

Vitamin E was discovered in 1922 (a deficiency caused fetal death and resorption in rats), and pure vitamin E was first isolated from wheat germ oil in 1936. For years, the medical establishment was laughed at it as a vitamin in search of a disease. Now we know it prevents us from having many diseases. Vitamin E deficiency is found mainly in premature infants, where it causes increased hemolysis of red blood cells and a decreased red blood half-life. In adults, it regulates platelet aggregation, prevents peripheral vascular disease, and modulates the immune system. These activities are all fundamental for good health.

There are eight naturally occurring forms of vitamin E; alpha tocopherol is one of the most active and the one generally used. Vitamin E is present in two forms, the d-form, which is the only one with biological activity, and the l-form, which has little activity. The synthetic preparation contains equal parts of the d- and l-form, labeled as dl-alpha tocopherol. The d-form is much more expensive because it is extracted from natural sources. There is still some debate about the relative merits of the d- versus the dl-form, but we are convinced that the d-form is more active. We have seen it help people when the same dose of the dl-form did not. One mg of dl-alpha-tocopherol is designated as 1 International Unit (IU); d-alpha-tocopherol is more active and 1 mg is equivalent to 1.49 IU.

> **Vitamin E has been found to be therapeutic for managing thrombosis, gangrene, indolent ulcers, thromboangiitis obliterans, thermal burns, radiation burns, cardiac disease, congenital heart disease, acute and chronic rheumatic fever, hypertensive heart disease, coronary heart disease.**

Vitamin E is a fat-soluble vitamin. It is absorbed into the walls of the intestine, there combined with other fats into chylomicrons and distributed throughout the body. It is almost all carried in the low density and high density lipoproteins. Its major role is its scavenger function of free radicals. Free radicals are highly reactive fractions of molecules, which, if allowed to remain, will damage cell membranes and amino acids rich in sulfur. Vitamin E is nature's best antioxidant for protecting cell surfaces. One vitamin E molecule will be used over and over and can protect against 1000 free radical molecules.

The history of vitamin E, its rejection for about 40 years and its increasing acceptance today, contains many lessons for physicians and for medical schools. In the 1940s, two Canadian doctors, the brothers Wilfred and Evan Shute, pioneered research in the therapeutic use of vitamin E, but found their work rejected in large by the medical community, chiefly because physicians at that time knew hardly anything about vitamins. At the end of their lives, they had some satisfaction from the recognition they received from orthomolecular physicians. They were the first doctors who had to face the unreasonable and unrelenting opposition of the medical establishment for their espousal of megadoses of a vitamin. This opposition was totally unscientific. Unless we learn from history, we are condemned to repeat this mistake.

Therapeutic Uses

Vitamin B-3 was the first vitamin used in megadoses in the 1930s, with doses of 600 mg given daily to prevent the symptoms of chronic pellagra from recurring, followed by Dr William Kaufman's work showing that this vitamin was therapeutic for the arthritides in doses of 3 to 6 g a daily. Vitamin E was the second vitamin used in these large doses.

The Shute brothers used 800 IU and more to treat large numbers of patients with circulatory problems and heart disease, and to accelerate healing after burns. They were subjected to powerful opposition from the medical establishment, especially in Ontario. Medical journals would not publish their papers, so they published in their own journal called *The Summary*. The December 1973 issue contained a report by Evan Shute, as well as letters, abstracts, and striking color photographs of the response of wounds caused by freezing, by diabetes, and by burns to the administration of vitamin E. Dr Shute described six therapeutic properties of vitamin E:

1. It is both an antioxidant and improves the ability of tissue to use oxygen.
2. It prevents the formation of emboli from clots and extension of the clot.
3. It is a vasodilator for the capillaries.
4. It improves damaged capillary fragility.
5. It resolves some scars.
6. It may improve muscle power in athletes and in animals.

Not surprisingly, vitamin E has been found to be therapeutic for managing thrombosis, gangrene, indolent ulcers, thromboangiitis obliterans, thermal burns, radiation burns, cardiac disease, congenital heart disease, acute and chronic rheumatic fever, hypertensive heart disease, coronary heart disease. Dr Shute refers to 57 published reports on the efficacy of vitamin E.

More recently, vitamin E has been shown to be valuable in the treatment of cardiovascular disease; premenstrual syndrome; and tissue ischemia (common in myocardial infarction, stroke, and renal failure). Vitamin E reduces ischemia and will be very important in dealing with these conditions. It has also been shown to be valuable in the prevention of cancer (studies show an inverse relationship between vitamin E status and the development or risk of dying from cancer.); in protection against environmental pollutants (it suppressed increased lipid peroxidation in cigarette smokers); and in enhancing immune functions.

It is clear that vitamin E will play an ever-increasing role in the prevention and treatment of disease. It is no longer a vitamin in search of a disease. It is now recognized as an antioxidant vitamin intimately involved in the biochemistry and physiology of the body and with a host of diseases. The lay vitamin literature is now well acquainted with vitamin E and its usefulness. In 1972 Dr E. Di Cyan, a friend of ours, wrote his excellent book *Vitamin E and Aging*, which today is still very up-to-date.

Heart Disease: In November 1992, *New York Newsday* carried a report that vitamin E decreases the risk of heart disease between one-third and one-half. Two studies were conducted at the Harvard School of Public Health. In one study, Dr M. Stampfer and colleagues found that during an 8-year follow up, women who had taken at least 100 IU of vitamin E daily for 2 years had a 46% lower risk of having a heart attack. This was based on a population study involving 87,245 women. The second study on men by Dr E. Rimm and colleagues, based upon 51,529 subjects, showed a 37% lower risk. Both research teams found that there was not enough vitamin E in food to reach these daily levels. Dr Stampfer was so convinced by the data that he is himself taking the vitamin. These findings corroborated the research conducted by Wilfred and Evan Shute on more than 30,000 patients.

Today, approximately 40% of all deaths in North America are caused by heart disease. Each day 2,000 people die from heart disease. Let us assume that the reduction in risk is exaggerated, and that in reality there is only a 10% reduction with therapeutic doses of vitamin E. This means that each day about 200 fewer people would die. It is difficult to calculate overall how many would have been saved if the medical establishment had examined the vitamin E claims in 1950 instead of waiting until 1992.

Two recent reports show that vitamin E also helps heart patients get well after by-pass surgery and angioplasties. Dr D.S. Sgoutas at Emory

University found that 35.5% of angioplasty patients taking vitamin E suffered from restenosis, while 47.5% of the control placebo group did. Dr T. Yau at The University of Toronto reported that presurgical supplementation of vitamin E helped the heart pump during the high-risk, 5-hour postoperative period. Controls did not do as well.

Psychiatric Disorders: Vitamin E may be working its way into psychiatry following reports that it had a slight effect in decreasing the symptoms of tardive dyskinesia in patients. This aroused some to consider its role there as an antioxidant and its possible effect in decreasing the oxidation of catechol amines to their oxidized derivatives. These are compounds like adrenochrome. It is an interesting hypothesis and corroborates our views published in the mid 1950s.

Oral Cancer: *The American Journal of Epidemiology* recently reported that people who took vitamin E regularly for at least 6 months had half the expected risk of oral cancer. This is based upon 1100 patients with oral cancer and 1300 normal controls. The amount of vitamin in multivitamins was not enough; they had to take pure vitamin E supplements, at least 100 IU per day. Several other similar studies are underway. The water-soluble succinate derivative has the best anticancer properties and is the one we have been using for the past 30 years.

Optimum Dose

Dr W. Shute and Dr E. Shute recommended doses from 400 to 8000 IU daily. The usual dose range was 800 to 1600 IU, but they report that they had given 8000 IU (about 8 g) without seeing any toxicity. We usually use between 400 and 1200 IU daily, but for Crohns disease, we have been giving 4000 IU and have not yet seen any side effects from vitamin E administration.

Dr Evan Shute advises starting with small doses for patients who have rheumatic heart disease. He starts with 90 IU and very slowly works up the dose. If too much is given at the beginning, the increased strength of the heartbeat may create some difficulty. The same applies to heart failure from hypertension. The initial dose should be small and gradually increased. If this is done, the final dose can safely reach 800 to 1200 IU.

Safety

Dr John Marks reports that adults can safely be given 100 to 800 IU, but excludes adults with alteration of vitamin K status or metabolism. Ingestion of 1200 IU has increased the coagulation defect produced by vitamin K deficiency or by warfarin treatment.

In a 2005 editorial published in the *Townsend Letter for Doctors & Patients*, Dr Alan Gaby described research that showed large doses of alpha-tocopherol to deplete gamma-tocopherol. He also discussed the more potent biochemical properties of gamma tocopherol over those of alpha-tocopherol that include: greater inhibition of nitric-oxide-derived free radicals; greater inhibition of platelet aggregation; and specific anticancer effects not possessed by the alpha-tocopherol form. In addition, Dr Gaby discussed how the positive effects of high-dose alpha-tocopherol might be negated by a reduction in gamma-tocopherol levels in the body.

For these reasons, it is highly recommended that mixed tocopherols be used (when possible) over the natural source or d-alpha-tocopherol form. Mixed tocopherols contain all four naturally occurring forms of vitamin E and likely produce more beneficial therapeutic effects than the single d-alpha-tocopherol form. The only issue with the mixed tocopherol form is that it is more expensive than natural source vitamin E. One should administer mixed tocopherols using the same dosages recommended for the alpha-tocopherol form.

Vitamin A, Beta-Carotene, and Mixed Carotenoids

Vitamin A is a fat-soluble vitamin stored in the body. It is found in two forms, as retinol in animal foods and as carotene in plant foods primarily.

Over 400 carotenoids are known in nature. They are the colored pigments widely found in plants. Beta-carotene is the most abundant and best known. One molecule can be converted into vitamin A. Only about 10% to 50% of the beta-carotene consumed is absorbed. The amount changed to vitamin A depends upon the vitamin state of the body. If the body has enough vitamin A, no more beta-carotene will be converted into the vitamin. Beta-carotene and other carotenoids may be stored in adipose tissue, the liver, and other organs, with the adrenals, testes, and ovaries having the highest concentrations.

Vitamin A is one of the three major antioxidants and is, therefore, receiving more and more attention in the treatment of cancer. It is non-toxic. Even with very high doses, the only side effect has been the deposition of the pigment into the skin, with the subjects becoming a bit carrot-like in color, especially on the palms and soles of the feet. This coloring is not necessarily the result of excessive dietary intake or supplementation; rather, it may be indicative of a deficiency in a necessary conversion factor (i.e., zinc, thyroid hormone, vitamin C, or protein).

> Vitamin A is one of the three major antioxidants and is, therefore, receiving more and more attention in the treatment of cancer.

The extra amounts over normal needs cannot be converted into vitamin A, nor can they lead to vitamin A toxicity. In other words, no amount of beta-carotene can lead to vitamin A toxicity. The only individuals who should avoid beta-carotene are those who smoke. The combined use of chronic smoking and beta-carotene has been shown to increase the risk of lung cancer in men; this association does not apply to non-smokers who want to take beta-carotene.

Therapeutic Uses

Cancer: Beta-carotene inhibits the formation of tumors in animals. In human subjects, the more beta-carotene there is in their body, the less risk there is of getting cancer. A 1984 study assessed the carotenoid content (including beta-carotene) of mammals, with the goal of evaluating if these compounds could extend lifespan. Since cancer and aging share a number of similar features, the researchers felt that the anticancer effects of carotenoids might also extend lifespan. They concluded that evolution appears to favor mammals that absorb carotenoids non-selectively (or more easily) from dietary sources. This non-selective absorption allows for higher concentrations of carotenoids to be stored in tissues of mammals, with human beings having the greatest capacity and thus the greatest potential to have an increase in lifespan. In other words, an optimal intake of beta-carotene and other carotenoids should not only prevent cancer, but should also extend lifespan.

By 1989 six studies on cancer of the esophagus showed there was a positive relationship, eight studies on stomach cancer were positive, and five studies out of 10 on colon cancer showed the same connection.

Heart Disease: There is a similar relationship between vitamin A and heart disease. A School of Public Health study showed that women who consumed more than 15 to 20 mg (25,000 IU) daily had a 40% less chance of having a heart attack.

Cataracts: Cataracts also are found more frequently in people with lower beta-carotene levels. The low beta-carotene group had five to seven times the risk of getting cataracts. Being an antioxidant, it should share with ascorbic acid and vitamin E the ability to be therapeutic for any disease characterized by an excess formation of free radicals.

Vision: Beta-carotene also has beneficial effects for the prevention of blindness when supplemented with other antioxidants and zinc. It is important for retention of normal vision, permitting formation of visual purple in the eye, counteracting night-blindness and weak vision.

In a landmark 2001 randomized controlled trial published in the *Lancet*, researchers found a significant reduction in intermediate age-related macular degeneration on vision loss. The treatment groups were given different combinations of nutrients. One group was only given 80 mg of zinc with copper (added to prevent associated copper deficiency). Another group was given an antioxidant combination of 500 mg vitamin C, 400 IU vitamin E, and 15 mg beta-carotene. A third group was provided with the zinc (with added copper) and the antioxidants. None of the patients in the groups knew whether they had received the nutritional treatments or placebo.

The zinc and antioxidant combination reduced the risk of developing advanced macular degeneration by 25% and the risk of central vision loss by 19%. Supplemental zinc by itself reduced the risk of advanced disease by about 21% and the risk of vision loss by about 11%. The antioxidants alone reduced the risk of advanced disease by about 17% and the risk of vision loss by about 10%.

In another randomized controlled trial, 90 patients were followed over 12 months. The patient were divided into 3 groups: Group 1 was given 10 mg of lutein (a carotenoid that prevents oxidative damage to the retina); group 2 was given 10 mg of lutein and additional broad spectrum supplementation with antioxidants, vitamins, and minerals; and group 3 was given a placebo. The results of this study were once again excellent, with lutein or the lutein/broad spectrum group having a marked improvement in visual function (positive changes in macular pigment density, Snellen visual acuity, and contrast sensitivity). Patients who were on placebo had no significant changes. These studies and many others show a clear clinical benefit from beta-carotene (with zinc and antioxidants) and/or lutein on visual function.

Women's Conditions: Beta-carotene and other carotenoids can reverse cervical dysplasia, aid the female reproductive system, and prevent yeast infections.

In the case of cervical dysplasia, a trial of 30 women with stage I or II of cervical intraepithelial neoplasia were supplemented with high dose beta-carotene. The use of beta-carotene was associated with regression of atypical cervical cells to normal in 70% of the women tested. These favorable effects persisted for 6 months following discontinuation of the beta-carotene as 30% of the patients continued to have negative (normal) Pap findings.

In an animal study involving cows, beta-carotene-deficient diets caused delayed ovulation and an increase in the number of follicular and luteal cysts. It would appear that beta-carotene has specific actions upon fertility, which is separate from its role as a precursor to vitamin A. Of all the organs, the corpus luteum (part of the ovarian follicle) has the highest concentration of beta-carotene. The carotene cleavage activity changes with each ovulation cycle, the highest activity occurring during the mid-ovulation stage. The proper ratio of carotene-to-retinol must be maintained to ensure proper corpus luteum function. Since the corpus luteum produces progesterone, inadequate corpus luteum function could have significant negative clinical effects on the health of the female reproductive system.

To prevent fertility issues, cysts, and PMS, it seems necessary to ensure an optimal daily intake of beta-carotene and other carotenoids. For the prevention of yeast infections, there might be a need for more beta-carotene since low beta-carotene levels have been found in exfoliated vaginal cells of women with yeast infections. Thus, a high supplemental or dietary intake of beta-carotene may be protective against frequent yeast infections.

Men's Conditions: Vitamin A can combat male infertility and prostate cancer. Lycopene is a carotenoid with interesting clinical uses. It provides twice the antioxidant effects of beta-carotene, and 10 times the antioxidant effects of vitamin E. Idiopathic male infertility is a significant problem that appears to be caused by an excessive amount of free radicals. Lycopene has been shown to concentrate heavily in the testes and seminal plasma of men,

> Based on these findings, it was speculated that dietary lycopene has a role in preventing oxidative damage of biomolecules and, most likely, in reducing the risk of prostate cancer.

but is apparently in lower concentrations among men suffering from infertility. Thirty men were given 2000 mcg (2 mg) of lycopene twice daily for 3 months. These results were very encouraging: 66% had an improvement in sperm concentration (statistically significant), 53% had an improvement in motility, and 46% had improvements in morphology (the shape of the sperm cells). Twenty-three percent of the men were able to conceive during the trial. The researchers recommended that all men with low sperm counts be given a therapeutic trial of lycopene for their infertility.

Prostate cancer is the leading cause of cancer in men (1 in 11 males will have prostate cancer during their lifetime). In a study assessing the dietary intake of tomatoes and tomato products containing lycopene, these carotenoids were shown to probably reduce the risk of prostate cancer. This study found that the status of lycopene, but not other carotenoids, in prostate cancer patients is different from that of controls. Based on these findings, it was speculated that dietary lycopene has a role in preventing oxidative damage of biomolecules and, most likely, in reducing the risk of prostate cancer. In a 2002 randomized controlled trial, researchers assessed the effect of 200 g of tomato sauce daily (containing 30 mg of lycopene) on DNA damage in men with prostate cancer. There were many notable benefits from the tomato sauce that yielded statistical significance, some of which included a 17.5% decrease in mean prostate specific antigen (PSA) levels, and a reduction in DNA damage in both leukocyte (white blood cell) and prostate tissue. The results of these studies indicate that lycopene or lycopene-containing foods can exert potent anticancer effects among men with prostate cancer. Lycopene is such a powerful agent that research shows it may also reduce the risk of other cancers involving the breast, cervical, skin, lung, and colon.

Osteoporosis: In a more recent study, lycopene was shown to reduce the loss of bone associated with osteoporosis. It is known that osteoclasts (cells that breakdown bone) can produce free radicals that stimulate bone loss (resorption). The group with the highest blood concentrations of lycopene had the least amount of bone resorption, as indicated by a specific laboratory marker (NTx). These results were statistically significant.

Other Conditions: Vitamin A (in the palmitate form) is also known as the anti-ophthalmic, anti-infective, and anti-acne vitamin. It maintains healthy mucous in the respiratory system and thus fights off infection and allergic symptoms. When supplemented at very high doses, it can effectively resolve acne in a few weeks time. Vitamin A also promotes protective sheathing around the nerve fibers, tissues, and organs internally and promotes healthy skin, hair and nails.

Optimum Dose

All of these studies indicate that one should consume high amounts of carotene-containing foods each day. They also point to a need of tissue-specific carotenes for the treatment or prevention of specific health conditions.

For optimal health and longevity, it is recommended to supplement with 15,000 to 25,000 IU of mixed carotenoids (includes beta-carotene and other carotenoids) daily. For problems of the female reproductive system, doses of 25,000 to 50,000 IU of beta-carotene should be taken. For the prevention of macular degeneration, the use of zinc, antioxidants, and beta-carotene seems very prudent.

In addition, the use of lutein should be provided at a dose of 5 mg two to three times each day. For idiopathic male infertility, 4 to 5 mg of lycopene daily seems warranted. For the prevention of prostate cancer, it is recommended that men consume plenty of lycopene-containing foods, and take 30 mg of supplemental lycopene daily. To reduce the loss of bone associated with aging, 5 to 10 mg daily should be sufficient.

For the treatment of acne, 50,000 to 150,000 IU of vitamin A (with vitamin E) can be given for several months. Once the acne clears, much smaller daily maintenance doses (15,000 to 25,000 IU) can safely be used for prolonged periods of time.

For acute infections (especially for influenza prevention), Dr Bradford S. Weeks recommends 100,000 IU at the onset of acute symptoms and another 100,000 IU prior to bed. If the ensuing infection has not resolved by the next morning, he recommends taking this twice-daily amount of vitamin A for no more than 1 week. There is truth to increasing the intake of vitamin A during an acute infection. It is known that the urinary excretion of vitamin A increases dramatically during an acute process. This results in a sharp decline of the vitamin A levels in the blood, necessitating an increased intake to combat the transient deficiency state.

Safety

Toxicity of vitamin A is a concern, and, therefore, therapeutic supplementation should only be done under the supervision of a healthcare professional. General vitamin A toxicity symptoms include dry fissured skin, brittle nails, alopecia (hair loss), gingivitis (swollen gums), cheilosis (chapped lips), anorexia (loss of appetite), irritability, fatigue, headache, and nausea. Prolonged toxicity can also lead to bone fragility and thickening of long bones. However, when high doses of vitamin A are administered with 800 IU of vitamin E, there is hardly any chance of toxicity. Vitamin E reduces vitamin A toxicity.

Doses as high as 50,000 IU can cause toxicity if taken for several years. Doses lower than this can also lead to toxicity if there are defects in vitamin A storage and transport due to health conditions, such as cirrhosis of the liver, hepatitis, and protein-energy malnutrition. In adults, toxicity of vitamin A usually occurs when daily doses of 300,000 IU are used for the treatment of skin conditions.

Once the vitamin is stopped, symptoms rapidly subside and complete recovery always results.

Women of childbearing age are at high risk for birth defects if their daily dose of vitamin A is 10,000 IU or greater. To be safe, women wanting to become pregnant should limit their vitamin A intake to 5,000 IU or less per day.

Accidental ingestion of a single dose of 100,000 to 300,000 IU of vitamin A in a child can lead to increased intracranial pressure with vomiting, headache, joint pain, stupor, and occasionally papilledema (edema and inflammation of the optic nerve).

The most recent concern about vitamin A supplementation is in post-menopausal women. A 2004 report in *Nutrition Reviews* speculated that long-term consumption of diets high in vitamin A stimulates bone resorption and inhibits bone formation, and may contribute to osteoporosis and hip fractures. This report caused many patients to discontinue supplementation with vitamin A. These concerns turned out to be unfounded. In a very large 2004 cohort study published in *Osteoporosis International*, 34,703 postmenopausal women were followed prospectively to determine if their supplemental vitamin A and dietary intakes were associated with increased hip fractures or all fractures. After subjecting all the data to rigorous statistical analysis, the results showed no association between vitamin A or retinol intake from food or supplements with an increased risk of hip or all fractures. The investigators concluded, "we found little evidence of an increased risk of hip or all fractures with higher intakes of vitamin A or retinol among a cohort of older, postmenopausal women." At present, there is really no reason why post-menopausal women should limit their vitamin A intake from foods or supplements unless medically indicated.

Vitamin D-3

Although we call it a vitamin, vitamin D-3 is made in the body by the action of ultraviolet light on the skin. By definition, vitamins cannot be made in the body. Humankind evolved in equatorial Africa, where exposure to sun is unavoidable, but as we expanded toward the polar regions, we no longer were able to get the right amount of ultraviolet light in sunlight. Thus, the further populations live from the equator, the more apt are they to suffer massive vitamin D-3 deficiency. In Canada, for example, there is enough ultraviolet in no more than 4 months out of each year. The rest of the year the ultraviolet is stripped from the light in its passage through the atmosphere. People living in the Arctic cannot expect ever to get enough vitamin D-3 from sunlight. Vitamin D-3 production also depends on the color of the skin. The more pigment in the skin, the more vitamin D-3 is made. Thus, the further we live from equatorial regions, the more dependent we are upon vitamin D-3 sources that are not endogenous, not made by our own skin.

> The further we live from equatorial regions, the more dependent we are upon vitamin D-3 sources that are not endogenous, not made by our own skin.

The pharmacology of this vitamin is very complex. Once it has been synthesized in the skin, it is converted into 25-hydroxy vitamin D and then into 1,25-dihydroxy vitamin D, which is the active hormone. The body can make 10,000 to 12,000 IU when exposed to sunlight containing enough ultraviolet light. This would appear to be the ideal dose; however, doses of 800 IU daily have been considered to be adequate until recently.

We have accepted the advice of dermatologists that ultraviolet light is very dangerous and that we should expose ourselves to the sun as little as possible because it is believed to cause skin cancer. While reducing our exposure to ultraviolet light, we need to take more vitamin D-3 to replace what is not being supplied by the sun. During the past few years, the role of vitamin D-3 in many reactions in the body has been seriously examined, and it has been found to be a very useful and even a remarkable nutrient needed in much higher dosages for optimum health.

Therapeutic Uses

Rickets and Subclinical Rickets: Childhood rickets is a vitamin D-3 deficiency disease. According to Dr J.T. Hart, although rickets was very common in Roman children in the first century, the disease was first described in 1650. Symptoms of subclinical rickets are head sweating, hair tenderness (noticed when hair is manipulated or brushed), and legs giving out (the child often wants to be picked up). Head sweating is the earliest sign in infants, and in Dr Hart's practice, 66% of new patients were found to have this symptom. These vanish when optimal doses of vitamin D supplements are given.

Deficient diets are caused by dairy allergy, strict vegetarianism, excessive use of sunscreens, and decreased sun exposure. Even in the developing world where there is ample sunlight, rickets still occurs. It was discovered that a lack of both dietary calcium and vitamin D-3 were responsible. The widespread use of fish oil supplements (cod and halibut) in school public health programs was very successful in preventing rickets, but recently this disease has returned and nearly 100 cases of rickets in children have been reported.

Osteomalacia (adult form of vitamin D deficiency): Supplementation with optimal doses of vitamin D can prevent osteomalacia, even in the absence of adequate sunlight. Osteomalacia causes softening of the bones and inadequate mineralization of the bone matrix. It is also associated with an acceleration of bone loss. Over time, it can cause muscle weakness or diffuse aches, and bone pain or tenderness. It is typically diagnosed following an acute fracture.

Osteoporosis: Seventy-five million persons in the United States, Europe, and Japan suffer from osteoporosis. In Canada, the prevalence is 15.8% for women aged 50 years or older. In this disease, bone density decreases, bones become fragile, and the risks of fractures are substantially increased. Many of these women will experience a fragility fracture at some point during their remaining years. Some of these patients will also experience a hip fracture, causing long-term disability, with a 20% chance of dying within one year of the fracture. Long-standing deficiencies of both calcium and vitamin D-3 significantly increase the risk of being diagnosed with osteoporosis. However, osteoporosis is completely preventable with naturopathic nutrition and nutrient supplementation, chiefly vitamin D-3 and calcium. If people were to follow the recommendations in this book before peak bone mass is achieved in late adolescence or early in the third decade, the chance of getting osteoporosis would be extremely rare.

Vitamin D-3 also boosts muscle strength and can improve balance among geriatric subjects, which would help reduce the chances of fracturing a hip or other serious injuries.

Multiple Sclerosis (MS): Evidence linking MS to vitamin D-3 deficiency is very persuasive. There is a clear but inverse relationship between the prevalence of MS and exposure to ultraviolet light. In 1952, we were asked to do a survey of MS in Saskatchewan. It was then known that the prevalence of

MS in Saskatchewan was four times as high as it was in New Orleans. The prevalence below Latitude 40 was much greater. This suggests that MS patients will do better if they move to sunnier climates. It is, of course, much easier to take supplements.

A few small clinical studies have confirmed that vitamin D is therapeutic, while the majority of studies show a strong relationship between vitamin D status and the clinical course of MS. For example, MS patients in one study were found to have lower bone densities than healthy controls. The researchers recommended that all MS patients should get adequate sunlight exposure and do specific strengthening exercises for their hip and back muscles to prevent debility and osteoporosis. In another clinical study, the blood levels of vitamin D were found to be lower during relapses. This was thought to play a role in regulation of clinical disease activity. One of our MS patients has been seeing us for over 10 years. His condition was stable, but he was still not well. We added vitamin D-3 to his orthomolecular program, 5000 IU twice daily. After a few months, he reported that he felt much better. We increased the dose to 6000 IU twice daily; at that dose, a skin problem he had always had cleared completely.

Mental Illness: The executive director of the Vitamin D Council proposes that a vitamin D-3 deficiency is also involved in the genesis of mental disease. The evidence arises from epidemiological studies, from decreased serum 25-hydroxy vitamin D levels, from significant comorbidity, from theoretical models, and from a few small studies showing that it is helpful.

Recently, we have routinely added vitamin D-3, 4000 IU daily, to the treatment protocol of our patients who are clearly more depressed in the winter than they are in the summer. It has been very helpful and can do no harm. Clinical studies do show that vitamin D-3 is very helpful in treating seasonal affective disorder, even more so than light therapy. Vitamin D-3 has also been shown to elevate mood in healthy subjects during the winter months. In a more recent study by Dr Vieth and his colleagues, they found vitamin D-3 to improve overall wellbeing when administered at doses of 4000 IU per day. These findings can probably be equally applied to chronically depressed and schizophrenic patients. Dr McGrath suggests that low prenatal vitamin D deficiency is a risk factor for schizophrenia.

Cancer: Vitamin D protects against some forms of cancer. For over 60 years, it has been observed that increased intake of calcium and vitamin D is inversely correlated with colon and colorectal cancer. It is also protective against prostate cancer. In one of our patients, whose PSA levels had begun to rapidly increase, the addition of vitamin D-3 at 3000 IU twice daily and selenium 1000 mcg daily to a comprehensive orthomolecular program precipitously brought the PSA level down to its previous lower level. The patient's previous program of nutrients had not been able to do so.

Inflammatory Conditions: Vitamin D-3 lowers inflammation. Since inflammation is an important problem in many chronic diseases, such as hypertension, heart disease, autoimmune disease, and diabetes, this finding is very important.

Optimum Dose

The optimum dose has not been established. Dr Vieth estimates that the desirable level of serum 25-hydroxy vitamin D should be 100 to 250 nmol/l. A daily dose of 4000 IU to 10,000 IU will provide this desirable level. These levels are considered safe since they have no pathological effects on calcium metabolism in the blood or urine.

In the United States and Canada, vitamin D-3 is considered a vitamin and is sold over the counter in 1000 IU pills, but in Europe, it is considered a prescription drug.

Safety

The toxic dose of vitamin D-3 starts at 40,000 IU daily, which is ten times the most recommended optimum dose. The popular idea that vitamin D-3 is toxic is based primarily on studies with vitamin D-2, which was added to milk and which is toxic.

MINERALS

All life originated in the seas, a vast solution of all the minerals known, mostly in very minute concentrations. Life adapted these minerals to its own needs, utilizing some that became essential and keeping some out that were toxic. Without these minerals, there can be no life.

As with vitamins and other nutrients, for each mineral there is an optimum requirement. Too little will inhibit many important reactions in the body and too much will be toxic. For most minerals, the useful range is much narrower than it is for vitamins – for some, it is very narrow indeed. Thus, minerals cannot be used with the same degree of freedom as vitamins. We have divided the key minerals into categories of absolutely essential, possibly essential, and non-essential.

Absolutely Essential

Sodium and Potassium

These two minerals need to be in balance. Both elements are involved in the transfer of energy in the body. Sodium remains in the fluid outside the cells, while potassium is held inside the cells. It requires work on the part of the cells to maintain this difference. Unprocessed foods contain much more potassium than they do sodium, but during processing, salt is added and this reverses the ratio.

Therapeutic Uses

Hypertension: The ratio of potassium to sodium is related to the development of hypertension or high blood pressure. This ratio is call the "K" factor and is determined by measuring the amount of sodium and potassium in the urine.

Hypertension affects one out of three people in North America. People with high blood pressure run the risk of dying from stroke, heart failure, or kidney disease. However, while it is developing, they will feel normal.

Blood pressure is considered high if the systolic (the upper reading) is equal to or greater than 140 or the diastolic (the lower) is greater than 89. Blood pressure increases with age. The old rule was that the systolic should not be higher than 100 plus the age – that is, if a person age 80 had a systolic pressure over 180, he was considered normal, whereas now this would be too high.

R.D. Moore and G.D. Webb, in their book *The K Factor,* concluded that high blood pressure arose from eating too little potassium (in some people too little magnesium or calcium) and too much sodium. Other factors affecting blood pressure are too little exercise and too much weight. In their book, they outline the four basic rules for maintaining normal blood pressure:

1. See your doctor.
2. Eat right. Their description of the right diet is exactly what we have been recommending as the naturopathic or orthomolecular diet, the diet our ancestors were forced to eat. For Moore and Webb, "the diet of our remote ancestors may be a reference standard for modern human nutrition and a model for defense against certain diseases of civilization."
3. Exercise.
4. Maintain normal weight.

There is tremendous value in adopting these healthy eating habits, and some value in lowering the amount of sodium consumed on a daily basis. A dietary approach for limiting salt intake has been the subject of a number of clinical trials over the past few years. The DASH (Dietary Approaches for Stopping Hypertension) diet has been developed for hypertension that emphasizes eating fresh fruits, vegetables, and low-fat dairy foods, as well as whole grains, poultry, fish, and nuts. It is reduced in fats, red meat, sweets, and sugar-containing beverages. In one clinical trial, participants were instructed to follow this diet with different intakes (high, intermediate, and low) of sodium. The results of the DASH-low sodium combination

> As with vitamins and other nutrients, for each mineral there is an optimum requirement. Too little will inhibit many important reactions in the body and too much will be toxic.

approach showed more significant decreases in lowering blood pressure than the diet combined with higher sodium intakes. However, a more recent study of the DASH-low sodium approach yielded inconsistent results because it was very difficult to determine which participants were salt-sensitive. Even the participants who were identified as being salt-sensitive did not have the most predicable response to the lowered sodium intake.

There is no doubt that an individual's daily salt intake should be limited, but the intake of other minerals seems to be more important. Magnesium and calcium also play a role in high blood pressure, while the direct role of sodium appears to be less important. The sodium chloride molecule appears to be more of a villain because the sodium ion alone is not that bad. The sodium in sodium ascorbate does not pose any risk.

It may be that with the right K ratio, increases in sodium are not as dangerous. In one study, giving sodium chloride increased systolic and diastolic pressure, whereas giving sodium citrate did not. In another study, a series of patients on hypertensive medication were given 1 g of calcium daily. After a few months, half of them no longer needed their medication. In areas where the drinking water is low in magnesium, there is a higher incidence of high blood pressure. Magnesium salts decrease elevated blood pressure. A study on 21,000 people showed a strong correlation between calcium intake and hypertension. It was the only nutrient that showed this high relationship.

A new classification scheme has recently been established for the aggressive drug management of all blood pressures considered to be abnormal. Some drugs will decrease the pressure, but they carry the risk of side effects. Most of the patients we see who are already taking blood pressure pills do not like the side effects and are keen to come off them. There is a concern that too many people are placed on medication unnecessarily.

Cerebral Hemorrhage (Apoplexy): Cerebral hemorrhage (apoplexy) is the second most common cause of stroke. The two most likely precursors are hypertension and abnormalities of the blood vessels. The factors involved in stroke are psychosocial, physiological, and nutritional, namely a deficiency of vitamin C, high salt diets, potassium deficiency, magnesium deficiency, selenium deficiency, excessive lead ingestion, and very low cholesterol levels.

Of all these nutritional factors, the most important single factor was a deficiency of magnesium. Five lines of evidence support this view, as Professor Harold D. Foster explains in his study, *Health, Disease and the Environment:*

1. Global mortality rates. Japan suffers from a very high incidence of stroke. Their soils and drinking water are very low in both calcium and magnesium. The Japanese also tend to have lower cholesterol levels because their intake of animal products and sugar is much lower. The combination of low cholesterol and low magnesium may be the cause. As the Japanese have increased their intake of animal foods, their cholesterol levels have risen and the incidence of stroke has fallen 60% between 1964 and 1983. Thailand and Egypt have the lowest stroke mortality rate. Their soils and drinking water are very rich in calcium and magnesium. The United States and Britain, areas characterized by high calcium and magnesium intake, have a lower incidence of stroke than areas where these minerals are deficient.
2. Declining stroke mortality in the developed world. This is due to the decrease in high cholesterol levels these people have been trying to achieve. There is also a decrease in the consumption of salt.
3. Gender factor. Men have more strokes because they lose magnesium faster than women. Alcohol also increases loss of magnesium.
4. Stroke increases with age. This is true in Western countries with the

high-tech diet. Diets of the elderly are much more prone to be magnesium deficient.
5. Strokes are more common in the winter. Magnesium is most often much less available in the winter, both in the drinking water and due to the decreased intake of fresh fruits and vegetables. Professor Foster made the useful suggestion that magnesium ought to be added to widely used foods, as is being done in Finland. In Finland, they are adding potassium and magnesium to salt. This decreases the sodium chloride to 65% of the mixture. There is already a decline in mean blood pressure in the study population.

The prudent diet to prevent stroke arising from high blood pressure and other causes is to consume much less salt, much more potassium (more vegetables and fruit and, if necessary, potassium supplements), much more magnesium, more calcium, much more vitamin C, and much less sugar – in short, the naturopathic diet, the diet to which we have been adapted.

If the cholesterol is elevated and will not come down by diet alone, then nicotinic acid will bring it down. Contrary to medical belief, nicotinic acid is not only a hypocholesterolemic (cholesterol-lowering) substance, but it also elevates the cholesterol if it is too low by increasing high density lipoprotein cholesterol. This provides an additional anti-stroke factor by elevating too low cholesterol levels.

Even though salt has been given a bad name, there are some circumstances where sodium might be therapeutic. Some patients with chronic fatigue syndrome or persistent fatigue suffer from an inability to regulate blood pressure properly when they change positions – from lying down to standing up, for example. This condition is called neural mediated hypotension (NMH) and is diagnosed by special testing with an upright tilt table. The patient is placed on a table that can change positions, forcing the blood pressure systems of the body to adapt. A patient who demonstrates swings of low blood pressure due to these positional challenges will be given the diagnosis of NMH.

Besides fatigue, NMH can also cause symptoms of lightheadedness, fainting, and general malaise. Some patients with NMH do benefit from increasing their salt intake since it helps to increase blood pressure and reduce other troublesome symptoms. It is disappointing that a 2003 clinical trial did not show any improvements among chronic fatigue patients provided with treatments to increase sodium levels in the body. Even so, we have treated several patients with chronic fatigue syndrome by increasing their daily sodium intakes, and have observed good improvements in their fatigue.

Optimum Dose

About 4 g each of sodium and potassium is required daily, but this varies tremendously due to a large number of factors.

Calcium and Magnesium

There is an inverse absorption rate between calcium and magnesium. If calcium is high, less magnesium is absorbed, and if magnesium is high, less calcium is absorbed.

Ninety-nine percent of the calcium in our body is in our bones and teeth. Each day 700 mg exchanges between bones and the rest of the body. The remaining 1% is very important in controlling many reactions, such as blood clotting, muscle function, nerve conduction, cell-wall permeability, and enzyme activity.

> There is an inverse absorption rate between calcium and magnesium. If calcium is high, less magnesium is absorbed, and if magnesium is high, less calcium is absorbed.

Only about 25% of the calcium in food is absorbed. Absorption is increased by vitamin D, protein, lactose, and an acidic medium. High phosphorus levels decrease its absorption, as does phytic acid, oxalate, and fiber. It is also decreased by excess fat, by alkalinity, and by stress.

The absorption of calcium from calcium citrate or calcium amino acid chelates is much more than what can be absorbed from calcium carbonate (the most common calcium preparation). Not all calcium supplements are well absorbed. Preparations that contain more calcium per unit weight are therefore preferable.

The body contains about 20 to 30 g of magnesium, half in the bones. The average diet contains about 150 mg per day, which is below the recommended dose. About one third of the magnesium ingested is absorbed. This is due to low magnesium in soils, in water, and in food due to processing. Other common reasons for too little magnesium are alcoholism, uncontrolled diabetes, excessive use of diuretics, and malabsorption syndromes. It is the mineral component of chlorophyll.

Therapeutic Uses

Osteoporosis: A deficiency of calcium is related to osteoporosis (though not directly) and an excess to the formation of kidney stones. Osteoporosis is the major disease linked to calcium. The most visible expression is the so-called dowager's hump. This disease affects between 15 and 20 million adults in North America. Of these, 1.3 million suffer fractures early. The bones are weakened by a decrease in the amount of calcium.

Bone mass loss is complicated, depending upon age, sex, race, hormones, nutrition, and activity. The general hypothesis is that bone loss is due to loss of estrogens after menopause, to a deficiency of calcium, and to a deficiency of fluoride. Other deficiencies are manganese, copper, zinc, and boron. Normal bone contains 150 mg per gram of calcium; osteoporotic bone only 114 mg. It also contains one quarter of the manganese levels found in normal bone.

It has been found that osteoporosis is more common in populations that consume very high protein diets and is much less common in populations that consume low protein diets. Apparently, the increased intake of protein demands more calcium, which is withdrawn from the bones. Too much protein increases the loss of calcium in the urine.

The ratio of phosphorus to calcium also determines what happens to calcium in bones and in the body. The high-tech diet is very rich in phosphorus, which comes from animal protein, soft drinks, preserved foods, food additives, and more. The optimum ratio is about 1:1. Animal protein has a ratio of 26:1 phosphorus to calcium. This disturbed ratio causes loss of bone calcium. Asians eat much less animal protein, much more vegetable protein, ingest about 500 mg of calcium daily, and do not have osteoporosis as a major problem. When Asians resettle in North America, within a short period of time, they develop heart disease, certain cancers, osteoporosis, and other health conditions due to the adoption of unhealthy, high-tech dietary habits.

Recent reviews of the research literature suggest that a combination of calcium and vitamin D will reduce the ravages of osteoporosis. Dr R. Heaney states that we know enough now to ensure that calcium and vitamin D are used to protect against this disease. Out of 43 studies on calcium intake and bone strength, 26 were positive and 16 were negative. In several studies, giving menopausal women 1000 mg of calcium each day reduced bone loss by one third to one half. In another study, these two supplements decreased non-vertebral fractures by 32% and hip fractures by 43%. A 20% reduction in hip fractures in United States would prevent about 45,000 hip fractures and save about $1.5 billion dollars in health costs.

Dr A.R. Gaby and Dr J.V. Wright, in their book *Nutrients and Bone Health*, describe the following compounds that can be used in treating osteoporosis:

1. Estrogens and calcium. These are only partially helpful. Estrogen in the context of hormone replacement therapy has been shown to have too many risks (e.g., stroke, blood clots, breast cancer) and is becoming a less than desirable option for post-menopausal women.
2. A naturopathic diet. This will not contain excess phosphorus.
3. Vitamin K. This is needed to make osteocalcin, found primarily in bone, that pulls calcium into the bone. The dose ranges from 5 to 10 mg daily.
4. Vitamin D-3. Very safe and the optimal dosage is equal to or greater than 1000 IU.
5. Magnesium. The optimum dosage is 250 to 750 mg daily.
6. Manganese. The optimum dosage is 15 to 50 mg daily.
7. Folic acid. Menopause is associated with folic acid deficiency. The optimum dosage is 5 to 15 mg daily. In Canada, a prescription is required.
8. Boron. The optimum dosage is 3 to 6 mg daily.
9. Strontium.
10. Silicon.
11. Vitamin B-6. A deficiency of this vitamin produced osteoporosis in rats. The optimum dosage is 250 to 500 mg daily.
12. Zinc. The optimum dosage is 25 to 50 mg daily.
13. Copper. The optimum dosage is 1 mg daily.
14. Ascorbic acid. The optimum levels, sublaxative, are 1 to 20 g daily.

There are other factors as well. Exercise is very important. Weight bearing is good for the spinal column. Very heavy people do not get osteoporosis as often. When walking it might be a good idea to carry a 5 lb item to increase the load on the back.

The naturopathic diet described will prevent most cases of osteoporosis. Treatment should include a normal diet not too rich in protein, with optimum amounts of all the trace elements, and enough calcium and magnesium. There is no advantage in gorging on calcium-rich foods, such as milk and cheese. To supplement this diet, you can use calcium 1 to 2 g, magnesium 500 to 1000 mg, zinc 10 to 50 mg, manganese 15 to 40 mg, boron 3 mg, and copper 1 to 2 mg all daily. As well, adequate vitamin D-3 should be obtained. The best sources are the fish oils – cod liver oil and halibut liver oil capsules.

We do not recommend fluoride since the best controlled studies have shown it has not had any therapeutic value and may be toxic. However, a recent report by Professor H.D. Foster adds evidence in favor of using fluoride. Fluoride is a natural antagonist to aluminum. It has been found that from one area in South Carolina that had the highest fluoride level in their water, the admission rate for Alzheimer's disease was only one fifth what it was from the area with the lowest amount of fluoride in their water. This epidemiological evidence leads to the conclusion that "because fluoride reduces the body's absorption of aluminum, it therefore reduces the risk of developing this form of dementia." The same relationship has been found between calcium in the water and Alzheimer's disease. Professor Foster concludes, "if the only significant gain from water fluoridation is reduced tooth decay in children, risks from fluoridation would seem to outweigh gains. However, if as suggested by the evidence presented in this article, because of its antagonism with both aluminum and calcium, moderate levels of drinking water fluoride are protective against Alzheimer's disease, osteoporosis and calcification of the arterial system, then the reverse may be true. Obviously, the great fluoridation debate can be expected to continue in earnest."

Magnesium Deficiency Disorders: There is no characteristic magnesium deficiency syndrome. The earliest symptoms are loss of appetite, nausea and vomiting, diarrhea, and mental changes. Hyper-irritability is common. It should be suspected if there is a potassium deficiency.

Other important symptoms of magnesium deficiency include fatigue and muscle spasms. The body's energy supply is in the form of adenosine triphosphate (ATP). Magnesium is required for the synthesis of ATP, and also facilitates the transport of potassium into cells. Since all the energy-producing reactions in the body require magnesium, it is an obvious treatment for fatigue. For patients suffering from unexplained fatigue, magnesium can be very helpful in returning energy levels back to normal. Magnesium is also a natural muscle relaxant because it prevents excessive muscular contraction and relieves spasms.

ADHD: Features of magnesium deficiency in children mimic attention deficit hyperactivity disorder (ADHD) and include excessive fidgeting, anxious restlessness, psychomotor instability, and learning disabilities. It is unfortunate that many children diagnosed with ADHD are deficient in this mineral, yet this relationship is hardly known by most doctors. A 1997 study published in *Magnesium Research* involved 116 patients (94 boys and 20 girls) with ADHD. Ninety-five percent of the patients had a magnesium deficiency when the levels were measured in their serum, red blood cells, and hair. Another study published in the same journal followed a group of 50 children with ADHD (aged 7 to 12 years) for 6 months. Each child was given 200 mg each day of magnesium. They were compared to a control group of 25 children who were not given magnesium, yet had a deficiency of the mineral. The study found the group supplemented with magnesium had a decrease in hyperactivity compared to the control group. These results suggest that the majority of children with ADHD are likely to be magnesium deficient, and that a deficiency of this mineral is associated with hyperactivity and possibly other behavioral problems. Of course, this is not that surprising given the poor dietary habits of most children.

Cancer: Magnesium plays a role in controlling growth of cells and may be useful in treating cancer. Green vegetables are usually recommended by alternative cancer treatments because they are high in magnesium in the chlorophyll.

Blood Pressure: Magnesium is also involved in controlling blood pressure. Rats on magnesium deficient diets suffer an increase in blood pressure.

Dr D. McCarron, Division of Nephrology and Hypertension, Oregon Health Services, has stated that "for too long we've assumed that the problems with blood pressure in humans are related to an excess of something. . . . Salt has been the culprit nailed repeatedly. But we are frankly amazed at how poor the data base is that links sodium intake to blood pressure." Dr McCarron concluded that a deficiency of calcium was much more important. The same could be said for a deficiency of magnesium. Dr McCarron recommends a ratio of calcium to magnesium of 2:1. Other authors recommend a ratio of 1:1. The naturopathic diet will provide over 500 mg of calcium. Supplements can be used to bring calcium up to 1000 mg and magnesium up to 500 to 1000 mg.

Optimum Dose

Calcium: Adults need about 500 to 1000 mg daily, while pregnant, lactating women, and post-menopausal women not on hormone replacement therapy need about 1500 mg. Milk products provide calcium. Two servings of dairy products will provide about 600 mg of calcium. Those who are dairy allergic will need to take supplements.

Magnesium: The normal diet will provide enough magnesium for most people. When supplements are needed, they should be balanced with calcium, already described. Magnesium in excess will cause diarrhea (thus the use of Epsom salts, high in magnesium, as a laxative). Common preparations are magnesium citrate (150 mg), magnesium amino acid chelate (100 mg), or magnesium oxide (420 mg).

Cal-Mag: A number of calcium-magnesium preparations are available. The best are the calcium/magnesium complexes providing a calcium to magnesium ratio of 1:2 or 1:1.

Safety

There has been some worry about lead in dolomite. In Canada, this is not a factor since quality control is good. About 6 mcg of lead has been found per tablet. But the daily food provides about 300 mcg daily. Since calcium decreases the absorption of lead, it probably adds nothing to the lead burden and may even decrease it. We recommend dolomite as an inexpensive preparation. The calcium magnesium (Cal-Mag) preparations are preferred over simple calcium salts.

Iron

The average adult has 3 to 4 g of iron in the body, of which 70% is in the hemoglobin. Red cells are recycled every 120 days. Iron is available from food, from which 10% is absorbed, 30% from meat. Absorption depends upon the amount in the food, on vitamin C levels, and on the amount of calcium. It is inhibited by phosphates, phytate, oxalate, and EDTA, a substance used as a preservative. It may be deficient in cases of malabsorption and after gastrectomy.

About one quarter of the female population is iron deficient. Women lose 50% more iron than men. Iron deficiency causes anemia, which is easily diagnosed. In men, there is danger of too much iron, which can cause hemochromatosis (a condition characterized by iron overload in the tissues). On the average, men need about 10 mg daily and women about 20 mg during the childbearing years.

Iron is one nutrient that is not used in large doses by naturopathic and orthomolecular physicians. It is difficult to rid the body of excess amounts, and in conditions where there is too much, the patient may have to be bled. It can also be removed by chelating it out with desferoxamine (an iron-binding drug) given intramuscularly.

Many years ago there was a vigorous debate over iron supplements when the U.S. Food and Drug Administration wanted to increase the amount of iron filings in flour to decrease the incidence of iron-deficiency anemia. Some physicians were already concerned by the over abundance of iron in flour. Luckily, it is unlikely any appreciable amount of the iron filings gets absorbed.

Therapeutic Uses

Iron-Deficiency Anemia: Iron deficiency is the most common cause of anemia worldwide. In children, the reason is usually due to an inadequate diet. In adults, blood loss can be responsible for the iron deficiency, and needs to be considered prior to the initiation of iron supplementation. Many people treat themselves with extra iron when they are tired, believing that fatigue is caused by anemia. However, it would be wise not to take any extra iron unless it has been shown that iron deficiency is present.

There is a very narrow optimum range for iron therapy. For the correction of diagnosed iron deficiency anemia, the daily replacement dose is 150 to 200 mg of elemental iron each day. Iron should be taken with vitamin C because this combination will improve the absorption of iron. To treat iron deficiency effectively, treatment is required for 4 to 6 months. The best way to assess if iron supplementation corrected the problem is to have a blood test for serum ferritin (the stored form of iron in the body) after 4 to 6 months, and assess if it has increased to an acceptable level. If the ferritin level has not reached the target and compliance is not an issue, other reasons for iron's lack of efficacy need to be explored (e.g., continued blood loss from menstruation, low stomach acid, Celiac disease, Crohn's disease).

Iron deficiency is the most common cause of anemia worldwide. In children, the reason is usually due to an inadequate diet.

Problems with iron treatment often include gastrointestinal complaints, such as nausea, constipation, diarrhea, and abdominal pain. To reduce these symptoms, timed-release iron preparations can be helpful or switching to different iron preparations, such as iron succinate or iron citrate. Common iron preparations, such as iron gluconate or iron sulphate, can be very irritating to the gastrointestinal system.

Sometimes, the best-tolerated form of iron is the one derived from liver extract. The liver is a good source of iron, and quality preparations deliver around 3 to 4 mg of heme iron per pill. Heme iron is the form found in meats (e.g., beef and liver) and is easily absorbed and even preferred by the body. To get an appropriate therapeutic response from liver extract, it is typically necessary to take 4 to 6 pills each day for at least 4 to 6 months. Recently, Japanese researchers demonstrated significant improvements in iron status (reflected by increases in serum ferritin levels) among 15,608 subjects given 45 mg each day of heme iron. The subjects were followed for 20 years, and the beneficial changes in iron status were associated with improvements in various conditions, such as fatty liver, chronic nephritis (inflammation of the kidneys), and peptic ulcer.

Heart Disease: Iron increases the formation of free radicals in the body. Very recently it has been implicated in the pathology of heart disease. Dr Salonen at the University of Kuopi, Finland, reported that high doses of dietary iron were associated with an increased risk of heart disease. Men with high ferritin levels (the best single measure of stored iron) over 200 mcg per liter were more than twice as likely to have heart attacks. Usually, iron overload is diagnosed when levels are over 400 mcg.

Dr Jerome L. Sullivan first proposed there was such a relationship after he observed that iron levels and heart disease risks rose with age in an identical pattern, but his hypothesis and research were rejected by the medical community until recently. The Finnish study has provided powerful support to Sullivan's hypothesis. Dr Sullivan has argued that the level of iron may turn out to be a more important risk factor than cholesterol or blood pressure levels. It could explain why women are safe from coronary disease until they stop menstruating and can accumulate iron, and why oral contraceptives increase the risk because they decrease menstrual blood flow. Jack Challem raised the possibility that it was not the overload of iron, but the deficiency of vitamin E that may have been the main factor. Vitamin E quenches free radicals and could overcome the deleterious effect of iron in increasing them. It is likely both factors are involved. It is prudent to prevent iron overload and also to take enough vitamin E.

Mental Disease: Iron overload will also cause mental disease. Dr Paul Cutler reported that iron overload has produced both neurological and psychiatric symptoms in patients with hemochromatosis. He began to look for iron overload in psychiatric patients resistant to treatment and found seven who showed evidence clinically for overload. They were given twice-weekly injections of deferoxamine, 10 mg per kg, intramuscularly until iron values became normal. There was significant improvement in anxiety, depression, obsessions, compulsions, and panic attacks.

Other Conditions: Other clinical indications for iron supplementation involve ADHD, restless leg syndrome, and excessive menstruation. A study published in *Neuropsychobiology* involved boys aged 7 to 11 years who were given an iron supplement, even though they were not anemic. The results showed significant improvements in the parents' Connors Rating Scale scores (used to assess the severity of ADHD) and significant increases in serum ferritin levels (from 25.9 +/- 9.2 to 44.6 +/- 18 ng/ml). Iron does play a role in the synthesis of dopamine and possibly other neurotransmitters within the brain. It is likely that the ADHD boys required extra iron due to biochemical needs that are different from the boys without a diagnosis of ADHD. The extra iron probably helped with the synthesis of important neurotransmitters, which favorably impacted behavior.

In restless leg syndrome and excessive menstrual bleeding, improvements from iron supplementation will occur, especially when the serum iron or ferritin levels were low prior to treatment. An effective clinical response will happen more frequently among patients having low serum iron or ferritin levels, even in the absence of anemia.

In other clinical situations, iron has proven to be therapeutically valuable due to its effect on increasing iron status in the body. Some of the other indications for iron supplementation include impaired cognitive function, hair loss, recurrent herpes simplex infections, decreased endurance, and impaired immune function.

Optimum Dose

For individuals with diagnosed iron deficiency anemia, the required dose is 150 to 200 mg of elemental iron for 4 to 6 months. There is some data demonstrating that elemental iron in dosages as low as 60 mg once or twice weekly can be beneficial in selected populations (elderly patients and patients requiring long-term iron replacement therapy). Testing of serum ferritin needs to be done to assess if the iron stores have normalized.

Adult men typically require around 10 mg daily to keep iron stores within a normal range, barring any absorption problems, or blood loss from peptic ulcers, inflammatory bowel disease, hemorrhoids, and even colorectal cancer. Lactating and non-lactating adult women require around 15 mg daily, but their needs increase with pregnancy to about 30 mg daily. Women with excessive menstruation may have to increase their iron intake to 30 mg or more daily. Children 6 months and older tend to require about 10 mg daily.

Safety

Iron supplementation should be restricted to those individuals with a diagnosis of iron deficiency anemia and to pregnant, lactating, and menstruating women. Adult men and non-menstruating women with no medical need for iron should avoid it in supplemental form because iron can increase the risk of cardiovascular events, such as heart attacks, and promote free radical damage. Dose depends on the degree of deficiency, to be determined by a healthcare professional. Iron supplementation treatments should be monitored by repeated laboratory tests.

All iron supplements need to be kept away from infants and children because iron poisoning can result in serious consequences, such as harm to the intestinal lining, nausea and vomiting, liver failure, shock, and even death.

Zinc and Copper

These minerals are best considered together because there is an inverse connection as measured by serum levels. Dr C.C. Pfeiffer has carried out the best research relating zinc and copper to human health and disease. We have found his book *Zinc and Other Micro-Nutrients* extremely valuable in deciding whether patients should be given extra zinc.

Most of the 2 to 3 g of zinc in the body is stored in the bones with a slow turnover. Serum levels range between 80 and 120 mcg. Zinc is one of the most important minerals. Deficiency is very common: it has been dissolved (leached) out of soils; it has been removed by centuries of cropping; it has been removed from grains by processing; it dissolves in cooking water; and it is removed by chelating agents, such as EDTA, added to food. Zinc deficiency causes a large number of symptoms, including stria, stretch marks in men and women, retarded growth of skin appendages, white areas in the nails, and acne. A deficiency of zinc interferes with the menstrual cycle (premenstrual tension), retards wound healing, and increases blood pressure, as well as causing joint pain, loss of taste and smell, psychiatric symptoms, and acrodermatitis enteropathica. A zinc deficiency is probably present if the subject finds a zinc sulfate solution, which normally should taste bitter, to have little or no taste at all.

Copper is needed for the formation of hemoglobin. The body contains about 125 mg. On the average, we ingest 3 to 5 mg, but we need only about 2 mg, so there is some accumulation. Dr Pfeiffer found no cases of deficiency in 20,000 patients examined. However, many vitamin and mineral preparations contain copper because of the widespread belief that copper deficiency is a serious problem. In certain areas where copper in soil is deficient and babies are fed cow milk, a copper deficiency may develop.

Copper deficiency is associated with the development of aortic aneurysms (an abnormal dilation or ballooning of a blood vessel), hypothyroidism, and high cholesterol. In one study, 13 autopsy subjects with aortic aneurysms and 13 autopsy control subjects were assessed for liver copper levels. The copper levels of the autopsy subjects were only 26% of the control subjects. Since copper is necessary for the proper cross-linking of collagen and elastin, deficiency of this mineral may cause weakened aortic tissue and greater susceptibility to aneurysms. Copper is also a necessary cofactor in the conversion of T_4 to the more potent thyroid hormone known as T_3 or triiodothyronine. If copper is deficient, this conversion will not be optimal, which can lead to under-functioning of the thyroid gland and increased total cholesterol levels.

Copper tends to accumulate if the diet is too low in zinc or where there is too much copper in the drinking water, usually due to copper plumbing and very soft water. Excess copper is associated with pregnancy problems, post partum psychosis, depression from birth control pills, and cancer.

The best measure of the copper and zinc status is the ratio of serum copper to zinc. The ratio is very high in cancer patients, and high ratios are associated with poor prognosis. Cancer patients with ratios under 1.75:1 have a much better outlook than when the ratio is higher. It has been suggested that the high ratio is also diagnostic. If there is a shadow in the lungs and the ratio is over 1.75:1, it is cancer with a 90% probability of being correct. If the ratio is under 1.75, it is probably not cancer.

Copper deficiency is associated with the development of aortic aneurysms (an abnormal dilation or ballooning of a blood vessel), hypothyroidism, and high cholesterol.

Dr Pfeiffer listed seven conditions where copper excess and zinc deficiency would occur: (1) during pregnancy, when growth and development require zinc; (2) during the first year when the newborn has excess copper and needs zinc to balance it; (3) during rapid growth; (4) from the 12th year when the maturing child needs zinc for normal pubertal growth; (5) during female adolescence (if zinc is low, premenstrual tension is common); (6) ages 15 to 20 for stress in general; (7) with stress in adults caused by illness, such as cancer, wounds, burns, hypertension, and in senile patients. Excess copper is also associated with a schizophrenic syndrome and with senility. We have found that copper levels increase substantially with age, and that presenile and senile patients have the greatest increase. Excess levels will be detected by dietary history, by blood tests, and by hair analysis.

Serum zinc levels tend to be very stable. A large series of patients we analyzed for the presence of copper and zinc showed that with increasing age there was no change in zinc levels, whereas copper levels went up significantly after age 50. Recently, we saw a patient, age 88, who has been coming to see us every year or two. We saw her first in 1986 when she complained she had lost her sense of taste, that food tasted awful, that she could not smell properly. She found eating almost intolerable, but knew she had to. She had been to see nearly 10 physicians, none of whom had been able to help her.

We suspected she had a zinc deficiency and started her on zinc supplements, using zinc sulfate 220 mg daily. After 2 years she was no better. One day, we asked her why she was still coming since we had not been of any use to her. We secretly hoped she would take that as a hint and not come again because we felt guilty whenever we saw her. She replied that at least we were willing to try to help. At this time, we gave her a liquid zinc and manganese preparation developed by Dr Pfeiffer (10% zinc sulfate and 0.5% manganese chloride). Two years later, she was much better. For the past 3 years, she has been well. She told us that she enjoyed eating. One of her new problems was she was a little too heavy. She was cheerful and relaxed and was still on the zinc manganese preparation.

Therapeutic Uses

Eating Disorders: Zinc deficiency is associated with eating disorders. Dr Schauss has summarized the research since 1934 establishing a relationship between zinc deficiency and eating disorders – specifically, obesity, pica, anorexia nervosa, and bulimia nervosa. Between 1985 and 1990, several studies showed that most eating disorder patients are low in zinc, and that when they are supplemented with liquid zinc 25 to 110 mg daily, they get better. Occasionally they had nausea, which was controlled by pretreating them with vitamin B-6. Dr Pfeiffer found that the combination of B-6 and zinc was more efficacious than either one alone. Rita Bakan, a psychologist at St. Paul's Hospital in Vancouver, found that adding zinc to the diet of anorexia patients helped them to regain weight. Vegetarians are more apt to be anorexic, and they are also more often low in zinc.

> Zinc deficiency is associated with eating disorders...specifically, obesity, pica, anorexia nervosa, and bulimia nervosa.

We find the connection between zinc and vitamin B-6 very interesting because it originated in some of our research in Saskatchewan, completed 35 years ago. We discovered a mauve staining substance in the urine of most schizophrenic patients when they were sick. If they recovered or went into remission, it disappeared from the urine. This was identified as kryptopyrrole. Dr Pfeiffer and his group at the Brain-Bio Center in Princeton discovered that too much of this compound caused a double deficiency of vitamin B-6 and zinc. This condition we had called malvaria, they termed, more appropriately, pyrroluria. The treatment included ample quantities of zinc and vitamin B-6.

While most schizophrenic patients have this factor, it is also present in a smaller proportion of non-schizophrenic patients suffering from depression, anxiety states, alcoholism, and behavioral disorders. It may be present in patients with eating disorders as well. We have described this in the section under vitamin B-6.

Epidermolysis bullosa: In Harrison's *Principles of Medicine*, an inherited zinc deficiency disease called epidermolysis bullosa is described. The symptoms and signs include severe chronic diarrhea, muscle wasting, and alopecia, as well as rough and thick ulcerated skin about the body orifices and on the extremities. Recently, we were consulted by a young man and his mother for help in the treatment of his severe intractable case of epidermolysis bullosa. His disease and his response to administration of zinc and a few other nutrients raises the possibility that his condition is a variant of a chronic zinc dependency.

A few days after this patient was born in June 1972, his skin, which had been under pressure from a forceps delivery, began to slough of. A few days later, lesions developed on his face, mouth, chest, and limbs, which later blistered. He was treated with topical antibiotics using sterile technique, but was no better. The lesions in his mouth made it impossible for him to feed, and he became anemic and hypoproteinemic. One month later, he was diagnosed with epidermolysis bullosa and started on vitamin E 600 IU daily, later increased to 800 IU. At age 4 months, 200 mg of ascorbic acid was added, and at age 6 months, he was given iron supplementation and the vitamin E was increased to 1000 IU. There was no response.

He was then admitted to hospital suffering from stomatitis, and later again for gastroenteritis and pneumonia. By now, he had multiple lesions and denuded areas on his legs, no nails, and adhesions between his fingers and his toes. In addition, he had been constantly constipated. His mother had to remove his stools manually daily.

In 1980, his parents took him to West Germany for 10 weeks to be treated by a biochemist who was using special skin salves and other treatment with some success. He was placed upon a vegetarian diet, supplemented with a moderate vitamin program, doses unknown. This regimen was helpful. They went back to Germany once more for 10 days and would have gone again, but they could no longer afford to do so.

When we first saw him, he appeared to be about 10 years old, very short and immature. Mentally he was normal; there were no perceptual changes, no thought disorder, and his mood was surprisingly cheerful and upbeat. The bullous lesions continued to erupt. He had lost all of his fingers and his toes. An attempt had been made to separate them surgically in Italy with no success. He told us that food did not taste normal. He was still severely constipated. Zinc deficiency will cause dwarfism, retarded wound healing, and loss of taste.

To test his sense of taste for a possible zinc deficiency, we gave him a teaspoon of a special zinc sulfate solution. He said it tasted like stale water, not bitter as it would to normal individuals. We could not order a blood test for zinc because all his superficial veins were gone and it would have required a cut down.

We advised him to start on the following supplements: niacinamide 500 mg twice daily, ascorbic acid 500 mg three times daily, pyridoxine 100 mg twice daily, cod liver oil 0.5 teaspoon daily, and 10 drops twice each day of a solution of zinc sulfate 10% and manganese chloride 0.5%, plus 1 teaspoon of linseed oil daily to increase his intake of omega-3 essential fatty acids.

Two weeks later, he was much improved. His mood remained normal, but his parents were much more cheerful. In that brief period, he had grown half of an inch in height, his skin was much healthier, and the lesions came on about one third as frequently. Those that did develop healed much more quickly. He gained 2 lb and was no longer constipated – he was able to have normal bowel movements for the first time in his life.

When we first saw him, his mother informed us that he was very sensitive to any tablets. Therefore, we had him start one nutrient at a time, and if there was no bad reaction, he was to proceed to the next. He had no bad reactions to any of the supplements. We increased his niacinamide to 500 mg three times a day and the ascorbic acid to 1 g twice a day. This patient's rapid response does not prove it was due entirely to the administration of the zinc. The other nutrients must also have played an important part, but we suspect that zinc was the main therapeutic variable. Single nutrient deficiencies are very rare. We could not in good conscience withhold the other nutrients since we were not certain that one alone might help. This can be determined later on by withdrawing one at a time to determine which are the most important. This family had already suffered too much and needed relief as quickly as possible.

Hypothyroidism: Zinc deficiency may also play a role in hypothyroidism, a condition characterized by an under-functioning thyroid gland. Zinc helps with the binding of T4 (thyroxine), which is one of the essential hormones produced by the thyroid gland that helps to optimize metabolism.

ADHD: Zinc probably plays an important role in correcting some of the biochemical abnormalities that lead to ADHD. Zinc helps the body and brain utilize essential fatty acids. A study published in the *Journal of Child Psychology & Psychiatry* in 1996 found that 48 children with ADHD had a mean serum zinc level far below normal. The investigators of this study were unsure if the decreased essential fatty acid levels were the principal cause of ADHD or if the disorder was the result of zinc deficiency. A recent randomized controlled trial has demonstrated another reason to supplement with zinc. The researchers discovered that taking a zinc supplement (15 mg per day of elemental zinc from 55 mg of zinc sulfate) with Ritalin (methylphenidate), significantly improved ADHD. Specifically, the Parent and Teacher Rating Scale scores improved with zinc sulfate over this 6-week trial. The results of these studies suggest that zinc is essential for the proper utilization of essential fatty acids, may improve the response to mainstream stimulant drugs, and can benefit children with ADHD.

Common Cold: Zinc lozenges are used to ward off the common cold and may be quite effective. Dr J.C. Godfrey and Dr B. Conant Sloane at Dartmouth College Health Service compared placebo against a zinc gluconate-glycine preparation for treating the common cold in a double-blind study using 23.7 mg of zinc. All symptoms disappeared in 4.9 days against the placebo 6.1 days. If treatment started after one day of the onset, the difference was greater, 4.3 days for the zinc group and 9.2 for the placebo control.

Optimum Dose

Zinc: Zinc is available in various tablets, such as gluconate, sulfate, citrate, succinate, and picolinate. There are also zinc chelates. Only a small percentage of the amount taken by mouth is absorbed. Liquid preparations are probably the most easily absorbed.

The optimum dose for adults is 30 to 50 mg of elemental zinc daily. Infants under 1 year need around 5 mg of elemental zinc each day, and children and adolescents need around 10 to 15 mg daily. It is very important that infants and children do get the optimal amount of daily zinc because it is essential for the attainment of maximum growth (that is, reaching one's genetic potential) for height and weight.

Copper: Copper is also available in various tablets, such as sebacate, citrate, picolinate, and amino acid chelates. The adult dose is around 1 to 3 mg daily of elemental copper. Infants and children need much less, typically less than 1 mg daily.

Safety

Zinc is water soluble and safe. It is very difficult to overdose, but there is no need to do so. Zinc sulfate doses of 220 mg taken three times per day have been recommended for arthritis, but usually doses one third that level are sufficient. Dr Pfeiffer described the case of a 16-year-old boy who took 12,000 mg over a 2-day period. He was drowsy for the next week, then recovered.

If high doses are taken for too long (> 150 mg per day of elemental zinc), it may drive copper levels too far down and lead to a depression of white blood cells and neutrophils (specialized type of white blood cells). This could be a major problem in areas where copper deficiency tends to be common. Soft water extracts copper from the plumbing in the average home.

Excess copper is treated by increasing the intake of zinc using Pfeiffer's solution, Zeman drops (10% zinc sulfate and 0.5% manganese chloride), ascorbic acid, high fiber diets, selenium, and, if necessary, copper chelators, such as penicillamine and EDTA.

Manganese

The body contains 10 to 20 mg of manganese. About 45% is absorbed from food, and 4 mg daily is excreted. The diet provides 2 to 9 mg.

Manganese deficiency is associated with growth impairment, abnormalities in bone, diabetic-like carbohydrate changes, incoordination, tardive dyskinesia, and convulsions. Zinc alone increases copper excretion in schizophrenics threefold; adding manganese increases the excretion even more. Giving zinc alone may induce a manganese deficiency.

Therapeutic Uses

Cerebral Function: Manganese plays a significant role in cerebral function, as it is a critical cofactor for glucose utilization within brain cells or neurons. Studies have shown this mineral to be useful in controlling seizure activity. It also has some antidepressant properties that may, in part, be explained by improvements in brain glucose metabolism.

HIV: Over the past few years, manganese has been studied for its potential effect on inhibiting an enzyme that helps to control HIV. Scientists at Johns Hopkins University have found that simply increasing manganese in cells can stop HIV's unusual ability to process its genetic information in reverse, and this might help to reduce the number of viruses that are replicated. To have any favorable effect on HIV, it is probably necessary to take enough manganese so that blood concentrations are higher than normal. In such cases, close monitoring by a healthcare professional would be necessary due the potential risk of manganese toxicity.

> Manganese deficiency is associated with growth impairment, abnormalities in bone, diabetic-like carbohydrate changes, incoordination, tardive dyskinesia, and convulsions.

Tardive Dyskinesia: Tranquilizers create a major toxic reaction called tardive dyskinesia, a motor disorder that can be irreversible. About 25% of patients on tranquilizers for long periods will suffer this disorder. The tranquilizers bind the manganese and are excreted, carrying the manganese with them and so cause a deficiency. Patients we have treated since 1955 with a naturopathic diet and orthomolecular medicine do not get this dreadful condition. Doses up to 30 mg are safe, but are seldom needed. We typically use less than 50 mg doses. If the drug companies would put 1 mg of manganese into every tranquilizer tablet, tardive dyskinesia would disappear. Good natural sources are tropical fruits and tea. British schizophrenics seem not to get tardive dyskinesia as often as America patients, perhaps because they drink much more tea.

Optimum Dose

Adults can safely take manganese in doses between 15 and 50 mg daily for therapeutic reasons. For adults with acute sports injuries (sprains, strains, and inflammation), manganese can be safely taken at a dosage of 200 mg daily for 2 weeks prior to resuming a lower daily dose. Infants require less than 1 mg daily, and children need 1 to 3 mg daily.

Manganese is best reserved for specific therapeutic reasons, when prescribed by a knowledgeable healthcare provider.

Safety

Manganese supplementation is very safe and has a low level of toxicity. The only real concern is that manganese can inhibit the absorption of iron, copper, and zinc – so extra attention should be given when supplementing with manganese to guard against a deficiency of these minerals.

Chromium

Glucose tolerance factor (GTF) contains one atom of chromium and two atoms of nicotinic acid. It has never been identified in humans and its structure has not been known until recently. Dr Walter Mertz suggested that it was a trivalent chromium atom attached to two niacin molecules and to four amino acids. Currently, the biologically active form of chromium is now considered to be a naturally occurring oligopeptide low-molecular weight chromium-binding substance (LMWCr). The LMWCr compound has been found in many different types of mammals, and is widely distributed in numerous tissues (e.g., liver, kidney, spleen, intestine, testicles, and brain). It comprises the amino acids glycine, cysteine, glutamic acid, and aspartic acid, with a multinuclear chromic assembly in which the chromic centers are bridged by the anionic ligands, oxide, and/or hydroxide.

Chromium deficiency is more likely than excess since it is present in the part of the grains commonly not used for food. Whole wheat contains about 1.7 mcg per gram, while white flour has only 0.14 mcg. The body loses more chromium when exercising and when consuming large amounts of sugar.

Therapeutic Uses

Diabetes: Chromium is an essential cofactor in the activity of insulin. It is thought to attach onto insulin and fasten it on the receptor. In a study involving 185 adult-onset diabetic patients, there were significant decreases in the concentration of fasting and 2-hour glucose levels, insulin, hemoglobin A_1C, and total cholesterol among patients supplemented with 1000 mcg of chromium picolinate compared to those on 200 mcg of chromium picolinate or placebo. Thus, chromium as part of the LMWCr should have the ability to improve glucose tolerance and increase insulin sensitivity in diabetic patients with poor glucose control.

Depression: Taking 500 mcg daily of chromium has antidepressant therapeutic properties. It is part of our natural program to treat mood disorders. It may act because it tends to stabilize blood sugar and decreases hypoglycemic episodes, which tend to aggravate depression and anxiety. A 1999 study published in the *Journal of Clinical Psychiatry* demonstrated that 200 mcg twice daily augmented conventional antidepressant therapy. In other words, combining chromium with standard antidepressant medication should increase the effectiveness of the drug treatment. A recent 2005 randomized control trial showed that 600 mcg of chromium improved atypical depression among patients with severe carbohydrate cravings.

Chromium deficiency is more likely than excess since it is present in the part of the grains commonly not used for food.

Other Conditions: Chromium in doses of 200 to 400 mcg daily has the following beneficial effects: decreases blood sugar; lowers cholesterol levels and elevates HDL; causes weight loss independent of exercise; and decreases body fat and increases lean body mass. It may be beneficial in preventing coronary disease. It decreases in tissues with age in societies where cardiovascular disease is very common. When given to rats, it prevented the formation of atheromatous lesions and increased life span. Chromium potentiated the hypocholesterolemic effect of nicotinic acid, and both taken together in small amounts improved glucose tolerance in elderly subjects, whereas either one alone had no effect. Given to rats it increased their life span by 1 year or 33%.

Optimum Dose

The RDA is around 100 mcg daily, but the average diet provides only 25 mcg. An optimum dose is 200 to 400 mcg daily, but sometimes doses as high as 8000 mcg daily are required (for example, in diabetes). The best food sources of chromium are brewer's yeast, sugar beet molasses, and meats, such as liver and beef.

Simple chromium salts do not have the same biological activity as GTF chromium. GTF chromium is absorbed better in the bowel and is more potent as an insulin potentiator, is better for improving impaired glucose tolerance, and is less toxic. Chromium polynicotinate (also called chromium nicotinate) is similar in properties to GTF.

Safety

Chromium has an exceptional safety profile. According to investigators, "there is no demonstration of general chromium toxicity in animals at a dose that would extrapolate to humans as 1050 mg daily." One of these investigators has even used 3000 to 4000 mcg of chromium as nicotinate given twice daily to adult-onset diabetic patients for months to years, resulting in tremendous reductions of glucose and lipid levels without any increases in blood urea nitrogen, liver enzymes, or other laboratory abnormalities. High supplemental doses of chromium would never come even close to 1050 mg per day.

Selenium

Once considered highly toxic, selenium is now known to be essential. When Dr Hoffer was working toward his M.S.A. in chemistry, he first studied selenium as a toxic component of wheat grown in South Dakota and in southwest Saskatchewan. For a while, there was some apprehension that wheat grown in these areas would be toxic to people. It was soon realized that wheat grown there, even if very high in selenium, would enter the huge main stream of wheat and would be diluted to the point it could do no harm.

Selenium-rich soils are found in the Great Plains and Rocky Mountain states. The Northeast, East, and Northwest of the U.S.A. are very low in selenium, as is southern British Columbia and Vancouver Island. On the Island, animals must be given selenium or they will not grow and thrive. Populations living on selenium rich soils have less cancer: southern Vancouver Island, low in selenium and carrying more mercury, has a very high incidence of cancer. In a recent study, it was also found that people had low selenium levels before they had a myocardial infarction.

Selenium promotes growth; protects against mercury, cadmium, arsenic, silver, copper, and other heavy metal poisoning; and protects against cancer. Selenium's most important property is its anticancer and antiviral properties. In spite of selenium's well-known preventive and therapeutic properties, it is not being added to our food, the amount in our soils is not being replenished, and ever more of our human population suffers the ravages of selenium deficiency.

Therapeutic Uses

Depression: Selenium has antidepressant properties, and for many people may be preferred to the major antidepressants. D. Benton and R. Cook found that subjects receiving 100 mcg of selenium improved mood over a five week period compared to placebo. In a double-blind cross-over study in *Biological Psychiatry,* 50 subjects received 100 mcg of selenium or placebo for 5 weeks. Subjects were given the Profile of Mood States to fill out during the study. They were also given a food frequency questionnaire that estimated their dietary intake of selenium. An adequate intake of selenium was correlated with a general elevation of mood and less anxiety. Those subjects with the lowest estimated level of selenium in their diets had a greater amount of reported improvements in symptoms of anxiety, depression, and tiredness following 5 weeks of supplementation. We have been giving our depressed patients 200 mcg twice each day when they do not want to take drugs and the results have been good.

Antioxidant: Selenium has very important biochemical properties with good clinical utility. One of the antioxidant enzymes in the body, known as glutathione peroxide, requires adequate selenium levels to function properly. This enzyme is a critical antioxidant enzyme that protects against free radicals (i.e., hydrogen peroxide and other lipid hydroperoxides). When selenium intake is insufficient, levels of the enzyme decrease, and clinical problems are more likely to arise.

Skin Conditions: Dr S.A. Levine and Dr P.M. Kidd, in their book *Antioxidant Adaptation,* cite a Swedish study that evaluated the levels of this critical enzyme in numerous patients with a variety of skin diseases. The study involved more than 500 patients with a diverse amount of dermatological conditions, and the levels of glutathione peroxidase were shown to be low in the majority of skin diseases. For example, eczema, atopic dermatitis, psoriasis, and dermatitis herpetiformis were found to have markedly decreased levels of the enzyme. Treatment with selenium and vitamin E for 6 to 8 weeks increased glutathione peroxidase levels and improved the majority of the skin diseases. We can recall one moderate case of eczema that completely cleared in 4 weeks from a mere 200 mcg of selenium daily. Selenium should be tried empirically for all skin diseases because the majority of them will show very good benefits from this mineral.

Thyroid Function: Adequate thyroid hormone function is also dependent on an adequate intake of selenium. Selenium is a cofactor for an enzyme that converts the thyroid hormones T4 to T3 in the liver. There is a thyroid condition, called underconversion hypothyroidism, where there is a problem with this conversion. Patients typically have normal thyroid blood tests, but can have a T3 test that is low or in the low-normal range. Some common symptoms of this condition are fatigue, difficulty losing weight, and mild depression. In a correspondence published in the *Journal of Orthomolecular Medicine* about selenium and hypothyroidism, Dr Hayashida stated: "Since being introduced to underconversion hypothyroidism, it is gratifying to see so many of our patients being cured of their low thyroid condition in the face of so-called normal thyroid laboratory tests. Many times just the addition of selenium (200 to 400 mcg daily) is enough to correct the hypothyroid condition."

> In spite of selenium's well-known preventive and therapeutic properties, it is not being added to our food, the amount in our soils is not being replenished, and ever more of our human population suffers the ravages of selenium deficiency.

Cancer: In his book *Selenium as Food and Medicine,* Richard A. Passwater described this vast importance of selenium. The amount of selenium in our soils is inversely related to the incidence of cancers of people living on those soils. Professor H.D. Foster reported that "there is a great deal of geographical and epidemiological evidence to suggest that cancer mortality tends to be depressed where environmental selenium levels are high. For cancer of the esophagus, the correlation coefficient was -0.55. Seldom are such high correlations found for biologic phenomena."

HIV/AIDS: Perhaps its most important role of selenium was missed until Professor Foster published his book *What Really Causes Aids.* An eminent student of catastrophes, he concludes that AIDS it is likely to become the greatest catastrophe in human history, predicting that by 2015 one-sixth of the world's population will have the disease. This is probably a gross underestimate for this major world pandemic.

According to Professor Foster, HIV/AIDS is caused by a deficiency of glutathione peroxidase, of which selenium is a component. Dr Taylor has likewise pointed out that selenium deficiency is a major factor and showed that HIV-1 encodes glutathione peroxidase. The virus cannot replicate without competing with its host for selenium. It has also been shown that AIDS patients are selenium deficient and that the greater this deficiency, the more apt they are to die. As the disease progresses, the deficiency increases. It is not surprising that poor nutrition increases susceptibility to the virus.

Selenium deficiency is a direct cause of the disease. HIV/AIDS produces a selenium deficiency in the body, and these patients die from this serious deficiency. The evidence is very powerful. In Senegal, there is a high level of unprotected sexual activity, yet in 1999, less than one per one thousand of the population of over 9 million had HIV/AIDS. In sharp contrast, in surrounding countries, such as South Africa, deaths from AIDS in 1999 were around 75 per 1000. Foster points out that in Senegal the soils are very rich in selenium, whereas in the neighboring countries they are not. In Finland, where selenium has been added to fertilizer since 1985, the incidence of HIV/AIDS has not increased in the past 10 years, while in the neighboring countries, where selenium is not added, it is twice as high.

The logical treatment of AIDS is to use selenium supplements, but also to ensure that the other components of glutathione peroxidase are available – the amino acids cysteine, glutamine, and tryptophan. Preliminary results confirm the therapeutic effect of these nutrient supplements.

Between 1900 and 1940, pellagra was one of the most serious pandemics in the Southern United States and around Mediterranean countries where corn was the staple food. The U.S. Public Health Service assigned the problem to Dr Joseph Goldberger. The favorite medical theory was that pellagra was an infection, but he soon deduced that it was a deficiency disease and showed how it could be prevented and cured. Dr Goldberger saved millions of people from the ravages of that dreadful disease and paved the way for the eradication of pellagra by the enrichment of flour with small amounts of niacinamide, starting about 1941 in the United States. A few pennies worth of vitamin saved billions of dollars worth of costs and the lives and health of the patients who would have gotten pellagra but for his work.

We think the situation with HIV/AIDS is similar, but with one major difference. HIV/AIDS is much more serious, is much more prevalent, and is present or will be present everywhere except in some areas where the soils are very rich in selenium, such as in Senegal. The preliminary therapeutic trials reported by Professor Foster support his hypothesis that this disease is caused by a deficiency of the components of glutathione peroxidase, of which selenium is a very important one. In Africa, the diet is so poor that amino acids deficiency must be common. In North America, this deficiency is not as marked, but selenium deficiency is still a major problem. It will be a major catastrophe if Foster's hypothesis is submerged by antiretroviral therapies and is not examined as quickly and fully as possible.

The logical treatment of AIDS is to use selenium supplements, but also to ensure that the other components of glutathione peroxidase are available – the amino acids cysteine, glutamine, and tryptophan.

The results of Professor Foster's preliminary trials are published in *What Really Causes AIDS*. AIDS is a nutritional disease, caused by a virus, he hypothesizes. Because HIV and humans both encode for the selenoenzyme glutathione peroxidase, the virus competes with its host for the four nutrients required to produce this antiviral enzyme: selenium, cysteine, tryptophan and glutamine. This means the symptoms of AIDS can prevented by supplementation with this trace element and three amino acids. What follows is supporting evidence for this hypothesis:

- In a series of open trials conducted in Africa, these supplements were administered to AIDS patients. Trials began in an AIDS hospice in South Africa, where five out of six AIDS patients greatly improved. Problems cases that had extreme diarrhea developed secondary deficiencies and could not absorb adequate nutrients. Another initial small trial took place in a Kenyan clinic, where patients here were weak and passing into AIDS. They soon recovered their energy and are now in much better health. None of the patients in either of these trials had ever taken antiretroviral drugs.
- Two larger open trials were set up. The first, in a Ugandan hospital, involved 40 HIV/AIDS patients. After one month, 77% reported a noticeable improvement in their health. These results were better than they seemed at first glance because seven of these patients also had tuberculosis and four also suffered from syphilis. Improvement continued

with the passage of time. In Zambia, the nutritional supplements were provided to a childcare and adoption society. The initial report from this organization was on 15 orphans and guardians who were HIV/AIDS patients. Several also had tuberculosis. Most people given the supplements improved within the first 2 weeks. A noticeable improvement started between the second and third week of taking the supplements. Their complexions, hair texture, and general outlook of their bodies improved. The supplements also gave them enough energy to move around, some have gained weight, and some who were bedridden started walking on their own.

Beyond such open clinical trials, Professor Foster has also collected considerable anecdotal evidence from North America AIDS patients that confirm the therapeutic value of selenium supplements given with these amino acids. Patients taking antiretroviral drugs as well as the four key nutrients seem to progress very well, showing that there is no antagonism with the conventional treatment.

In addition, R. Kupk and colleagues have reported in *The Journal of Nutrition* on the relationship between death from AIDS and plasma selenium levels in pregnant women in Tanzania. Blood was collected from 949 pregnant women and saved for 5.7 years, by which time 306 of them had died. Statistical analyses showed that the lower her original plasma selenium level, the more likely the woman was to have died of AIDS. This selenium-death relationship was statistically significant.

Optimum Dose

The therapeutic dose is between 200 and 600 mcg daily. Patients have taken up to 2000 mcg daily, though we do not recommend this.

Safety

Selenium toxicity is extremely rare. When taken for long periods of time (more than a few years), intakes above 900 mcg daily can produce toxicity signs and symptoms, such as depression, nervousness, nausea and vomiting, and a garlic-breath odor. However, toxicity is extremely rare and unlikely because many patients (especially those with cancer) have used doses as high as 2000 mcg for years without any problems or evidence of toxicity.

Possibly Essential Minerals

Fluoride

Fluoride has been used a supplement for preventing dental caries and studied as a treatment for osteoporosis. In both cases, the reviews are mixed, even controversial.

Therapeutic Uses

Dental Caries: The controversy over the addition of fluoride to the public water supply still rages. Proponents of fluoride maintain that it is an important public health measure for decreasing the number of carious teeth in children, and that the only way to ensure it will be used universally is to place it in our water so we will have no choice. They maintain that this means of supplementation is safe.

Opponents maintain that the improvement in the teeth of children is not proven and that there is the same decrease in carious teeth over time in children in areas where the water was never fluoridated. They also maintain that its safety has not been proven; that, in fact, it is toxic, causing an increase in the incidence of cancer, mottling of teeth, and other undesirable changes. They maintain that if parents want their children to receive the benefit of fluoride, they can use fluoride toothpaste and have their dentists apply it. They claim that the main reason for the massive use of fluoride today is the desire of the chemical companies to dispose of their excess fluoride by dumping it into our drinking water.

The anti-fluoridationists seem to be slowly winning the battle as communities are reversing their stance and making it illegal to use fluoride. *The Medical Tribune* recently carried the headline: "60% of Drinking Water Fluoridated, but Tide Turns."

Osteoporosis: Fluoride has been examined as a treatment for osteoporosis. However, the results of several clinical trials have shown that it is not helpful. There is an increase in bone density, but the bones become much more brittle. Dr Lawrence Riggs at the Mayo Clinic reported the results of a 4-year study, in which he gave to 202 postmenopausal women with osteoporosis and vertebral fractures 75 mg of sodium fluoride or placebo. They all received 1500 mg of calcium as well. There was an increase in bone density and a redistribution of bone. Each group suffered the same number of new fractures, but the number of nonvertebral fractures at the hip was higher in the fluoride group. Fluoride users also had more fractures of the femur. Two-thirds of the users suffered severe side effects. He concluded that fluoride increased bone density, but made the bones too fragile.

Except for the prevention of dental carries (controversial), supplementation with sodium fluoride is not recommended because there are much better and safer ways of effectively treating osteoporosis.

Optimum Dose

In very few cases, sodium fluoride is given as a treatment for osteoporosis at a dosage of 25 to 40 mg twice daily. When supplementing with fluoride, one must also take optimal doses of calcium to prevent bone loss at the appendicular skeleton. Except for the prevention of dental carries (controversial), supplementation with sodium fluoride is not recommended because there are much better and safer ways of effectively treating osteoporosis.

Safety

It is best to not supplement with extra fluoride, except when it is obtained in small amounts from the daily brushing of the teeth or from using mouthwashes. Fluoride supplementation is not that safe. It can weaken parts of the skeleton, encourage the development of various cancers, and cause neurological and behavioral (for example, hyperactivity) impairments. When taken at high supplemental doses (75 to 100 mg daily over several years), it has been associated with nausea and vomiting, organ damage, and bloody diarrhea.

Lithium

Lithium should probably be considered an essential mineral. It has diverse biochemical and clinical effects that can help a variety of medical maladies. It appears that lithium is an important essential mineral, particularly among individuals living in areas with little or no lithium in the water supply.

Therapeutic Uses

Bipolar Disorder: The lithium carbonate drug has proven very valuable in stabilizing bipolar patients.

Mood Disturbances and Violent Behavior: A sub-optimal intake of lithium might be a predisposing risk factor for mood disturbances, violent behavior, and possibly even incarceration. Lithium might have a favorable effect on the prevention of violence and other associated crimes. In a 1990 study by G.N. Schrauzer and K.P. Shrestha, the drinking water of 27 Texas counties was analyzed for its lithium content. Normally, lithium in drinking water should range from 70-170 mcg/L. In the Texas counties with the lowest lithium content (< 70 mcg/L), there were higher incidences of rates of robbery, burglary, and theft. In the counties with low water lithium content, there was also significant increases in the incidences of arrests for possession of opium, cocaine, and their derivatives (morphine, heroin, and codeine). These investigators hypothesize that lithium has a moderating influence on criminal and deviant behaviors. The addition of lithium to water supplies might be an important therapy for the reduction of crime, suicide, and drug-dependency at the individual and community level.

Herpes: This mineral also helps in the prevention and treatment of oral and genital herpes infections. Lithium has been shown to inhibit the herpes virus replication (both HSV-1 and HSV-2 types) in both in vitro and in vivo studies. This may be due to enhanced immune function, and/or from some type of interaction between magnesium-dependent enzymes. It is effective when applied topically to the herpes lesions in the forms of lithium succinate (8%) or lithium chloride solutions. To speed the recovery from a herpes infection, lithium can also be supplemented at a dose of 5 to 10 mg, two to three times daily.

Other Conditions: Lithium also increases the uptake of vitamin B12, and enhances the transport of folic acid into cells. This is of interest due to the clinical usefulness of lithium therapy for depression.

Optimum Dose

There is no established RDA for lithium. The RDA for lithium would probably be in microgram doses. The mean daily intake for adults in one study was 730 mcg each day. This value was based upon the average hair lithium concentrations among 2,648 predominantly American adults.

> It appears that lithium is an important essential mineral, particularly among individuals living in areas with little or no lithium in the water supply.

Good over-the-counter forms of this mineral are lithium aspartate, lithium orotate, or lithium from vegetable source. For a herpes outbreak, 5 to 10 mg two to three times daily of lithium aspirate or orotate can be used until the lesions resolve. For bipolar disorder, lithium carbonate is useful at dosages of 300 to 900 mg daily, but can have significant side effects. For the treatment of mild mood disturbances, 5 mg per day of lithium aspartate or orotate might be helpful. Even smaller microgram doses of vegetable source lithium might help to prevent mood disturbances and violent tendencies.

Safety

Nutritional doses of lithium will not increase blood levels like the carbonate form. However, nutritional doses can increase the concentration of lithium in the hair. All forms of lithium (except small microgram doses) can potentially increase the excretion of sodium from the kidneys and lead to sodium depletion. For this reason, anyone supplementing with lithium should not be on a salt-restricted diet. Lithium carbonate can also induce low thyroid function and can cause tremor, kidney toxicity, or even visual loss. The real safety concerns are primarily with the carbonate form of lithium. Supplementing with sunflower, safflower, or flaxseed oils may ameliorate some of the side effects from the carbonate form, but more research is needed to substantiate this.

Non-essential Toxic Minerals

Six metals are toxic – aluminum, mercury, cadmium, silver, gold, and lead. Aluminum is present in our food, in drinking water, in cooking utensils, in cosmetics, and in preservatives. Mercury is present in our water and food (especially in certain fish), and along with silver and gold is used in dental amalgams. Cadmium is present in the air around tires that are being worn down by use. Lead was used in gasoline and paint for many years and is still used in some cooking utensils.

While the toxicity of cadmium, silver, gold, and lead is now universally accepted, aluminum and mercury are still the subject of debate between proponents who maintain they are safe as used and those, like us, who maintain that they are toxic and ought not to be used. The aluminum and mercury debates recall the controversy raged over lead added to gasoline to prevent the motor from pinging and to paint to improve adhesion, used in shot gun pellets and lead sinkers for fishing, and used in glassware (leaded glass) and cookware because of its weight and pliability. The debate over lead illustrates very clearly how high-tech societies have approached innovation. Toxic minerals are added to products because they give them a quality that is desirable commercially. When these metals

> While the toxicity of cadmium, silver, gold, and lead is now universally accepted, aluminum and mercury are still the subject of debate between proponents who maintain they are safe as used and those, like us, who maintain that they are toxic and ought not to be used.

were introduced, little thought was given to the effect they would have on the health of the population. After they were used on a large scale, there was a slow, tedious, and costly accumulation of research data showing they were toxic. Finally, after extreme counter pressure, governments, with great reluctance, forced the removal of these products. The procedure seems to be threefold: add the product without concern for the health consequences; prevent any serious examination of the effect on health as long as possible; give way as slowly as possible on the plea that it would be too expensive to change these dangerous practices quickly. Meanwhile millions will have suffered from the exposure to these products.

Aluminum

Organic forms of aluminum are more toxic than aluminum salts. Thus, aluminum hydroxide is absorbed poorly from the gut, while aluminum citrate passes rapidly into the blood. The aluminum in drinking water is inorganic and also in salt form. In one study of aluminum in drinking water, 52% was aluminum hydroxide, 29% was associated with organic material, and 19% was a fluoride complex.

Toxicity

Alzheimer's Disease: The evidence pointing to aluminum as one of the causes of Alzheimer's disease is powerful and becoming stronger. Professor D.R. Crapper McLachlan, Director of the Centre for Research in Neurodegenerative Disease at the University of Toronto, concluded that public health efforts to reduce exposure to aluminum would reduce the incidence of Alzheimer's disease. He reviewed four lines of evidence. Aluminum impaired learning and memory performance in animals. Aluminum induced neurochemical changes in the brain. It interferes with over 65 different reactions in the body. It deposits in four sites in the brain – in the neurofibrillary tangles, in the amyloid cores of senile plaques, in the ferritin extracted from the brain, and in the chromatin fractions. Even moderate increases of aluminum in the blood are toxic. Many epidemiological studies support the hypothesis. If aluminum is removed using desferoxamine, there is less deterioration compared to a control group. This substance binds aluminum and reduces the amount in the body.

Dr McLachlan made the following suggestions. Exposure to aluminum should be minimized, but this will be difficult since it is found in food and added to drinking water, many processed foods, cosmetics, toothpaste, and a variety of other cosmetics. Public action is necessary. Aluminum content should be listed on packages and in cosmetic products. Municipal processed water should be regulated so there is less than 50 mcg per liter and eventually less than 10 mcg. Daily intake should be lowered to 3 mg or less.

Two orthomolecular treatments – malic acid and silic/silicon – might have some value in treating clinical conditions where aluminum is suspected as causing damage. Malic acid is found in high concentrations in apples and in many other fruits and vegetables that are preserved by fermentation. When supplemented at doses of 1500 to 2400 mg per day, malic acid is a very effective method for chelating aluminum and, possibly, for lowering brain aluminum levels as well. It also prevents aluminum from binding to cellular lipid membranes, thus reducing /preventing cellular toxicity.

Sources of silica include high-fiber cereal grains and root vegetables. By taking 5 mg of silica with meals, the aluminum that might be present in foods or liquids would bind to the silica, forming a non-absorbable compound, known as aluminosilicate. This silica-aluminum compound prevents aluminum from being absorbed from the gastrointestinal tract, thus reducing aluminum availability to the brain and other tissues. An acceptable daily amount of silica is between 5 to 20 mg.

Mercury

Mercury amalgams in dental practice are easy to install and aluminum chemicals add certain qualities to food and cosmetics that are seen to be desirable. Mercury is a highly toxic liquid mineral with a relatively high vapor pressure, which, therefore, vaporizes very easily.

Toxicity

Psychosis: Mercury has been known for many years as a brain toxin that will cause psychosis. The "mad hatters" of Europe were mercury-intoxicated hat makers. Mercury vapor will rarely be a factor today. However, about 20 years ago we saw two men in 1 month, both with the schizophrenic syndrome caused by prolonged contact with liquid mercury. Eliminating the mercury also eliminated the psychotic condition.

> Contrary to the view put forward by the dental profession, mercury is not harmless when present in the amalgam with other metals; rather, it gradually disappears from the amalgams and seeps into the rest of the body.

Intoxication: The major source of intoxication from mercury comes from the mercury amalgams dentists have introduced into our mouths. The mercury is thereafter absorbed both from the vapor and from direct contact with tissue in the gums. However, this view is stoutly attacked by the dental and medical professions. This debate is as vigorous as it was for lead and as it still is for fluoride.

While Dr Hal Huggins is one of the early and strongest critics of the use of mercury amalgams, the sharpest scientific attack comes from Dr Murray

J. Vimy, Clinical Professor in the Department of Medicine, University of Calgary, and Dr D. Shwartzendruber, Chair of the Biology Department, University of Colorado. Dr Shartzendruber presented evidence to the Washington State Dental Disciplinary Board during a hearing on a proposed restriction regarding dentists making statements against the use of mercury amalgams. He noted that mercury amalgams contain over 50% mercury, 35% silver, 13% tin, and lesser amounts of copper.

Contrary to the view put forward by the dental profession, mercury is not harmless when present in the amalgam with other metals; rather, it gradually disappears from the amalgams and seeps into the rest of the body. It is released as vapor, which is increased by chewing. The amount released accumulates daily. The mercury lodges in the tissues, is absorbed by the lungs and intestinal tract, and accumulates in the brain and other organs. Methyl mercury is absorbed from the mouth and goes directly to the brain.

Dr Shartzendruber added that as a general toxin it affected all tissues. There is no safe level except zero. He pointed up that the World Health Organization had determined that amalgams were the prime source of human mercury exposure. In his view, people in general looked upon mercury toxicity as being as serious as asbestos and DDT poisoning, more serious than lead paint and auto emissions, and slightly less serious than PCBs and uranium mining.

Dr Vimy also reported the results of his studies with sheep to the Washington State Dental Disciplinary Board Public Hearing. He placed mercury amalgams in sheep and studied what happened to the mercury. Within 30 days, substantial amounts of mercury were taken into their tissues. The same occurred with monkeys. Sheep lost 50% of their ability by their kidneys to recycle sodium, and the secretion of albumin decreased. He then referred to studies showing that Alzheimer's patients have five to eight times more mercury in their brains than the normal population. The greatest amount was found in those parts of the brain where the Alzheimer's lesions were present. He concluded that mercury is released from amalgams; it is released continuously when we chew; it is taken up into the tissues in animal models, particularly the liver, gastrointestinal tract, and kidneys; and it can induce pathology in sheep. Removal of the mercury improves kidney function. It is linked to Alzheimer's disease and to the development of antibiotic resistant bacteria. The board eventually decided not to bring in their pernicious recommendation.

In a recent paper, Dr A. Summers, Professor of Microbiology at the University of Georgia, reported that mercury fillings weakened the effectiveness of antibiotics against bacteria. This means that for some patients the usual amount of antibiotic will be inadequate, and they will have to be given much higher doses. For others, the antibiotic will be ineffective at any dose. The implications are chilling. Some bacteria were resistant to six antibiotics.

Recently, Dr Siblerud found that a very significant deterioration of psychological health occurred in people with mercury amalgams and an improvement occurred when these fillings were removed. Fifty subjects with fillings had 1.43 ppm in their hair and 3.70 ppm in urine, compared with 50 with no fillings who had 1.13 in hair and 1.23 in urine. The amalgam group was more depressed, had less peace of mind, and had more problems in concentration. They had more than twice as many complaints, such as sudden outbursts of anger, depression, irritability, and anxiety. They craved sweets more, smoked more, and drank more coffee and alcohol. A further study on subjects after the mercury was removed showed that 80% felt much better. They were less nervous, less depressed, felt more confident, and their memory was better.

Recently, one of our female patients had all her amalgams removed. She had been depressed for many years and had failed to get well after 2 years of psychiatric treatment, but within a few weeks after the mercury was removed, she was free of depression. Higher levels of lead and mercury have been found in the hair of emotionally disturbed children.

Not everyone will need to have amalgams removed, even though this would be ideal. But whenever a person has any physical or mental problem for which there appears to be no cause and which has remained untreatable, it is important to examine the question whether mercury amalgams might be an important factor. More dentists are familiar with mercury toxicity and have developed methods for helping determine whether there is a problem. They take special precautions not to expose themselves to mercury. Even their associations, who stoutly defend the use of mercury, advise their members not to be exposed to it. They think it is all right to maintain continuous exposure in one's mouth but not in their offices. Even undertakers now have to be careful. So many bodies being cremated contain mercury, there is a great danger that the mercury vapor will injure them while they are working. Dentists will want mercury analysis of blood and urine and will do certain conductivity tests in the mouth plus their personal examination of the teeth. Everyone should insist that mercury amalgams not be used and gradually replace existing mercury amalgam fillings with other material. When the demand for other safer compositions becomes noticeable, the manufacturers will surely meet the demand and dentists will learn the needed skills to work with these materials.

Detoxification

The final diagnosis of metal toxicity for aluminum and mercury, as well as for cadmium, silver, gold, and lead, is made by laboratory tests, namely blood analysis, urine analysis, and hair analysis. Once toxicity is diagnosed, the source of the toxic mineral must be determined and withdrawn. Then the naturopathic diet should be instituted.

Removing additives decreases the toxic burden on the body and adding fiber increases the excretion of toxic minerals. Then chelating compounds are used. The safest is ascorbic acid, which should be given in optimum doses. The three other chelating compounds that bind minerals and remove them are penicillamine for copper, desferoxamine for aluminum and iron, and EDTA for iron and other compounds. This is called chelation therapy when it is given by vein in a series of treatments.

Finally, natural antidotes should be used, such as selenium against mercury and cadmium, malic acid against aluminum, zinc and manganese against copper, and zinc against cadmium. There is also some clinical utility for compounds that impair gastrointestinal absorption and/or enhance excretion through the feces – these are silica to prevent aluminum absorption and alkylglycerols to increase fecal and urinary removal of mercury. Some effective strategies to remove mercury include selenium and shark liver oil.

Selenium is an effective chelator of mercury. It has been shown to reduce pubic hair mercury levels in just 4 months of continued use. Shark liver oils contain compounds known as alkylglycerols, which reduce the tissue deposition of metallic mercury and increase excretion through the urine and feces.

⑬ AMINO ACIDS

Eight of the 22 amino acids that have been identified are considered essential supplements because they cannot be made in the body and adequate amounts must, therefore, be present in the food. These are isoleucine, leucine, lysine, methionine, phenylalanine, threonine, tryptophan, and valine. The other 14 amino acids are inter-convertible in the body, and for this reason, have been labeled non-essential. These include arginine, tyrosine, glycine, serine, glutamic acid, glutamine, aspartic acid, taurine, carnitine, cystine, histidine, proline, alanine, and gamma-aminobutyric acid (GABA). They are all *essential*, however, and if there is a metabolic problem resulting in a deficiency of any of the 22, the results would be devastating to the body.

The amino acids available over the counter usually come in the L-form, which is the most physiologic or natural composition that exists in the body. Other forms are also occasionally available – the D-form or DL-form – but are not as physiologically natural.

In the last decade, there has been much more interest in studying the clinical applications of many of the amino acids, including ones from both the essential and non-essential groups. In this chapter, the clinical uses of tryptophan and 5-hydroxytryptophan, tyrosine and phenylalanine, arginine, carnitine, glutamine, and the main inhibitory amino acids (GABA, glycine, and taurine) will be discussed.

Tryptophan and 5-Hydroxytryptophan (5-HTP)

Tryptophan and 5-HTP are used clinically to increase the production of serotonin in the brain. Serotonin is involved in controlling mood and sleep, with a deficiency causing anxiety, depression, and insomnia. It is implicated in numerous other neuropsychiatric conditions. Tryptophan is also a precursor of vitamin B-3 in the form of nicotinamide adenine dinucleotide (NAD). Most of the tryptophan proceeds down the pathway that leads to NAD, but only 1 mg of it is produced from 60 mg of tryptophan. Pellagra is caused by a deficiency of tryptophan and vitamin B-3. The usual pellagra producing diet was rich in corn and very deficient in high-quality protein-containing foods. It had too little tryptophan, too little vitamin B-3, too little isoleucine, and too much leucine. 5-HTP is the immediate precursor to serotonin, whereas tryptophan is not. Unlike tryptophan, 5-HTP is not converted into NAD and is more potent than tryptophan for clinical applications.

Therapeutic Use

Tryptophan is used for treating depression, as well for controlling manic-depressive mood swings. It may be used alone or in combination with other antidepressants, such as the amine oxidase inhibitors, tyrosine, and lithium. We have used tryptophan for at least the past 30 years, but primarily for patients with insomnia. It is very helpful to 50% of the patients, and they awaken in the morning without hangover. They much prefer it to hypnotics.

5-HTP has also been shown to benefit depression, fibromyalgia, obesity, insomnia, and chronic headaches. It can reduce pain, improve fatigue, mitigate carbohydrate cravings, and enhance sleep quality and REM sleep, which explain the value of using this amino acid for the treatment of many clinical conditions.

Optimum Dose

Tryptophan requires a prescription for use, whereas 5-HTP is available over the counter as an extract from the African seed plant, *Griffonia simplicifolia*.

Tryptophan: Tryptophan is used in doses of 500 mg to 12 g daily. For insomnia, the dose is 1 to 3 g taken before bed on an empty stomach. If it is taken with food, it has difficulty passing into the brain and, therefore, has no effect on the serotonin levels. When taken on an empty stomach, it does not have to compete with other amino acids. For depression, we have been using 3 to 6 g daily, as well as for manic depression (bipolar disease).

5-HTP: 5-HTP can be taken with food since it is not affected by the ingestion of other amino acids. It is more potent than tryptophan, and the initial dose should be 50 mg, three times daily. If no response occurs after 2 weeks of use, the dose can be increased to 100 mg three times daily, or 300 mg at bedtime for the treatment of insomnia. 5-HTP can cause nausea, so the dose needs to be increased gradually.

Safety

Toxicity: In the United States, tryptophan was not available for some time because many feared it is toxic; however, it is now available again. In Canada, it was available from health food stores and also by prescription. The health food store preparation has been withdrawn, but the prescription product called Tryptan is freely available.

In October 1989, several people in New Mexico became very tired with sore muscles. Their white blood cells were increased. All had taken the amino acid tryptophan. This condition was later called eosinophilia-myalgia syndrome (EMS) and was reported in Europe and elsewhere in America. Symptoms included pain, swelling of the extremities, and severe muscle symptoms involving nerve damage. The eosinophil (a type of white blood cell) count went high. By August 1990, more than 1500 cases had been reported with 27 deaths. In November 1989, tryptophan supplements were recalled, and a few months later, all products containing tryptophan were also recalled.

The Center for Disease Control suggested, however, that the problem was caused by a contaminant. Six companies in Japan made all the tryptophan used in the United States. In October 1990, K. Sakimoto isolated and identified an impurity from tryptophan, which, in acid fluid, as in the stomach, broke down into tryptophan and a toxic chemical. Even though tryptophan was thus proven safe and effective, the FDA has still not removed its ban on its use. The health food industry believes that this is a political decision, not based upon scientific data, and is fighting back.

> **Tryptophan is used for treating depression, as well for controlling manic-depressive mood swings.**

Serotonin Syndrome: The use of 5-HTP or tryptophan with antidepressant medications may cause an overproduction of serotonin, leading to a condition known as serotonin syndrome. Although many healthcare professionals have combined these treatments, careful monitoring is necessary. Serotonin syndrome is usually a medical emergency, characterized by agitation, confusion, delirium, tachycardia (excessive heart rate), sweatiness, and blood pressure changes.

Phenylalanine and Tyrosine

Phenylalanine is partially converted in the body into tyrosine. Tyrosine is a precursor to catecholamines (noradrenaline/norepinephrine, etc.) and to thyroid hormone. It is also the precursor to melanin, a major pigment in the body. It has antidepressant properties, probably because it acts in the same way in the body as does phenylalanine.

Therapeutic Uses

When the body cannot make any tyrosine, it causes a condition known as phenylketonuria. Untreated, it leads to mental retardation, which may be very severe. These children have to be on special phenylalanine-free diets. Phenylalanine is used as a treatment for depression since it increases the production of noradrenaline. The DL-form of phenylalanine is helpful in controlling pain since it inhibits the breakdown of endorphins (natural painkillers) made in the body.

   Dr Priscilla Slagle uses a combination of tryptophan with phenylalanine and tyrosine as a treatment for depression. She was depressed herself for many years, did not respond to the usual treatment, but recovered on the program she developed, as she describes in her book *The Way Up From Down*. She recommends that people suffering from depression take tyrosine 500 to 3500 mg on rising in the morning and again mid-afternoon. These should be taken without high-protein food. One starts with 500 to 1000 mg daily for one week, then the dose is increased gradually, depending upon the response. After several weeks or months, if the response is not adequate, she adds phenylalanine to the program.

She also recommends tryptophan, 500 to 6000 mg at bedtime, taken on an empty stomach or with carbohydrate, not with protein; B complex (50) at breakfast and again after dinner at night; ascorbic acid, up to 4 g daily; and a good multi-mineral preparation providing calcium 250 to 1000 mg, magnesium 125 to 599 mg, manganese 10 to 30 mg, zinc 15 to 30 mg, selenium 50 to 200 mcg, and chromium 50 to 200 mcg. Dr Slagle also prescribes dietary changes to improve this. The results are probably as good, if not better, than the results using antidepressant drugs. If the full program is not followed, one could try individual doses of these amino acids.

When the body cannot make any tyrosine, it causes a condition known as phenylketonuria. Untreated, it leads to mental retardation, which may be very severe.

Optimum Dose

In Canada, tyrosine is readily available, but phenylalanine (at present) is not. In the United States, both are available over the counter. Phenylalanine can be found in several different forms (L-form, DL-form, or D-form), and each form has similar clinical uses.

The dose of tyrosine should be slowly increased over several weeks until 100 mg/kg/day is reached. The dose of DL-phenylalanine is 150 to 200 mg per day (helpful for both pain and depression), and for D-phenylalanine it is 350 mg/day but may need to be increased to have any antidepressant effects. For the L-form of phenylalanine, the dose can be increased over several weeks, from an initial dose of 500 mg per day, eventually to 14 g per day if necessary.

Side Effects

It is important to monitor for side effects, such as insomnia, restlessness, anxiety, and agitation, when supplementing with these amino acids.

Arginine

Arginine is really a semi-essential amino acid because many physiological processes require it, namely, the immune, endocrine, and cardiovascular systems. Arginine gets into the body primarily through dietary means, although it can be synthesized in the body from glutamine, glutamate, and proline. The absorption of arginine is excellent, with some 50% of it being converted into ornithine after absorption. Although arginine has been used for numerous clinical conditions, it is best reserved for the treatment of cardiovascular diseases, erectile dysfunction (ED) and male infertility, and improving athletic performance.

Therapeutic Uses

Cardiovascular Diseases: Arginine helps a variety of cardiovascular diseases because it dilates blood vessels by increasing the production of nitric oxide (NO), causing blood vessels to relax and open-up. In angina pectoris, the arteries supplying the heart are compromised, resulting in a lack of oxygen and the production of symptoms (varying in intensity and duration), such as chest pain, anxiety, and shortness of breath.

> Although arginine has been used for numerous clinical conditions, it is best reserved for the treatment of cardiovascular diseases, erectile dysfunction (ED) and male infertility, and improving athletic performance.

A number of clinical trials using doses in the range of 6 to 15 g of arginine per day have demonstrated improvements in blood flow through the coronary arteries, quality of life, and exercise tolerance. Not all of the studies have shown favorable therapeutic results, but the addition of arginine to standard angina treatment is probably a very good idea. At 6 g daily, arginine was shown to lower blood pressure in a very small trial with hypertensive patients refractory to standard ACE-inhibitor and diuretic therapies. In doses ranging from 5 to 15 g daily, arginine can also help congestive heart failure patients by improving blood flow, arterial compliance, functional status, exercise tolerance, and kidney function. Recently, a sustained-release arginine has become available in the United States and is probably more effective than the immediate-release arginine. By lasting longer in the bloodstream, sustained-release arginine should allow for a longer duration of blood vessel dilation at smaller dosage levels.

Erectile Dysfunction: Arginine is also useful for erectile dysfunction (ED). In fact, problems with penile endothelial arginine are thought to be responsible for part of the pathogenesis of ED. In a small clinical trial involving men with ED, 40% of the treatment group on 2.8 g of arginine daily for 2 weeks demonstrated improvements compared to no improvements among men in the placebo group. In a larger trial, 50 men with ED were given 5 g of arginine per day or a matching placebo for 6 weeks. There was a subjective improvement among 31% of the men in the arginine group. Another study combined 1.7 g of arginine with increasing doses of pycnogenol in a 3-month trial involving 40 men with ED. All the men took 1.7 g of arginine during the first month, and then during the second month were given 40 mg of pycnogenol twice daily with the same dose of arginine. During the third month, the dose of the pycnogenol was increased to 40 mg three times daily with the same dose of arginine. At the end of the second month, 80% reported a normal erection, and by the end of the third month, this therapeutic response increased to 92.5%. Other benefits that were noted included a quicker erection in response to stimulation and an increased duration of erection.

Male Infertility: Arginine also has some benefit for the treatment of male infertility. In some trials, the use of arginine has increased both sperm counts and motility, resulting in more successful pregnancies.

Athletic Performance: Another common use of arginine is for improving athletic performance. Arginine can increase growth hormone and have a tissue building or anabolic effect in some populations, but it is not exactly known how it accomplishes this. In a few trials, arginine has been combined with ornithine and the results have been encouraging. When doses in the range of 500 to 1000 mg of each are used, there can be decreases in body fat and improvements in strength and lean muscle tissue. That is why body builders and athletes looking for an "edge" over their competition commonly use arginine.

Other Conditions: Arginine has also been used for diabetic patients, burn injuries, compromised immune function in cancer patients (debatable value), select gastrointestinal disorders (gastritis, ulcer, and GERD), interstitial cystitis, and catabolic conditions.

Optimum Dose

For cardiovascular disease, the optimum dose is 6 to 15 g. For ED, the dose should be in the range of 1.7 to 5 g daily to have any positive effects. The optimum dose for infertility is 500 mg per day, while doses in the 5 to 10 g per day range are effective for improving athletic performance.

Safety

Arginine should be used with caution in patients with renal (kidney) or liver disease. It should not be used for patients with herpes infections or with a history of herpes since it can potentially cause an outbreak or replication of the virus.

Carnitine

This amino acid helps to shuttle fatty acids into parts of cells called mitochondria, which is where fat is oxidized for cellular energy production. Carnitine is made in the body from the methylation of lysine and obtained from meat sources in the diet. It is absorbed from the intestine by passive and active mechanisms, and its absorption is variable and rather unclear since studies have demonstrated a range of absorption between 16% to 18% and 54% to 87%.

Therapeutic Uses

Carnitine can benefit a number of clinical conditions, such as anorexia nervosa, various cardiovascular diseases, diabetes, fatigue (cancer-related and CFS), HIV-positive infection, hyperthyroidism (overactive thyroid), male infertility, kidney failure, and respiratory distress in premature infants. It can improve athletic performance and promote weight loss.

In a study of cancer patients, 15 of 18 were deficient in carnitine. These patients were given 250 mg each day, which was increased to 3 g daily. By the end of one week of carnitine supplementation, there were positive changes in depression, fatigue, and sleep quality. In another study, patients with hyperthyroidism were given 2-gram and 4-gram doses of the amino acid. Carnitine was shown to ameliorate typical hyperthyroidism symptoms and even benefit bone mineralization. Other studies have shown carnitine to help patients who are on dialysis with renal failure by treating the associated anemia, heart dysfunction, insulin and lipid abnormalities, and excessive oxidation (free radicals).

Optimum Dose

The optimum dose is in the range of 1 to 2 g, two to three times each day (total dose 2 to 6 g daily).

Side Effects

Gastrointestinal symptoms (abdominal cramps and diarrhea) can occur from using this amino acid, but generally it is well tolerated without significant side effects. Since some medications (anticonvulsants and antiretrovirals) deplete carnitine, it should be taken concurrently to prevent deficiency problems, such as muscle weakness, loss of muscle tone, fatigue, and cardiomyopathy. There are some negative drug interactions with carnitine, so a healthcare professional should be consulted prior to taking it.

Glutamine

Glutamine is made from glutamic acid, one of the so-called non-essential amino acids, but still very essential. Glutamic acid does not pass readily across the blood-brain barrier, but glutamine is more successful. It is found in the highest concentrations in human blood because the cells readily synthesize this amino acid. The skeletal muscle, lungs, liver, brain, and stomach tissue contain high concentrations of this amino acid. Under situations where there is an increased breakdown (catabolism) of body tissues, the need for glutamine is much greater than what could be obtained from diet alone. Clinical situations, such as injury, sepsis, prolonged stress, endurance training, gastrointestinal disease, cancer, surgery, trauma, and HIV-positive/AIDS, require large amounts of glutamine to replenish what is lost.

Therapeutic Uses

Alcoholism: Dr Roger Williams used glutamine many years ago to decrease the use of alcohol by rats. Studies with alcoholics showed a similar therapeutic effect. It also decreased craving for alcohol. The dose to use in order to reduce craving for alcohol is 2000 mg each day.

Intelligence: There have also been a few studies using glutamic acid and glutamine to enhance I.Q. The dose varies between 500 to 4000 mg per day. Dr Newbold recommends increasing it slowly.

Gastrointestinal Disease: For gastrointestinal diseases, glutamine is very useful because it provides fuel to the cells of the small intestine, known as enterocytes. Many gastrointestinal diseases are marked by increased intestinal permeability, which causes the intestinal cells to be 'leaky', allowing large protein molecules, bacteria, fungi, and other toxins to gain entrance into the systemic circulation. The consequences of this may include food allergies, joint pain, and a worsening of bowel problems associated with irritable bowel syndrome, ulcerative colitis, and Crohn's disease. Glutamine can significantly improve or even reverse the intestinal permeability dysfunction of the small intestine. By improving the gut barrier, glutamine can improve immune function and reduce the frequency of relapses in gastrointestinal diseases in which the small intestine is involved. Doses in the range of 2 to 4 g daily are sufficient for gastrointestinal diseases.

Under situations where there is an increased breakdown (catabolism) of body tissues, the need for glutamine is much greater than what could be obtained from diet alone.

Healing Wounds and Injuries: In wound healing from surgery, trauma, or injuries, glutamine can hasten recovery by speeding the healing process and encouraging the growth of cells. The therapeutic dose for wound healing is the same as the dose recommended for the treatment of gastrointestinal diseases. The addition of arginine and omega-3 EFAs should provide additional support for the recovery process. By contrast, individuals under large amounts of stress (for example, endurance athletes) tend to have increased rates of infection, have much lower glutamine levels in their blood, and a greater demand for even large supplemental doses of glutamine.

AIDS: HIV-positive patients seem to have a glutamine deficiency induced by the HIV virus, which results in muscle wasting, increased intestinal permeability, and malabsorption. All of these negative effects worsen when the clinical situation progresses to AIDS.

Cancer: Some research shows that growing tumors of cancer patients concentrate glutamine and steal it from muscle sources, and may even use it as a fuel source to increase tumor growth. There is debate and controversy over the use of glutamine for cancer, and the guidance of a healthcare professional is essential if glutamine is to be considered during cancer treatment.

Optimum Dose

The optimum dose is 2 to 4 g daily for alcohol craving, cognitive enhancement, intestinal support, and for general wound healing. The dose required for prolonged stress, HIV-positive/AIDS patients, and possibly cancer is 10 to 40 g per day in divided doses.

Side Effects

No notable or important side effects have been associated with the use of glutamine.

Main Inhibitory Amino Acids: Glycine, GABA, and Taurine

Glycine, GABA, and taurine are considered to be inhibitory amino acids because they increase membrane permeability to chloride ions, producing an inhibitory postsynaptic potential (IPSP) and preventing action potential generation. In other words, these amino acids calm the central nervous system. They are useful for various related conditions, such as anxiety, mania, and hyperactivity. These amino acids work similarly to the benzodiazepine group of drugs, but do not have any significant side effects.

Therapeutic Uses

Receptors for glycine are found in the vertebrate CNS, spinal cord, and brain stem areas, and are equally distributed throughout mammalian tissues. The highest concentrations of glycine are found in the thalamus, amygdala, substantia nigra, putamen, and globus pallidus. The unique aspect of glycine's mechanism of action has to do with its presumed antagonism of norepinephrine (NE). The neurons for NE are located in a part of the brain stem called the locus coeruleus, from which the NE neurons branch out to touch as many as half of all the cells in the brain (probably several billion) in the cerebral cortex.

When an individual experiences anxiety or panic, NE is released from the locus coeruleus and affects a part of the brain known as the nucleus accumbens, leading to feelings of anxiety and panic. Glycine antagonizes the release of NE from the locus coeruleus and the ensuing signals to the nucleus accumbens, thus mitigating anxiety and panic, as well as feelings of over-arousal. Glycine is also part of the phase two biotransformation pathways in the liver, which helps to detoxify salicylates. Studies do show that a sub-population of children with ADHD may have a reduction in their symptoms when salicylates are removed from their diets. Supplementing with glycine may be an easier way to improve salicylate tolerance as opposed to removing salicylates from the diet.

GABA might also help with anxiety, but there is uncertainty if GABA can cross the blood-brain barrier when administered orally. GABA might have a therapeutic effect comparable to benzodiazepine medications and might be useful for patients addicted to them as well. In a case report, a 40-year-old female patient with a history of severe anxiety was able to stop her diazepam and replace her lorazepam with 200 mg of GABA four times each day.

Taurine calms the brain and spinal cord in a manner similar to GABA and glycine. Taurine reduces anxiety by stabilizing nerve cell membranes. It can be used to enhance the effectiveness of other natural anti-anxiety therapies. It also has many side-benefits. It has been shown to be of value in epilepsy and retinal degeneration. It reduces blood pressure, it protects the heart, and it helps with cholesterol excretion. Taurine may also slow down the progression of neurodegenerative diseases, such as Alzheimer's disease or Parkinson's disease. Taurine may take the edge of many of the symptoms of ADHD due to its calming properties.

> These amino acids work similarly to the benzodiazepine group of drugs, but do not have any significant side effects.

Optimum Dose

Glycine: The best way to administer glycine is sublingually so that the gastrointestinal route is bypassed. This allows for quicker absorption, a faster onset of action, and swift entry to the CNS. It is very palatable and sweet tasting, making it easy to administer sublingually.

At least 2 to 10 g are required in order to stop a panic attack. We have our patients place 2 g under their tongue at the onset of an acute panic attack. They can take another 2 g every few minutes until the panic attack subsides. It usually works within a matter of a few minutes.

GABA: This amino acid should be prescribed at 2 to 3 g per day away from meals to aid with sleep, induce relaxation, and control symptoms of anxiety.

Taurine: The recommended dose range for taurine is 500 to 3000 mg daily. Children require less taurine and can benefit from 250 to 1000 mg daily.

Side Effects

Glycine: Side effects are very rare when high doses are administered. There is one report that 14 g given to a 70-kilogram adult male produced nausea. However, 15 to 30 g have been given to two manic patients producing no side effects except for cessation of the manic episode and calmness within one hour of supplementation. We have never found glycine to work better than the vitamin, niacinamide, for daily use. It is best reserved for acute panic attacks or acute periods of anxiety.

GABA: Even though side effects are rare, there is one report of neurologic tingling, flushing, transient hypertension, and tachycardia in a subject taking very high oral doses (10 g on an empty stomach) of GABA. Smaller oral doses (1 to 3 g daily) of GABA were reported to cause neurologic tingling and flushing in several volunteer subjects.

Taurine: Taurine is considered very safe and side effects are rare, but can include itching in psoriasis patients, and nausea, headache, dizziness, and gait problems among epileptic patients. There was one study showing some serious side effects when taurine was administered to patients with a medical condition known as adrenocortical insufficiency, but these patients were not responding well to standard treatments either. This is the only known contraindication to the use of taurine.

(14) ESSENTIAL FATTY ACIDS

During the past 40 years, there has been a marked change in medical opinion in the use of nutrients as supplements. In the early 1950s, it was generally believed that nutrition played a very minor, if any, role in the practice of medicine. Nutrition was not taught in medical schools, and physicians allowed non-clinical nutritionists and dietitians to take over the whole field. In 1955, the first paper was published that introduced the concept that large doses of vitamins could be used therapeutically for treating conditions not known to be vitamin deficiency diseases. The period from 1970 to 1980 marked the beginning of the megavitamin decade. The following decade saw the introduction of mineral supplements on a larger scale. The 1990s could be called the essential fatty acid (EFA) decade. Dr David F. Horrobin has been one of the foremost investigators who have brought these essential fatty acids to medical attention.

There has been an enormous rise of interest in the roles these fats and oils play in a large number of diseases, especially cardiovascular disease and the connection between cholesterol and other fats and a large number of the chronic diseases. Like essential vitamins, amino acids, and minerals, EFAs are essential nutrients that play a major role in our health and well-being.

There are two series or classes of essential fatty acids, omega-3 and omega-6 series. Omega-3 essential fatty acids are highly reactive fatty acids, some of which are converted in the body into the essential prostaglandins. They are needed for growth, for many metabolic roles, for the integrity of the cell membranes, and for preventing skin from drying and flaking. One of the best sources is linseed oil made from flax seed. Linseed oil used to be a very popular and widely consumed oil, but now is mostly available in health food stores. It is very rich in omega-3 oils, up to 60%. Omega-3 fatty acids are also found in seafood. The common vegetable oils have a lot of the omega-6 fatty acid, but are deficient in the omega-3 type.

Like essential vitamins, amino acids, and minerals, EFAs are essential nutrients that play a major role in our health and well-being.

The omega-3 group are chemically more reactive than the omega-6 group, have lower melting points (they are more liquid at room temperature), and are made in cold climate plants to make them more resistant to freezing. However, they must be in balance with omega-6 fatty acids. The omega-6 essential fatty acids play an equally important role in maintaining health. They are made in the body by adding one double (unsaturated) bond to linoleic acid. Omega-6 fatty acids are found mainly in plant seeds, notably in evening primrose, borage, and black currant. The omega-6 series has two main functions: to provide flexibility to cell membranes and control behavior of membrane bound proteins; and to control a large number of rapid reactions in the body.

Both series of EFAs began to disappear from our diet about 75 years ago. Only 20% of our needs are available in the average diet today. Dr D. Rudin and Dr C. Felix call essential fatty acids the nutritional "missing link." They have presented convincing evidence that this missing nutrient is one of the main factors in producing much of the illness we have to contend with in our modern high-tech society.

Therapeutic Uses

GLA Affected Conditions: EFAs assist the body in making gamma linolenic acid (GLA). Dr Horrobin lists the following conditions that have been helped by GLA: atopic eczema, diabetic neuropathy, premenstrual syndrome, breast pain and prostatic hypertrophy, rheumatoid arthritis and other forms of inflammation, systemic sclerosis, Sjögren's syndrome, dry eyes associated with contact lenses, gastrointestinal disorders, viral infection and post-viral fatigue syndrome, endometriosis, schizophrenia, alcoholism, cardiovascular disease, renal disease, cancer, and liver disease.

GLA is clearly not a specific treatment for any one condition, but has an enormous importance in the general health of the body. It helps repair biochemical problems that have helped create these pathological diseases. The simplest way of getting GLA is by taking evening primrose oil and other GLA-rich oils. The dose range varies from under 1 gram per day to 10 g for very serious conditions.

Prostaglandin Affected Conditions: *Fats and Oils* by Udo Erasmus is one of the best books describing the chemistry and biochemistry of the two series of essential fatty acids. In the body, EFAs are converted into prostaglandins, which help regulate the entire body. When there is a deficiency, digestion is compromised and healing is retarded. There are about 25 important reactions in the body that depend upon having the right amount and kind of prostaglandins. The conversion to prostaglandins requires a large number of cofactors, such as vitamins and minerals. Minerals, antioxidants, and B-vitamins (especially pyridoxine), in conjunction with optimal amounts of omega-3 EFAs, produce the necessary prostaglandins.

Dr Rudin and Dr Felix suggest that pellagra is due to the deficiency of these prostaglandins and that this may occur for two reasons: (1) a deficiency of these cofactors, such as vitamin B-3, the best known cause of pellagra; and (2) a deficiency of the essential fatty acids so that even in the presence of these cofactors not enough prostaglandins can be made. The first type of pellagra is the cofactor pellagra (vitamin B-3, vitamin B-6, tryptophan) and the second type is a substrate pellagra. The two pellagras are responsible for many of the chronic illnesses, including both mental and physical illnesses.

Dr Rudin considers the production of these prostaglandins to be absolutely required in order to improve or reverse the clinical presentation of substrate pellagra. In one of the early published reports on EFAs, Dr Rudin proposed that an omega-3 essential fatty acid deficiency may lead to "substrate pellagra" even when the diet contains adequate amounts of tryptophan and B-vitamins. Bearing in mind that the modern diet hardly contains 20% of omega-3 EFAs, substrate pellagra may develop in susceptible individuals. Substrate pellagra is characterized by alterations in thought (schizophrenia), in mood (manic-depressive psychosis), and in neurotic fears (agoraphobia). It is also marked by symptoms of irritable bowel syndrome, dermatitis, tinnitus, and fatigue. In his report, 3 of 4 patients with a history of agoraphobia for 10 or more years improved after supplementing with flaxseed (linseed) oil for 2 to 3 months. The dose of flaxseed oil ranged from 2 to 6 tablespoons daily and contained 50% alpha-linolenic acid.

Cardiac Arrhythmia: Fish oils have largely replaced the use of flaxseed (linseed) oils for many clinical conditions, including cardiovascular disease and mental illness. The best way to manage and/or prevent cardiac arrhythmias is through daily supplementation with fish oil. In a randomized, double-blind, placebo-controlled trial, 65 patients with cardiac arrhythmias (without coronary heart disease or heart failure) were followed for 6 months and divided into two groups. One group was given 3 g daily of encapsulated fish oil (equivalent to 1 g daily of omega-3 EFAs), whereas the other group was given 3 g daily of olive oil as placebo. In the fish oil group, there were considerable lipid-modifying benefits that included a decrease of serum triglycerides, total cholesterol, low-density lipoprotein cholesterol, plasma free fatty acids, and thromboxane B2, as well as an increase in high-density lipoprotein cholesterol. The subjects in the fish oil group also had 46.9%, 67.8%, 71.8%, and 100% fewer incidences of the four types of arrhythmia (irregular heartbeat) monitored in this study (atrial premature complexes, ventricular premature complexes, couplets, and triplets). Unlike the fish oil group, no positive changes occurred in the placebo group. The results of this study demonstrated that fish oil supplementation has anti-arrhythmic effects, and can reduce the incidence of fatal myocardial infarction (heart attack) and sudden cardiac death.

Cardiac Mortality: In a recent meta-analysis of fish oil supplementation, the pooled results of many clinical trials showed a dramatic 32% reduction in cardiac mortality (deaths due to heart diseases) and a 23% reduction in overall mortality (death from all causes) among individuals ingesting therapeutica amounts of fish oils. These results were superior to those obtained from the statin drug group. Based on the results of numerous studies, all individuals wanting to prevent deaths from cardiovascular and non-cardiovascular diseases should take fish oil supplementation on a daily basis. It should also be given to individuals at risk or who currently have cardiovascular disease. The simple reasons are that fish oils have therapeutic effects upon all major cardiovascular causes of death (stroke, heart attack, and arrhythmias).

Mental Illness: Omega-3 fatty acid deficiencies cause a wide range of adverse central nervous system effects, which involve decreased dopamine content in specific brain regions, decreased serotonin receptor density in the frontal cortex, reduced glucose uptake by the brain, compromised blood-brain integrity, and decreased membrane fluidity. In fact, low blood levels of omega-3 EFAs have been associated with various mental disorders, including ADHD, Alzheimer's disease, schizophrenia, and depression. There are numerous published reports demonstrating the benefits of supplementation with individual or combination omega-3 EFAs for many of these mental disorders as well as borderline personality disorder, conduct disorder in children, and bipolar disorder.

Although it is unclear as to what are the exact mechanisms that explain the benefits of omega-3 EFAs, it is known that they do play an integral role in the functioning of the brain and neurons. Docosahexaenoic acid (DHA) is the predominant omega-3 fatty acid in the brain, and eicosapentaenoic acid (EPA) is involved in reducing inflammation. Both DHA and EPA are involved in numerous neuronal functions that include proper neurotransmitter function for dopamine and serotonin, normal membrane fluidity, ion channel and enzyme regulation, and gene expression.

Optimum Dose

Here is the EFA supplement program recommended by Dr Rudin and Dr Felix:

1. Select the best oil you can; ideally, this is linseed oil. However, this oil tends to become rancid and develops a very bad flavor so it should be stored cold. Other good oils are soybean oil, walnut oil, and wheat germ oil.
2. A 100-pound person can start with 1 tablespoonful of linseed oil daily and a 200-pound person with 3 to 4. It is important not to take more than is needed as the extra oil can cause some side effects.
3. Be sure your diet is vitamin and mineral rich. Magnesium, biotin, zinc, pyridoxine, calcium, and ascorbic acid are needed for normal EFA formation. Vitamin B-3 is needed for the conversion to prostaglandins. Fiber is also very important.
4. Maintain the program by adjusting the amounts. One's health is used as the measure, looking at such things as your skin texture and feeling of well-being. The amount of supplementary oil should be the smallest amount for maintaining good health.
5. Balance the two series, the omega-3 and omega-6. This is done by using both linseed oil and some of the other oils. During the winter season, you will need more of the omega-3 and during hot weather, less. Fish oils are very good, as is evening primrose oil, which contains important omega-6 fatty acids.

For individuals who are vegetarians and want to take omega-3 EFAs for mental health reasons, the dose of flaxseed oil should be similar to what Dr Rudin had his patients take (2 to 6 tablespoons daily).

Despite the clinical utility of flaxseed oil, it is not biologically equivalent to other types of omega-3 EFAs, such as those found in fish. Fish oils are preferable since they contain biologically more potent sources of omega-3 EFAs, which include EPA and DHA. Fish oils have a greater spectrum of cardiovascular and neurobehavioral effects and are more efficacious than flaxseed oil.

For the treatment of mental disorders, the daily dose of fish oil should provide a minimum of 1000 mg of EPA daily, but better results might be more achievable with higher daily doses containing both EPA and DHA. In terms of the optimum dosage for cardiovascular protection and treatment, the daily amount of fish oil should provide 450 to 1000 mg of both EPA and DHA (the minimum effective daily dose is 400 mg of EPA and 200 mg of DHA).

Side Effects

Supplementation with flaxseed oil can cause side effects, such as hypomania, mania, or other behavioral changes, in a very small percentage of individuals (about 3%). Other more common side effects from flaxseed oil include loose stools or diarrhea.

The most common side effects from fish oil supplements are gastrointestinal and consist of mild indigestion, belching, increased flatulence, diarrhea, or a fishy aftertaste. Side effects can be minimized when taken with food or by taking an enteric-coated fish oil preparations.

Oil Quality

Obtaining the correct oils is not always simple. In his book *The Facts about Fats,* John Finnegan discusses some of the problems in the preparation of the commercial oils and fats. If we are to use these essential nutrients with skill and safety, it is important that we understand their chemistry and know how these oils are made.

They are very unstable; they have double bonds in them, which are avid for oxygen. This is why linseed oil is used to make a base for paint. For the same reason, once the oils have been extracted, they will not store very well. During their deterioration or oxidation, the oils are changed to products that are of no value and may be harmful. Manufacturers have tried to avoid some of these changes by using what is called a cold pressing process, which is supposed to avoid the use of heat. Heat increases oxidation and deterioration. But even when the oil is cold pressed, there is a lot of heat generated in the process, unless the oil is pressed so slowly that the heat has a chance to dissipate. This means that the cold pressed oils are little better than the heat-treated oils.

Finnegan recommends that high quality oils must be produced by pressing at temperatures below 118ºF using light and oxygen excluding methods, then bottled in containers that prevent exposure to light that causes the oil to go rancid. He also recommends that the oils should be produced from third-party, certified organically-grown seed. Currently, there are many reputable manufacturers who produce high-quality flaxseed and fish oils, which have independent third party analysis (when requested), are cold pressed, and are properly sealed with nitrogen.

NUTRITIONAL THERAPY
CASE STUDIES

15 | NUTRITIONAL THERAPY CASE STUDIES

Case studies may best illustrate the effects of nutrient deficiency and dependency upon health – and the effectiveness of nutrients for preventing and treating various disease conditions and common illnesses. The following case histories are taken from our files, with the names of the patients removed, of course.

Nutrient Dependencies

Case 1: Prisoner of War Malnutrition

All good food to which anyone has adapted is both preventive and therapeutic. It prevents the diseases that will inevitably occur if the food is deficient in quantity or quality, and if the diet of a person that had made him sick is corrected, it will help restore his health. There is a major exception to this principle. This is the case where the deficient diet has been the main diet for such a long time that there is permanent damage to the body or to its biochemistry.

A combination of severe stress and starvation will lead to permanent impairment of the nutritional biochemistry and only the administration of very large amounts of some of the vitamins will allow that person to function adequately. This is happening now in those countries where there is major starvation, but when it is combined with stress, as it is in Africa, with war and brutality, the impact on the population is going to be even worse.

We have already described the effect of an inadequate diet on rats. There was a steady deterioration in their health until the eighth generation after which it remained bad. This was on a diet that was the same each year. If the diet continues to deteriorate each year, the effect on the health of the animals would be even worse. When they were placed on a good diet, it required four generations to recover their original state of health. It is possible that these rats, if given the right vitamins as supplements, might have regained their health faster.

During the Second World War, human population experiments were carried out by the Germans and by the Japanese. I will not discuss the impact of the concentration camps on the survivors, except to point out they too became vitamin dependent and responded when they were given large doses of niacin. My experience with the impact of the Japanese experiment came from the Canadian soldiers imprisoned in Hong Kong who came to me for help long after this war was over. The first one was Mr George Porteous, later Lieutenant-Governor of Province of Saskatchewan.

I first met Mr Porteous when I was doing a study on the effect of niacin upon elderly people living in a nursing home of which he was director. I had explained to him how the people might react to the niacin so that he would be familiar with the flushing effect. He asked me whether he could himself take the niacin. He wanted to experience first hand the flush so that he could be more reassuring to them.

About 6 months later, in the fall of 1960, he came to see me at the University Hospital. He told me that he was a Hong Kong Veteran and that he had been a prisoner of war in a camp in the Far East for 44 months. He described the horrible conditions he and the other Canadian soldiers had to endure. It was an extraordinary combination of stress, brutality, and starvation. The death rate was very high. At the end of the war when they were liberated, one quarter of the soldiers who had been captured were dead. They all suffered from diarrhea, pellagra, scurvy, beri beri, and almost every nutritional deficiency known.

He described his health from the time of his release to the time he began to take the niacin, 3 g daily. He had lost one third of his body weight. On the hospital ship coming back to Canada, the doctors gave the soldiers the only vitamin supplements they then had, mostly rice bran polishings. Mr Porteous regained his weight but not his health. From that moment on, he was anxious, tense, very sensitive, fearful, physically weak, and suffering from arthritis. He could not lift his arms over his shoulders. He continually consulted the doctors of the Department of Veteran Affairs, who treated him with amphetamines in the morning and barbiturates at night to help him sleep. Eventually, on the very flimsiest of evidence (hearsay from another person), he was diagnosed neurotic and sent to a psychiatric ward. He came back even worse because his self-esteem had dropped even further. He then received sympathetic psychotherapy in Saskatoon and regained the state he was in before he was admitted to the psychiatric ward. He told me he could not tolerate either heat or cold.

All good food to which anyone has adapted is both preventive and therapeutic. It prevents the diseases that will inevitably occur if the food is deficient in quantity or quality, and if the diet of a person that had made him sick is corrected, it will help restore his health.

But a month or so after he had started to take the niacin, he became normal. All the symptoms vanished. His favorite opening gambit when he saw his family doctor was to stretch his arms to the ceiling and say, "See that." Previously he could not raise them over his shoulders. Mr Porteous wanted me to know about this miraculous response to niacin. Two years later he went with his son to the mountains for 2 weeks. He forgot to take his niacin with him. By the time he came home, all the symptoms he had suffered previously were coming back. He never forgot to take them thereafter and remained well until his death when he was Lieutenant-Governor.

This aroused my interest in the fate of the Hong Kong veterans. About 2,000 soldiers were freed from the camps, but never recovered their health, unlike their siblings who had served in Europe and in other areas during the same war. They continually demanded that something be done for them, and eventually the Canadian government appointed a commission that examined their claims for a special pension. The commission found that they were, in fact, very ill. They had a very high death rate, a high rate of cardiovascular disease, and about 25% suffered from neurosis, psychoses, and neurological diseases. All the Hong Kong veterans were awarded a special pension.

Mr Porteous told his fellow POWs about his success with niacin therapy, and within a few years I treated a dozen Canadian vets and some POWs from the United States. Later, the information spread to other POWs. Without exception, veterans who went onto the vitamin program recovered fully or enough so that they were pleased with their new health.

After my experience with the veterans and after reading the literature, I concluded that 1 year in the camps had aged the veterans by 4 years. A prisoner in camp 4 years would come back having aged the equivalent of 16 years. Other investigators had come to a similar conclusion. By this time I was familiar with the concept of vitamin dependency. I have concluded that severe food deprivation combined with stress experienced long enough will cause a vitamin B-3 dependency, and that these individuals will never be well until their increased need for niacin is recognized and they start taking 3 g or more daily.

For these patients made ill by their food, restoring the food is therapeutic, although it may not be enough for those made vitamin dependent. The natural diet is thus both preventative and therapeutic. [Dr Hoffer]

Case # 2: Improved I.Q.

Single nutrients are seldom used for prevention and for treatment, with the exception of niacin, which we discovered lowered total cholesterol when it was given alone in large enough doses. It is recognized that on our modern high-tech diets any nutrient deficiencies are usually multiple and involve both vitamins and minerals. This is one reason why the B complex preparations have become so popular and also the multi-vitamin and multi-mineral preparations. Almost all the patients treated by naturopathic doctors or orthomolecular therapists are advised to take more than one vitamin, although it is not necessary to give them individual pills containing these nutrients separately. I will discuss two conditions where multi-vitamin and multi-mineral preparations were used and yielded valuable results.

In 1988, David Benton and Gwilym Roberts reported in the British medical journal *The Lancet* that vitamin and mineral supplements increased intelligence of school children not considered to be nutritionally deprived. D. Benton and R. Cook completed a double-blind experiment on 60 children. Thirty were given a vitamin-mineral supplement containing the following: bioflavonoids 50 mg; biotin 100 mcg; choline bitartrate 70 mg; folic acid 100 mcg; inositol 30 mg; niacin 50 mg; pantothenic acid 50 mg; para-aminobenzoic acid 10 mg; pyridoxine 12 mg; thiamin 3.9 mg; riboflavin 5 mg; vitamin A 375 mcg; vitamin B-12 10 mcg; vitamin C 500 mg; vitamin D-3 3 mcg; vitamin E 79 IU; vitamin K 100 mcg; calcium gluconate 100 mg; chromium 0.1 mg; magnesium 7.6 mg; manganese 1.5 mg; molybdenum 0.1 mg; iodine 50 mcg; iron 1.3 mg; and zinc 10 mg. Thirty were given placebo.

On our modern high-tech diets any nutrient deficiencies are usually multiple and involve both vitamins and minerals.

After 8 months, there was no significant difference between the groups on verbal intelligence scores. However, only the supplemented group increased non-verbal intelligence scores. Non-verbal I.Q. increased from 111 to 120, while with placebo it remained unchanged at 109. Verbal intelligence is a measure of an individual's unique cultural, educational, and environmental experiences. Non-verbal intelligence is considered to be innate or biologic in nature; the answers do not require general information and vocabulary. The growth curve of non-verbal intelligence parallels other physical factors, such as brain weight. Improved nutrition would be expected to affect non-verbal I.Q. first, but later with the interplay of an enriched environment, verbal I.Q. would also be expected to rise. In a recent report, Benton and Cook confirmed their earlier findings on a different population. Intelligence was increased by 7.6 points, while on placebo, there was a decline of 1.7 points.

C.F. Harrell and colleagues reported similar findings when mentally retarded children were given vitamins and mineral supplements plus thyroid. This paper stirred up a hornets' nest, so much so that seven attempts have been reported to repeat the Harrell study, yet none of the seven repeated it successfully. However, they used a different type of population of children and did not use thyroid. It seems too difficult for critics to really repeat work of which they are critical.

These two studies lead to two conclusions: (1) even normal children on the usual diet are more intelligent after they are given very moderate doses of vitamins and minerals; and (2) mentally retarded children need more vitamins and minerals. During the past 45 years, I have treated about 1500 children with vitamins and minerals. I have no doubt that there is a major improvement in their intelligence performances following their recovery. I don't think any one can perform at their best when they are ill, depressed, have poor concentration, or difficulty with memory. [Dr Hoffer]

Case # 3: Adolescent Schizophrenia

In 1960, a doctor from California called me. He was very depressed and cried as he told me about his son, then 12 years old, who was in a university psychiatric hospital in Palo Alto. He had just been advised by his son's psychiatrist that he would never recover and that the only thing left for him would be to transfer him to a mental hospital. After that frightening advice, he began to read as much as he could in the medical library and discovered the first paper we had published in 1957, where we described the use of vitamin B-3 for the treatment of schizophrenia.

I recommended he obtain nicotinic acid and give his son 1 g three times each day. In 1960, no company was making these large-sized doses. The smaller 100 mg tablets were useless because they contained so much filler that the correct dose, 30 tablets daily, would make anyone sick from the fillers. The physician contacted a drug company that agreed to make the 500 mg tablets for him.

When his supply arrived, he took it to the hospital and asked the psychiatrist to start his son on it. The psychiatrist became very angry and promptly came back with two lies. He told the father that they had tried the vitamin and that it had not done any good, then added that it would "fry" his brain. He concluded by warning the father that if he insisted his son would be discharged. He was too psychotic to be discharged.

The father then decided he was going to have his son take the vitamin without the psychiatrist's knowledge. He ground up each tablet and placed one gram on a slice of bread. This he covered with jam. Each day he appeared at the hospital to visit his son and to feed him jam sandwiches. After a few weeks, he became worried that the psychiatrist might find out because his son said to him, "Daddy, whenever I eat that sandwich I turn red." He promptly changed the nicotinic acid to nicotinamide.

After 12 weeks, the boy said he wanted to go home. He was discharged and completed high school in the top 95 percentile for the United States. He went to university, took medicine, graduated, and is now a research psychiatrist. Had he not been on this vitamin the state would have faced enormous costs, as would his family, and he would be a chronic patient today. Instead he is a normal productive psychiatrist doing research and paying income tax.

How does one compare these two results? It is very simple. The vast majority of schizophrenics never do recover. However, a large proportion of early schizophrenic patients do when they are treated by naturopathic nutrition and orthomolecular medicine. I know personally 17 men and women practicing medicine and psychiatry who were all teenage schizophrenics. On the orthomolecular regimen, they have recovered. Several have academic appointments. One was the president of a major psychiatric association for one year. [Dr Hoffer]

Case # 4: Down Syndrome Treatment

Down syndrome, at one time considered an excellent example of a disease caused by bad mothering, is one of the genetic diseases and, therefore, considered untreatable by many physicians and psychiatrists.

Dr Henry Turkel was the first physician to think otherwise. He began to treat cases of Down syndrome more than 40 years ago using a combination of vitamins, minerals, and hormones. He began to see major recoveries among the patients he treated. The parents of the children he treated were very enthusiastic about his treatment, but his views were so outrageous to the establishment that no one paid any attention to him. The FDA tried to suppress his work and eventually he was permitted to treat only patients in his own state of Michigan. He used every technique known to disseminate his views in medical journals, but he was rejected by the editors and their committees. He did have some of his work published in a journal I was editing, and, more recently, he published a book called *Medical Treatment of Down 'Syndrome'*, where he presents individual case histories and photographs of the children before and after treatment.

Few doctors in North America have shown interest in these amazing results. As Professor Linus Pauling comments in his introduction to this book, "The work of Dr Henry Turkel provides a striking example of the way in which this opposition operates to the detriment of the health and well being of a large number of people. Dr Turkel has developed, over a period of decades, a treatment of mentally retarded children with the use of vitamins, minerals and cerebral stimulants, and other substances. He has gathered together a convincing body of clinical observations showing the genetic condition of mental retardation need not be accepted as inevitably leading to permanent defect and inability of the individual to function in normal society. Dr Turkel has indeed provided new hope for the mentally retarded and for members of their families, hope that a great improvement in functioning can be achieved."

"If I were the parent of a child with Down syndrome, I would move heaven and earth to have the child placed under Dr Turkel's treatment."

In the same book Dr Bernard Rimland wrote, "Government-sponsored research designed to thoroughly evaluate the Turkel treatment should have been started 30 years ago. Perhaps, if the readers of this book write to their representatives in Congress in sufficient numbers, such research may yet be done. In the meantime, what of the millions of retarded children whose treatment could have begun years ago but for FDA opposition? . . . The thought is appalling. If I were the parent of a child with Down syndrome, I would move heaven and earth to have the child placed under Dr Turkel's treatment."

Dr Allan Cott has seen similar recoveries in his large series of children he treated with orthomolecular methods, and I have seen the improvement in a few whom have been referred to me. [Dr Hoffer]

Case #5 Attention Deficit Disorder (ADD)

Children today suffer from a large number of serious behavioral and learning disorders, which are caused primarily by the food that they eat. There is a pandemic of sick children suffering from these conditions usually called attention deficit disorder (ADD) or attention deficit hyperactivity disorder (ADHD). About 20% of all boys entering public schools and about 5% of girls suffer from these diseases, a remarkable statistic given that in 1950, when I first started to practice psychiatry, there were hardly any cases of ADD.

One evening, early in 1962, my friend George called me at home to say he was very worried about his youngest son, Ben. Then 9 years old, Ben had become a behavioral problem. He could not learn to read and was making so little progress in school the teaching staff had advised he be prepared for a school for slow learners or for the 'retarded'. However, he had tested 120 on an I.Q. test. This was not only very disturbing, but extremely puzzling. I asked my friend to bring Ben to my office in the research department of the University Hospital, where I was then Director of Psychiatric Research, so I could examine him.

Ben was a good-looking, apparently healthy youngster. He was normal at birth, sat up at 7 months, walked at 14 months, and began to speak clearly by 20 months. He denied he had any problems at school or at home. I was then inexperienced in interviewing children and could not elicit any symptomatology. As I found out later, a large proportion of these children are not aware there is something wrong with their health or behavior and tend to blame their environment for any problems that arise. Only after they are well do they recall how different they once were. They develop retrospective insight for their illness.

Ben's parents considered him to be an ideal child until he was 7 years old in Grade 2. In late 1960, his mother became concerned by a slight change in his behavior. He became anxious. Ben could not fall asleep at night and he awakened frequently after he fell asleep. His mother discovered she could overcome some of the sleep difficulty by feeding him just before bed. This relaxed him. He continued to change, however, and school became very difficult for him. The family moved to a new home, and Ben was enrolled in a different school. He became more upset. This was attributed to his difficulty in making new friends. It is a common fallacy to confuse cause and effect. Late that year, his parents were shocked by his poor and erratic school performance. The teachers said he seemed to be in a shell. Reading and spelling were very poor.

In July 1961, he was referred to a mental health clinic for evaluation. He had completed Grade 3 with a D average in spite of a lot of tutoring and drilling at home by his mother, herself a teacher. When he was being taught, he seemed to understand, but soon after he could not remember what he had learned. He balked at his mother's tutoring. His mother reported that he reversed letters, had little knowledge of phonetics, and his eyes skipped back and forth or up and down so much so she used a ruler to guide his eyes on a line. He received extensive investigation from the clinic. His difficulty was again attributed to the move or sibling rivalry with his older brother. The clinic noted his habits of thumb sucking, nail biting, and bed-wetting. They recommended remedial reading, which he received for several months with little improvement.

I ordered a mauve factor (kryptopyrrole) urine test, expecting it would not show anything. To my surprise, the following morning the special area on the paper chromatogram specific for this compound was almost blood red. Ben was excreting large quantities of this factor. That evening, I called his father and opened the conversation by saying, "George, you are in luck, Ben has schizophrenia." George wanted to know why that made him so lucky. I replied that the majority of schizophrenics excreted this factor, as did a minority of non-schizophrenic patients, and that any patient with this factor, irrespective of the diagnosis, responded to vitamin B-3 treatment. I advised him to start Ben on nicotinamide 3 g daily.

Children today suffer from a large number of serious behavioral and learning disorders, which are caused primarily by the food that they eat.

A few months later, George called me again. He wanted to know whether I would be interested in his son's response. He then told me that they were no longer worried because Ben was normal. Two months after he started on the vitamin, the clinic giving him remedial reading discharged him as well. He had not responded to their program the previous 6 months. He had spent that summer happily reading books and enjoying them.

I received a report from a teacher who had been especially interested in Ben's case. Prior to receiving vitamin B-3 treatment, she recalled that Ben had not done well in school and had a reading problem. Students called him "stupid." He had developed such an inferior feeling that he would not answer questions.

Following treatment, she reported that "Ben is no longer shy. He has a sparkling personality; not afraid to speak up. He has started to show an interest in sports, in which he excels. He now gets along with the children at school and at camp. He will assume leadership and organizational duties. Ben can now read with eye-reversal not noticeable in reading and seldom in writing. Ben has gone up on the stage to sing, say a speech, and read the morning scripture to the whole student body and staff. All these things he did well with little nervousness and tension noticeable. Ben also reads books without being told and enjoys reading them.

Ben's teacher also reported many other improvements, physically,

> If we do not try to improve the nutrition of our children, not only of children clearly suffering from ADD, but also of almost every child in our high-tech society, we can look forward to another millennium of chronic illness, perhaps so severe as to threaten the species.

socially, and emotionally. He took pride in the fact that his mother was a teacher and started to mention his father and brother in class discussions.

Early in 1966, his father told me that Ben had completed Grade 7 with A's and B's. In Grade 9, he went to a track meet, participated in extra curricular activities, and worked as a stage manager for a high-school play. His parents considered him to be normal. I examined him for the last time in August 1970. He was well.

Since then Ben has remained normal. He is an outdoors professional, fully employed in a permanent position, and happily married with two children.

Although Ben was one of the first children I tested for mauve factor (KP) and advised to take large doses of niacinamide, he is an excellent example of what can be done for these children with so-called learning disabilities and behavior disorders if they are examined, diagnosed, and treated with the correct naturopathic or orthomolecular approach. Ben's treatment and response to a vitamin in megadoses is a prototype of what can be achieved through diet and nutrient supplements, not only for 'ill' children like Ben, but also for 'healthy' children.

Since then, I have diagnosed and treated over 1,500 children under the age of 14 suffering some learning disability, behavior disorder, or chronic disease with a regimen of a sugar-free naturopathic diet and optimum doses of vitamins, minerals, amino acids, and essential fatty acids. This treatment regimen is described fully in my book, *Healing Children's Attention and Behavior Disorders*, where I chronicle 120 more case studies.

If we do not try to improve the nutrition of our children, not only of children clearly suffering from ADD, but also of almost every child in our high-tech society, we can look forward to another millennium of chronic illness, perhaps so severe as to threaten the species. [Dr Hoffer]

Niacinamide Therapy for Anxiety Disorders

Anxiety disorders are the most common psychiatric disorders in North America. They are extremely debilitating. Patients have greater chances of developing other medical illnesses, such as chronic obstructive pulmonary disease, diabetes, and hypertension. The underlying anxiety that exists in these patients also tends to prolong the course of any additional medical illnesses that they may develop.

Anxiety disorders are classified into various categories, such as generalized anxiety disorder (GAD), obsessive-compulsive disorder (OCD), panic disorder (PD), post-traumatic stress disorder (PTSD), and social phobia/social anxiety disorder (SAD). The conventional approach to severe anxiety involves pharmacotherapy with benzodiazepines, selective serotonin re-uptake inhibitors (SSRIs), or other medications, such as buspirone, imipramine, or trazodone.

Here, I report on four cases where the use of optimal doses of nicotinamide considerably improved the symptoms of anxiety. In each case, frank symptoms of pellagra were absent, even though neuropsychiatric and gastrointestinal manifestations were present.

Case#1: Young Doctor with Severe Anxiety

A 33-year-old Caucasian male presented with a history of anxiety for the past 20 years. When the patient was 13, his homeroom teacher would embarrass him every week by having him stand up in front of the class and remain standing until he was noticeably red in the face, at which point the teacher would comment about how red he was. The entire class would laugh at this. Over time, this patient became increasingly nervous and fearful about social situations and involvement in activities that could draw attention to him. Throughout junior high and high school, the patient would have pronounced anxiety and panic when making presentations and conversing with his peers, friends, or girls. Typically, his symptoms were facial flushing, profuse sweating, increased heart rate, muscle tension, burning in the stomach, and the need to get away.

These symptoms persisted throughout university, and when the patient was 22, he finally sought professional help for his anxiety. The clinical psychologist diagnosed the patient with social phobia, panic disorder, and mild agoraphobia. The patient underwent once- or twice-weekly sessions of psychodynamic and cognitive-behavioral therapy for the next 6 months. During this time, the patient's symptoms improved only slightly, but the patient somehow convinced the psychologist that he was completely cured and that therapy was no longer necessary.

> **Optimal doses of nicotinamide considerably improved the symptoms of anxiety.**

By the time he was 24 years old, he entered medical school and his anxiety worsened. He was so upset by his inability to just "go with the flow," or "feel comfortable in my own skin" that he again sought the help of a psychiatrist. This time the psychiatrist assessed and diagnosed him with social phobia, panic disorder, dysthymia, and mild agoraphobia. He was started on Zoloft (sertraline HCl) 50 mg daily. After the first 2 weeks, the patient's anxiety slightly improved, but he had noticeable side effects from the medication, such as lethargy, apathy, and anorgasmia. After 4 weeks of use, the Zoloft seemed to work fairly well; the patient had some days without any anxiety. His dose of Zoloft was increased to 100 mg daily. The patient was also put on 5 mg of Buspirone (BuSpar) three times each day. After 3 months of use, the patient had no significant improvement, and his anxiety symptoms continued to be debilitating. He found his tendency to avoid social situations increased due to severe fears of blushing. He also avoided interactions with his professors and peers as much as possible. He preferred to stay at home and only go out when necessary. At this point he discontinued both the Zoloft and BuSpar due to their apparent ineffectiveness.

From age 25 to 28, the patient investigated a variety of natural approaches for the treatment of his anxiety. From his readings, he decided to take the following nutrients daily: 6 to 12 g of vitamin C; 800 IU of vitamin E; 50 mg of zinc; a B-complex containing 100 mg of each of the B vitamins; 1000 mg of calcium; and 400 mg of magnesium. Although he followed this plan diligently, his anxiety did not lessen. After 6 months of the vitamin plan, he added a standardized extract of Kava two to three times each day. Within

2 weeks, his anxiety symptoms were markedly improved. He was able to be in stressful social situations without blushing or appearing nervous.

However, by the fourth week of continual Kava use, he experienced pronounced depression. The depression became so unbearable that he felt it necessary to discontinue the Kava. After a few days of discontinuing the Kava, the patient's depression completely lifted. In an attempt to see if the Kava was the problem, the patient resumed taking Kava. Once again, the anxiety significantly improved, but his depression came back. He discontinued the Kava, and shortly thereafter the depression lifted once again. By the time the patient was 28, he had also tried St. John's wort, adrenal extract, constitutional homeopathic medicine, and amino acids, such a gamma-aminobutyric acid (GABA), inositol, and L-taurine. None of these natural approaches helped.

Just before he turned 29, the patient's anxiety worsened. Even though he did not notice any reduction in anxiety, he continued to take the following nutrients daily: 6 to 12 g of vitamin C; 800 IU of vitamin E; 50 mg of zinc; a B-complex containing 100 mg of each of the B vitamins; 1000 mg of calcium; and 400 mg of magnesium. During his medical residency, he purposely avoided his assigned patients, his condition significantly interfering with his ability to perform. Due to the urgency that he felt, he once again sought the help from a medical doctor, who prescribed 0.5 mg of Ativan (lorazepam) twice daily. Within 2 days, all of his anxiety symptoms resolved and the patient felt normal for the first time in his life. He could function and perform with confidence. His anxiety did not interfere or prevent him from completing the residency program.

From ages 29 to 33, the patient continued with the benzodiazepine medication. At one point, his medical doctor changed the Ativan to Klonopin (clonazepam, 0.5 mg twice daily) since he was told that this preparation was better for long-term use. He had no more anxiety symptoms, but never felt good about taking the benzodiazepine medication. When he was 32, he went off the Klonopin for 1 month. During the first week, he experienced severe insomnia at night, and during the day, he experienced recurrent bouts of panic and anxiety. Almost 2 weeks later, the insomnia resolved, but his anxiety returned to its pre-treatment state. He was completely debilitated. He resumed the Klonopin and once again felt complete relief.

When he turned 33, he did somewhat of a literature search on anxiety and found intriguing information on niacinamide. He informed his psychiatrist of his plan to wean himself off the Klonopin and take niacinamide. The psychiatrist encouraged the patient to do so, but wanted the patient to contact him if he were to experience withdrawal symptoms, such as recurrent anxiety, insomnia, and irritability. For the first week, the patient took 0.5 mg of Klonopin every morning along with 500 mg of niacinamide, 500 mg of niacinamide at lunch, and 1000 mg at bedtime. He experienced no recurrences of his anxiety or insomnia during the first week of weaning. In the second week, the patient discontinued the Klonopin and took 1000 mg of niacinamide in the morning, 500 mg at lunch, and 1000 mg at bedtime. The patient felt great and could not distinguish between taking Klonopin and niacinamide. The patient was completely free of benzodiazepine medication as of August 1, 2002. The psychiatrist was impressed with the outcome and commented that it gave him hope that a patient could actually go off benzodiazepine medications and not chronically depend on them.

As of November 7, 2003, this 33-year-old patient has been able to practice as a doctor without any impairments or restrictions, and continues to do very well approximately 15 months after stopping the Klonopin. He no longer feels that anxiety is a problem, and believes that the niacinamide is equally as effective as benzodiazepine medication, but is potentially safer to take for long-term use. [Dr Prousky]

Case #2: Panic Disorder and Social Phobia

An 11-year-old girl first presented to my office on November 10, 2003. Her chief complaints were nervousness, anxiety, and excessive worrying. The onset of her symptoms occurred when her father tragically died in September 2003.

She reported anxiety when she had to sit for examinations and when she was around her classmates. The most concerning symptom was her fear of being kidnapped, which was instigated by a well-publicized kidnapping of a young Asian girl in the city where she lives. She also reported having approximately two panic attacks each month since September. She had learned to deal with them by "leaving the situation to get air." Other symptoms that were reported included some facial acne, frequent blushing, stomachaches, and sweatiness. Her past medical history was unremarkable, except for asthma that was diagnosed approximately 1 year ago. The asthma was not a concern since her symptoms were reported to be mild with the rare use of an inhaler as needed. Apart from the inhaler, she was on no other medications at the time of the visit.

A complete physical examination was performed, and all findings were within normal limits. The only notable sign was some acne along her cheeks and chin. She was diagnosed with PD, with some elements of social phobia. She was prescribed a daily multiple vitamin/mineral preparation, 25 mg of zinc, 100 mg of pyridoxine, 400 mg of magnesium, and 500 mg of niacinamide twice daily.

A follow-up appointment occurred on December 13, 2003. The patient reported a slight improvement with her anxiety. She did not like taking all the supplements and agreed to continue with just the multiple vitamin/mineral preparation, zinc, and niacinamide. She also agreed to increase the dose of niacinamide to 1000 mg twice daily. No side effects were reported.

A second follow-up occurred on February 7, 2004. The patient, now 12-years-old, reported a striking improvement with her anxiety. She did not always take her pills daily, but was happy with the results. Her panic attacks completely stopped, and her acne was much improved as well.

In a recent e-mail from the patient, she reported to be taking only the 1000 mg of niacinamide twice daily. Her anxiety remained much improved and was no longer interfering with her ability to engage in a regular life. [Dr Prousky]

Case #3: General Anxiety Disorder (GAD)

A 28-year-old woman came to my private practice with a chief complaint of GAD on May 10, 2004. She had been struggling with this anxiety disorder for the past 12 years. She is a high school teacher, and noted that her anxiety was more pronounced during the academic year. Her anxiety was worse in the morning, with symptoms of frequent muscular tension, the passing of flatus, and chest pain. She reported a fear of smelling bad when she needed to expel gas. The anxiety also made it difficult for her to concentrate and focus on things.

When she experienced anxiety symptoms, she would feel the need to isolate herself from others. The same isolating need would also occur when she simply thought about possibly feeling nervous and expelling gas. She also reported fears of embarrassment and worried about being criticized from others. She had been on paroxetine for 1 year, but had not noticed any improvement. She reported feeling depressed due to the anxiety and would get apathetic when her anxiety was at its worst.

Baths, lying in bed, walking, and exercising helped to reduce her anxiety slightly. She was unable to correlate any of her symptoms with foods. This patient also had a history of thrombocytopenia for the past 5 years, for which she was being regularly monitored by her family physician. She did report easy bruising, but did not have any history of widespread bruising and bleeding. The rest of her past medical history was insignificant.

In her words, "I take the niacinamide and I'm fine afterwards."

Physical examination revealed a well-nourished woman with normal vital signs. All her systems were within normal limits. She was subsequently diagnosed with GAD (with some social phobia) and thrombocytopenia. Lab tests were requisitioned, and she was prescribed niacinamide at an initial dose of 500 mg three times daily for 3 days, and then was instructed to increase it to 1000 mg every morning, 500 mg at lunch, and 1000 mg at dinner. She was also prescribed 5-hydroxytryptophan (5-HTP) at a dose of 100 mg twice daily for her mild depression, and 2000 mg of vitamin C to be taken daily for the thrombocytopenia.

The patient had a follow-up appointment on May 31, 2004. She had difficulty swallowing the niacinamide pills due to their bitter taste. Despite this, she was taking the recommended dose of 2500 mg per day. Her anxiety was much improved and she had experienced only three minor panic attacks since the initial visit. Prior to the treatment, her anxiety was chronic, occurring daily, with the sensation or need to pass gas. The patient continued to complain of depression, which she felt was more pronounced prior to menses. Her complete blood count was normal, except that her platelets were low at a value of 79 (reference range, 150-400 X 10^9/L). The patient was unsure if the treatments were working due to her time away from teaching. We agreed that she would discontinue all prescribed treatments, except for the vitamin C, until June 14, 2004. After this date, the patient would resume the 5-HTP and niacinamide, take 250 mg of vitamin

B-6 and 400 mg of magnesium. The vitamin B-6 and magnesium were prescribed for the premenstrual symptoms of depression.

On June 4, 2004, I received an urgent telephone call from the patient. Since discontinuing the prescribed treatments on June 1, her anxiety symptoms returned promptly and she had difficulty functioning. She agreed to resume only the niacinamide tablets.

On July 2, 2004 the patient e-mailed me with an update. She discontinued all the prescribed treatments, except for the niacinamide. She found her anxiety and depression to be much relieved due to being at home and not teaching during the summer months. When she felt anxiety, she would take niacinamide and it would help. In her words, "I take the niacinamide and I'm fine afterwards." [Dr Prousky]

Case #4: Panic Attacks

A 42-year-old woman first presented to my private practice on May 16, 2004, for chief complaints of constipation and anxiety. About 3 weeks before, her father was diagnosed with advanced carcinoma of the stomach. For 3 days following his diagnosis, the patient experienced very soft stools once or twice daily. For her entire life, she had been constipated, requiring regular laxatives in order to have a daily bowel movement. The patient reported additional gastrointestinal symptoms of bloating, gas, and right-sided abdominal pain. She had taken fiber therapy in the past, but had never stayed on it long enough to see the benefits. She was not concerned about the constipation since she had been having at least one-to-two soft stools per day.

Since her father's diagnosis, she had been feeling very anxious with symptoms of shakiness, light-headedness, numbness of the extremities, and balance problems. Her medical doctor had her do a 24-hour holter monitor and the results were normal. She was unable to correlate her anxiety with feelings of hunger. In the past, she would have the same kind of anxiety symptoms when stressful events occurred. Her medical doctor felt that the patient's anxiety was related to hyperventilation.

On physical examination, the patient was well-nourished but slightly overweight, with normal blood pressure and normal heart sounds. All other systems were within normal limits. Even though her mother currently has heart disease, the rest of her family history was unremarkable. She was diagnosed with panic attacks, dyspepsia (possible irritable bowel syndrome), and mild obesity. She was advised to continue with her liquid multiple vitamin/mineral preparation, to take 500 mg of niacinamide three times each day for 2 days, and to increase the dose to 1000 mg twice daily. Two capsules of *Lactobacillus acidophilus* were prescribed every morning upon rising.

A follow-up visit occurred on May 26, 2004. The patient felt a little better during the first week on niacinamide. However, she felt jittery, and related this to her father's grim prognosis. Her sleep was unaffected, even though she did wake up once each night to go to the bathroom. Overall, she felt much more under control. She was advised to increase the niacinamide to 1000 mg three times each day.

On July 12, 2004, she came in for another visit. She had cut back on the niacinamide since she felt that it caused her to have feelings of not being "present." Instead of 3000 mg daily, she lowered the dose to 2000 mg per day. Her constipation was not a problem, and she was having one bowel movement daily. Her anxiety was much improved on this dose, and the previous shakiness had completely resolved. In fact, she had not experienced any episodes of shakiness since the last visit. She was told to continue the prescribed treatments and to take a B-complex vitamin preparation and 1 mg of folic acid each day. [Dr Prousky]

Schizoaffective Disorders

Schizoaffective disorder is a combination of thought disorder (or other psychotic symptoms) and a mood disorder (depression or mania). It is best viewed as a psychiatric disorder with features of both schizophrenia and bipolar disorder. In the United States, the lifetime prevalence is in the range of 0.5-0.8% (slightly less than schizophrenia).

The following case report is an excellent example of the effectiveness of naturopathic nutrition and orthomolecular medicine. The patient was eventually able to discontinue most of his mainstream treatments (except for risperidone) and fully recover from his diagnosis of schizoaffective disorder.

Case # 1: Schizoaffective Disorder

The patient, a 24-year-old Hispanic male, first presented to my private naturopathic practice on November 13, 2004, with chief complaints of schizoaffective disorder and obesity. He described a history of being unwell emotionally since the age of 15. His symptoms became more severe at the age of 16 when he started hearing messages from billboards, spent countless hours surfing the Internet, felt emotionally very flat, and believed that 100% of the bible was true and that the devil was forcing him to do things. He read excessively and did report some occasional thoughts of violence. Due to his moods, he had participated in a hospital-based program for depression that helped very much.

His past medical history included a suicide attempt at the age of 21, for which he was hospitalized and released shortly thereafter. Review of systems illuminated other problems that consisted of glaucoma, mild musculoskeletal complaints, obesity, and shortness of breath. His weight was about 200 pounds in the year 2000. Since being prescribed risperidone in 2001, his weight increased to 260 pounds. His current prescription medications were risperidone (3 mg daily), olanzapine (20 mg daily), and bupropion hydrochloride (150 mg daily).

The patient's family history revealed some genetic predisposition to schizophrenia, as his paternal grandmother was diagnosed with this disorder at 60 years old. On physical examination, the patient was well nourished, clinically obese, with high to normal blood pressure and mild tachycardia. All of his main systems were within normal limits. He was prescribed vitamin B-6 (250 mg daily), niacinamide (1000 mg three times daily), vitamin C (1000 mg three times daily), chromium (1000 mcg three times daily), liquid fish oil (1 teaspoon twice daily) providing close to 2 g of EPA, and zinc (50 mg daily). He was told to discontinue all dairy and milk products. Regular use of dairy and milk products can be associated with psychosis and depression.

On December 13, 2004, the patient returned for a follow-up. He reported an increased sense of alertness and vigor from the treatments. He also described symptoms of social anxiety where he would feel scared to talk to people and would even avoid teachers and classmates while completing his auto mechanic program. He did have some depression since the last visit, and experienced suicidal ideation on three separate occasions since the initial visit. His vitals were within normal limits. The patient was given the Beck Anxiety Inventory (BAI) and the Beck Depression Inventory (BDI) to fill-out. His BAI score was 33, indicating moderate anxiety. His

BDI score was 26, indicating moderate depression. Laboratory tests showed a normal CBC, normal fasting plasma glucose, and an abnormal lipid profile showing the patient to be at an "above average risk" for coronary heart disease. The patient was switched from the niacinamide to niacin at a dose of 1500 mg three times daily to help control his psychiatric symptoms and to have a favorable impact on his lipid profile. He was also given L-glycine for his symptoms of panic, at a dose of 2000 mg sublingually as needed. An intramuscular injection of vitamin B-12 (1500 mcg) was also provided.

The patient was given the Hoffer-Osmond Diagnostic (HOD) test to determine the severity of his schizoaffective disorder. The patient's HOD test was received and scored on December 17, 2004. For a patient with a pre-established diagnosis, the HOD test can also be used to evaluate the severity of mental disturbances and assess a patient's response to treatment. In this patient's case, his total score did indicate that he was symptomatic. If his total scores were to decline over time, it would be an indication of improvement.

Patient's First Set of HOD Results

HOD Test Items	December 2004 Results
Total Score (TS)	40
Perceptual Score (PerS)	4
Paranoid Score (PS)	2
Depression Score (DS)	10
Ratio Score (RS)	4
Short Form (SF)	1

About six weeks later, on January 26, 2005, the patient returned for another appointment. He felt that he was no longer symptomatic in terms of his diagnosis of schizoaffective disorder. The niacin caused the patient to vomit, so he reduced the dose to 1000 mg three times daily. He did not like the taste of L-glycine, so he never really tried the treatment. He did feel that his anxiety had improved about 10%. The patient was given another intramuscular injection, but the dose was different as it now contained folic acid (0.5 ml or 2.5 mg) and had a greater concentration of vitamin B-12 (1 ml or 5000 mcg). He was asked to retry the L-glycine and return in another 5 to 6 weeks.

On March 7, 2005, the patient felt that his diagnosis was better described as social anxiety disorder with some symptoms of schizoaffective disorder. He did not try the L-glycine as he was instructed to do. In terms of his anxiety, he felt about 20% to 30% better than the last visit. He was given another intramuscular injection of folic acid (2.5 mg) and vitamin B-12 (5000 mcg).

The patient returned for another appointment on April 20, 2005. He had seen a new psychiatrist, who recommended that the patient complete a series of cognitive behavior therapy for his social anxiety disorder. The patient was also attending a weekly group for patients with social anxiety disorder. The psychiatrist prescribed 20 mg of citalopram and took him off the olanzapine. He was sleeping less since discontinuing the olanzapine. The psychiatrist also instructed the patient to continue with risperidone (4 mg at bedtime) and bupropion hydrochloride (150 mg daily). The patient did report a better sense of well being, even though he felt more depressed during the previous week. His only problem was fear. He was unable to look at people when riding the subway because of the way people looked back at him. He also thought that people were judging him. For his anxiety, the patient was prescribed L-taurine at a dose of 1500 mg twice daily to be taken away from food. He was also prescribed ginkgo biloba extract (180 mg daily) to help with depression, for the side effects of risperidone, and for erectile dysfunction. Another intramuscular injection of folic acid (2.5 mg) and vitamin B-12 (5000 mcg) was given to the patient.

The patient had one more follow-up on June 27, 2005. He had reduced the risperidone to 2 mg daily on his own. He also discontinued the citalopram and bupropion hydrochloride. He did not feel worse than before and, in fact, indicated that he was more alert and required less sleep. He did not complain of any withdrawal symptoms from discontinuing the medications. His social anxiety seemed much improved. He was able to cover for his father as a courier and interact with people. This would not have been possible just a few months previously. He had just completed his auto mechanic program and was excited about going to college in the fall for accounting. He also remarked that his paranoid thoughts were gone, and were much better since stopping the two medications. The patient was instructed to stay on the nutrient and botanical treatments. He was also advised to continue avoiding all milk and dairy products. I assured him that as long as he remained consistent with the program, he had very little chance of a relapse.

I received the patient's final set of HOD results on June 30, 2005. As evident, the patient's scores improved significantly. [Dr Prousky]

Patient's Final Set of HOD Results

HOD Test Items	June 2005 Results
Total Score (TS)	5
Perceptual Score (PerS)	0
Paranoid Score (PS)	0
Depression Score (DS)	1
Ratio Score (RS)	5
Short Form (SF)	0

Niacin Therapy for Low Stomach Acid

Low stomach acid can impede the absorption of nutrients needed to maintain our health and fend off toxins. Once normal stomach acid levels are restored, often minor and even serious health conditions are resolved. One of the following cases comes from the files of Dr Melvin R. Werbach.

Case # 1: Fatigue and Constant Abdominal Bloating

In 2001, a 28-year-old Caucasian male of Jewish descent presented to my private office at the Canadian College of Naturopathic Medicine (CCNM) with complaints of fatigue and constant abdominal bloating after meals. These symptoms had persisted for 3 months. He began to take niacin at incremental dosages of 100 mg, eventually working up to 1200 mg per day. Within 3 days of supplementation, there was a noticeable increase in energy and a significant decrease in abdominal bloating. Occasionally, no abdominal bloating occurred.

The patient remained on 1200 mg per day of niacin for 2 months. When the patient went off the vitamin (due to the holiday of Passover), he experienced diarrhea, blood in the stools, and abdominal pain. After Passover, he resumed niacin at a dosage of 750 mg per day and these symptoms quickly abated. He continued on 750 mg per day of niacin for 2 more months with a significant relief of his symptoms. Occasional episodes of abdominal bloating and belching still occurred. [Dr Prousky]

Case # 2: Gastroesophageal Reflux Disease (GERD)

In 2001, a 28-year-old Caucasian male of European ethnicity presented to my private office. He reported a history of frequent abdominal bloating of at least 15 years duration, occasional abdominal pain, regurgitation of stomach contents, and repeated belching. He was previously diagnosed with gastroesophageal reflux disease (GERD). Despite trying various standard medical treatments for the past 7 years, his symptoms had not significantly abated. When he came to see me, he was experiencing about four flare-ups of GERD-related symptoms every month. Only Zantac and Gaviscon supplementation gave him symptomatic relief.

I recommended a trial course of oral niacin. Soon after taking 2000 to 3000 mg per day of niacin, his stomach regurgitation ceased and no more flare-ups occurred. The patient also reported a 50% reduction in his symptoms of belching and abdominal bloating. I followed this patient for almost a year after initiating niacin treatment and he continued to do well. During that time, he did not have another flare-up of his previous gastroesophageal reflux symptoms. [Dr Prousky]

Case # 3 Maldigestion

A 39-year-old Caucasian male presented to my office at The Robert Schad Naturopathic Clinic with chief complaints of bloating, intermittent diarrhea, gas, chronic throat irritation, perianal swelling, and back pain related to maldigestion. The gastrointestinal complaints had persisted for the previous 10 years, reaching a peak 4 years ago. At this time, the patient quit smoking and regular coffee drinking. These dietary changes improved his symptoms, but did not completely resolve them.

The patient works as a custodian at a church and reports that there is little stress in his life. He has no family history of gastrointestinal disease. He had seen numerous family physicians for his complaints, but was never prescribed any medications. Physical examination revealed a well-nourished male, with normal vital signs, and normal heart sounds. His skin was dry and pale, most notably along his face, upper thorax, and legs. There was also mild right-lower quadrant tenderness without rigidity or rebound signs.

> Low stomach acid can impede the absorption of nutrients needed to maintain our health and fend off toxins. Once normal stomach acid levels are restored, often minor and even serious health conditions are resolved.

The patient returned a week later for three consecutive fasting Gastro-Tests, with each test administered 15 minutes apart. The first test revealed a fasting gastric pH of 7, indicating severe low stomach acid. A second Gastro-Test was administered following a challenge with 500 mg of non-sustained release niacin. The distal 5 cm of the string showed a pH of 3. A change of 4 pH points since the first Gastro-Test clearly indicates that gastric pH can be made more acidic by taking oral niacin. A third Gastro-Test was performed with an additional 1000 mg of non-sustained release niacin. This time the result again demonstrated a pH of 7. It is unclear why the pH reverted to a 7. Perhaps the parietal cells could no longer respond to the addition of more acid with the third Gastro-Test.

The patient was then prescribed 1000 mg of non-sustained release niacin, three times each day. It was also recommended that he reduce his intake of fried foods, especially bacon and fast-food hamburgers. He was further instructed to have one salad daily in addition to increasing his intake of fruits and vegetables (no exact amount was specified).

Two days after commencing the dietary and niacin treatment, the patient felt a sense of improved well being and increased energy, with significant improvement in his throat irritation and perianal swelling. However, by the end of the first 2 days of treatment, the patient experienced a superficial rash with swelling and pruritus along the upper thorax, with the axilla and inner thighs being the areas most affected. He went to the emergency room of a local hospital and was given an oral antihistamine. He also was also told to discontinue the niacin. Within 24 hours the superficial rash completely cleared.

The patient resumed his niacin treatment the next day, but was switched to the IHN form to reduce the potential for flushing. Each IHN capsule contains 150 mg of inositol and 500 mg of niacin. He was instructed to take one capsule, three times daily. He came back to the clinic for a fasting Gastro-Test. The patient fasted 7 hours, and during the day of the test, he did not take any IHN. He drank as much water as he desired during the fast, but did not consume any food. The Gastro-Test showed a pH of 1 at the distal 8 cm of the string. The patient noticed a reduction in gastrointestinal bloating and claimed to have better-formed stools. The patient also reported an increase in energy. Objectively, the patient appeared more upbeat and his skin had less dryness and more of a pinkish color compared to our initial evaluation. The patient also remarked that his skin looked better.

The patient returned to the clinic for a repeat Gastro-Test. The patient fasted 6 hours, and during the day of the test, he did not take any IHN. The Gastro-Test showed a pH of 3 at the distal 6 cm of the string. The patient once again remarked on his improved health and almost complete absence of gastrointestinal symptoms. [Dr Prousky]

Case # 4: Alopecia (Hair Loss)

A 38-year-old woman came to my office complaining of generalized hair loss. She first began losing excessive scalp hair 15 years earlier when she went on a low-carbohydrate diet (<40 g daily). She stopped the diet and the excessive hair loss also stopped.

Four years earlier, she went on the Cambridge (liquid) diet along with salad and additional protein and lost 30 pounds in 30 days. Once again, she began to lose scalp hair. She also had palpitations and was very tired. A medical work-up at the time revealed mitral valve prolapse. She stopped the Cambridge diet after 2 months, but continued to note intermittent excessive hair loss. Her condition failed to improve despite nutritional supplements, a food elimination diet, and a trial of spironolactone.

In the year prior to her consultation, she counted her lost hairs daily and was unable to find any consistent pattern, although sometimes there was no significant hair loss for up to 4 days. She noted that her hair seemed less "lively and healthy" than it used to be. Every time she dyed her hair, her cervical lymph nodes would swell up; however, she continued to use a hair dye.

She also noted the recent onset of occasional burning sensations in her scalp. Her family had a history of hair loss: her mother wore a wig due to severe alopecia, and her two sisters also complained of excessive hair loss.

On March 13, she was started on betaine hydrochloride 10 grains with pepsin following each meal and was told to increase the dosage gradually as tolerated. On March 18, she was up to 2 tablets with meals. On May 12, she reported that her hair loss began to reduce about 1 month earlier and was now no greater than normal. On August 25, she reported that her hair was "doing fine." [Reprinted by permission from Melvin R. Werbach, *Case Studies In Natural Medicine,* Tarzana, CA: Third Line Press, 2002: 24-25. All rights reserved.]

Case # 5: Bowel Changes

Kathy, a 25-year-old female, presented to my private naturopathic practice with worrisome bowel changes. The onset of her symptoms occurred after she undertook a "cleanse" sometime in March 2002. This cleanse involved eating fruits and vegetables, followed by the elimination of all meals. Eventually, she was not consuming any foods, but was substituting all meals with a nutritional shake. Two days after initiating the cleanse, she started to note changes in her bowel functioning.

For the next 7 months, her bowel movements became thinner and were less formed with occasional mucous. She would cycle between loose stools and very hard ones. Daily fiber supplementation was necessary in order to have a daily bowel movement. After every meal, she would always have uncomfortable gas. She reported a bothersome white coating on her tongue, but denied any changes in weight, fatigue, or other symptoms. She had no family history of digestive disorders or diseases. Physical examination revealed a healthy female.

She was prescribed supplemental stomach acid, in the form of betaine hydrochloride. A follow-up visit showed marked improvements. She was taking 4 capsules (2000 mg) of betaine hydrochloride with large meals and 2 capsules (1000 mg) at smaller meals. She remarked that the gas had improved following meals, the white coating on her tongue had gone away, and her bowel movements were normal in appearance and form. Daily fiber supplements were discontinued, and she was having at least one bowel movement daily. No mucous was visible and she felt great. [Dr Prousky]

THE NUTRIENT CONTENT
OF COMMON FOODS

THE NUTRIENT CONTENT OF COMMON FOODS

It is always best to acquire all of the daily allotment of nutrients you need from the nutritional quality of foods eaten. The following list of the vitamin and mineral content of many foods will help you tailor your eating to your specific dietary needs. Use the listing to identify foods that are good sources for the particular vitamin or mineral you are interested in.

While the values given in these lists can be useful in comparing nutritional content in foods, the absolute values for food nutrients will vary, depending on such factors as the condition of the soil where the food was grown (or what type of nutrition an animal received), the amount of processing or refining, and the method of preparation.

The serving size of each food in the lists has been standardized to 100 grams. This was done to provide a more appropriate comparison between the relative amounts of nutrients in foods and allows them to be ranked from highest to lowest. Remember, however, not all foods are consumed in 100-gram quantities, especially if they are highly concentrated, like kelp, dulse, wheat germ, and brewer's yeast. Such foods often appear at the top of the list, indicating that they are concentrated nutritional sources. To get an idea of what 100 grams of a food represents, it may be helpful to consider what it is equivalent to in common measurements. A 100-gram serving size is approximately equal to any one of the following:

- about ⅜ cup fluid measure
- about ¼ cup dry measure
- 3¼ ounces of milk or yogurt
- slightly more than 1 cup leafy vegetable
- ¾ cup root vegetable
- 5½ ounces nuts, seeds
- ⅔ cup of sliced fruit
- ½ cup cereal grain, uncooked
- 7 tablespoons cooking oil
- 5 tablespoons honey, molasses

The following lists indicate the amounts of important nutrients available in 100-gram portions of various foods.

Bad Food

The following foods contain large amounts of sodium chloride, added during processing, and should generally be avoided.

Canned or frozen vegetables	Packaged spice mixes
Cured, smoked,	Bouillon cubes
or canned meats	Canned fish
Commercial peanut butter	Salted crackers
Potato chips, corn chips, etc.	Canned or packaged soups
Processed cheeses	Commercial salad dressings
Luncheon meats	Meat tenderizers
Salted nuts	

Vitamins

Vitamin A (Carotene)

I.U. per 100-gram (3.5 oz) portion		I.U. per 100-gram (3.5 oz) portion	
50,500	Lamb liver	43,900	Beef liver
22,500	Calf liver	21,600	Peppers, red chili
14,000	Dandelion greens	12,100	Chicken liver
11,000	Carrots	10,900	Apricots, dried
9,300	Collard leaves	8,900	Kale
8,800	Sweet potatoes	8,500	Parsley
8,100	Spinach	7,600	Turnip greens
7,000	Mustard greens	6,500	Swiss chard
6,100	Beet greens	5,800	Chives
5,700	Butternut squash	4,900	Watercress
4,800	Mangos	4,450	Peppers, sweet red
4,300	Hubbard squash	3,400	Cantaloupe
3,300	Endive	2,700	Apricots
2,500	Broccoli spears	2,260	Whitefish
2,000	Green onions	1,900	Romaine lettuce
1,750	Papayas	1,650	Nectarines
1,600	Prunes	1,600	Pumpkin
1,580	Swordfish	1,540	Whipping cream
1,330	Peaches	1,200	Acorn squash
1,180	Eggs	1,080	Chicken
1,000	Cherries, sour red	970	Butterhead lettuce
900	Asparagus	900	Tomatoes, ripe
770	Peppers, green chili	690	Kidneys
640	Peas	600	Green beans
600	Elderberries	590	Watermelon
580	Rutabagas	550	Brussels sprouts
520	Okra	510	Yellow cornmeal
460	Yellow squash		

Vitamin A from animal source foods occurs mostly as active, preformed vitamin A (retinol), while that from vegetable source foods occurs as pro-vitamin A (beta-carotene and other carotenoids) that must be converted to active vitamin A by the body to be utilized. The efficiency of conversion varies among individuals; however, beta-carotene is converted more efficiently than other carotenoids. Green and deep-yellow vegetables, as well as deep-yellow fruits, are highest in beta-carotene.

Vitamin B-1 (Thiamin)

I.U. per 100-gram (3.5 oz) portion		I.U. per 100-gram (3.5 oz) portion	
15.61	Brewer's yeast	14.01	Torula yeast
2.01	Wheat germ	1.96	Sunflower seeds
1.84	Rice polishings	1.28	Pine nuts
1.14	Peanuts, with skins	1.10	Soybeans, dry
1.05	Cowpeas, dry	.98	Peanuts, without skins
.96	Brazil nuts	.93	Pork, lean
.86	Pecans	.85	Soybean flour
.84	Beans, pinto and red	.74	Split peas
.73	Millet	.72	Wheat bran
.67	Pistachio nuts	.65	Navy beans
.63	Veal heart	.60	Buckwheat
.60	Oatmeal	.55	Whole wheat flour
.55	Whole wheat	.51	Lamb kidneys
.31	Garbanzos	.48	Lima beans, dry
.46	Hazelnuts	.45	Lamb heart
.45	Wild rice	.43	Cashews
.43	Rye, whole grain	.40	Lamb liver
.40	Lobster	.38	Mung beans
.38	Cornmeal, whole	.37	Lentils
.36	Beef kidneys	.35	Green peas
.34	Brown rice	.33	Walnuts
.30	Pork liver	.25	Garlic, cloves

.25	Beef liver	.24	Almonds, ground
.24	Lima beans, fresh	.24	Pumpkin and squash seeds
.23	Brains, all kinds	.23	Soybean sprouts
.22	Peppers, red chili		

Vitamin B-2 (Riboflavin)

I.U. per 100-gram (3.5 oz) portion		I.U. per 100-gram (3.5 oz) portion	
5.06	Torula yeast	4.28	Brewer's yeast
3.28	Lamb liver	3.26	Beef liver
3.03	Pork liver	2.72	Calf liver
2.55	Beef kidneys	2.49	Chicken liver
2.42	Lamb kidneys	1.36	Chicken giblets
1.05	Veal heart	.92	Almonds
.88	Beef heart	.74	Lamb heart
.68	Wheat germ	.63	Wild rice
.46	Mushrooms	.44	Egg yolks
.38	Millet	.36	Peppers, hot red
.35	Soy flour	.35	Wheat bran
.33	Mackerel	.31	Collards
.31	Soybeans, dry	.30	Eggs
.29	Split peas	.29	Beef tongue
.29	Brains, all kinds	.26	Kale
.26	Parsley	.25	Cashews
.25	Rice bran	.25	Veal
.24	Lamb, lean	.23	Broccoli
.23	Chicken, meat and skin	.23	Pine nuts
.23	Salmon	.23	Sunflower seeds
.22	Rye, whole grain	.22	Navy beans
.22	Beet and mustard greens	.21	Beans, pinto and red
.22	Lentils	.22	Pork, lean
.22	Prunes	.21	Mung beans
.21	Blackeyed peas	.21	Okra
.13	Sesame seeds, hulled		

Vitamin B-3 (Niacin)

I.U. per 100-gram (3½ oz) portion		I.U. per 100-gram (3½ oz) portion	
44.4	Torula yeast	37.9	Brewer's yeast
29.8	Rice bran	28.2	Rice polishings
21.0	Wheat bran	17.2	Peanuts, with skins
16.9	Lamb liver	16.4	Pork liver
15.8	Peanuts, without skins	13.6	Beef liver
11.4	Calf liver	11.3	Turkey, light meat
10.8	Chicken liver	10.7	Chicken, light meat
8.4	Trout	8.3	Halibut
8.2	Mackerel	8.1	Veal heart
8.0	Chicken, meat only	8.0	Swordfish
8.0	Turkey, meat only	7.7	Goose, meat only
7.5	Beef heart	7.2	Salmon
6.4	Veal	6.4	Beef kidneys
6.2	Wild rice	6.1	Chicken giblets
5.7	Lamb, lean	5.6	Chicken, meat and skin
5.4	Sesame seeds	5.4	Sunflower seeds
5.1	Beef, lean	5.0	Pork, lean
4.7	Brown rice	4.5	Pine nuts
4.4	Buckwheat, whole grain	4.4	Peppers, red chili
4.4	Whole wheat grain	4.3	Whole wheat flour
4.2	Mushrooms	4.2	Wheat germ
3.7	Barley	3.6	Herring
3.5	Almonds	3.5	Shrimp
3.0	Haddock	3.0	Split peas

Pantothenic Acid (a B vitamin)

I.U. per 100-gram (3.5 oz) portion		I.U. per 100-gram (3.5 oz) portion	
12.0	Brewer's yeast	11.0	Torula yeast
8.0	Calf liver	6.0	Chicken liver

3.9	Beef kidneys	2.8	Peanuts
2.6	Brains, all kinds	2.6	Heart
2.2	Mushrooms	2.0	Soybean flour
2.0	Split peas	2.0	Beef tongue
1.9	Perch	1.8	Blue cheese
1.7	Pecans	1.7	Soybeans
1.6	Eggs	1.5	Lobster
1.5	Oatmeal, dry	1.4	Buckwheat flour
1.4	Sunflower seeds	1.4	Lentils
1.3	Rye flour, whole	1.3	Cashews
1.3	Salmon	1.2	Camembert cheese
1.2	Garbanzos	1.2	Wheat germ, toasted
1.2	Broccoli	1.1	Hazelnuts
1.1	Turkey, dark meat	1.1	Brown rice
1.1	Wheat flour, whole	1.1	Sardines
1.1	Peppers, red chili	1.1	Avocados
1.1	Veal, lean	1.0	Blackeyed peas, dry
1.0	Wild rice	1.0	Cauliflower
1.0	Chicken, dark meat	1.0	Kale

Vitamin B-6 (Pyridoxine)

I.U. per 100-gram (3.5 oz) portion

3.00	Torula yeast	2.50	Brewer's yeast
1.25	Sunflower seeds	1.15	Wheat germ, toasted
.90	Tuna	.84	Beef liver
.81	Soybeans, dry	.75	Chicken liver
.73	Walnuts	.70	Salmon
.69	Trout	.67	Calf liver
.66	Mackerel	.65	Pork liver
.63	Soybean flour	.60	Lentils, dry
.58	Buckwheat flour	.58	Lima beans, dry
.56	Blackeyed peas, dry	.56	Navy beans, dry
.55	Brown rice	.54	Garbanzos, dry

.53	Pinto beans, dry	.51	Bananas
.45	Pork, lean	.44	Albacore
.43	Beef, lean	.43	Halibut
.43	Beef kidneys	.42	Avocados
.41	Veal kidneys	.34	Whole wheat flour
.33	Chestnuts, fresh	.30	Egg yolks
.30	Kale	.30	Rye flour
.28	Spinach	.26	Turnip greens
.25	Beef heart	.26	Peppers, sweet
.25	Potatoes	.24	Prunes
.24	Raisins	.24	Sardines
.24	Brussels sprouts	.23	Elderberries
.23	Perch	.22	Cod
.22	Barley	.22	Camembert cheese
.22	Sweet potatoes	.21	Cauliflower
.20	Popcorn, popped	.20	Red cabbage
.20	Leeks	.20	Molasses

Folic Acid (a B vitamin)

I.U. per 100-gram (3.5oz) portion		I.U. per 100-gram (3.5oz) portion	
2022	Brewer's yeast	440	Blackeyed peas
430	Rice germ	425	Soy flour
305	Wheat germ	295	Beef liver
275	Lamb liver	225	Soybeans
220	Pork liver	195	Bran
180	Kidney beans	145	Mung beans
130	Lima beans	125	Navy beans
125	Garbanzos	110	Asparagus
105	Lentils	77	Walnuts
75	Spinach, fresh	70	Kale
65	Filbert nuts	60	Beet and mustard greens
57	Textured vegetable protein	56	Peanuts, roasted
		56	Peanut butter

53	Broccoli	50	Barley
50	Split peas	49	Whole wheat cereal
49	Brussels sprouts	45	Almonds
38	Whole wheat flour	33	Oatmeal
32	Dried figs	30	Avocado
28	Green beans	28	Corn
28	Coconut, fresh	27	Pecans
25	Mushrooms	25	Dates
14	Blackberries	7	Ground beef
5	Oranges		

Vitamin B-12 (Cobalamin)

I.U. per 100-gram (3.5 oz) portion		I.U. per 100-gram (3.5 oz) portion	
104	Lamb liver	98	Clams
80	Beef liver	63	Lamb kidneys
60	Calf liver	31	Beef kidneys
25	Chicken liver	18	Oysters
17	Sardines	11	Beef heart
6	Egg yolks	5.2	Lamb heart
5.0	Trout	4.0	Brains, all kinds
4.0	Salmon	3.0	Tuna
2.1	Lamb	2.1	Sweetbreads
2.0	Eggs	2.0	Whey, dried
1.8	Beef, lean	1.8	Edam cheese
1.8	Swiss cheese	1.6	Brie cheese
1.6	Gruyere cheese	1.4	Blue cheese
1.3	Haddock	1.2	Flounder
1.2	Scallops	1.0	Cheddar cheese
1.0	Cottage cheese	1.0	Mozzarella cheese
1.0	Halibut	1.0	Perch, fillets
1.0	Swordfish		

Biotin (a B vitamin)

I.U. per 100-gram (3.5 oz) portion		I.U. per 100-gram (3.5 oz) portion	
200	Brewer's yeast	127	Lamb liver
100	Pork liver	96	Beef liver
70	Soy flour	61	Soybeans
60	Rice bran	58	Rice germ
57	Rice polishings	52	Egg yolk
39	Peanut butter	37	Walnuts
34	Peanuts, roasted	31	Barley
27	Pecans	24	Oatmeal
24	Sardines, canned	22	Eggs
21	Blackeyed peas	18	Split peas
18	Almonds	17	Cauliflower
16	Mushrooms	16	Whole wheat cereal
15	Salmon, canned	15	Textured vegetable protein
14	Bran	13	Lentils
12	Brown rice	10	Chicken

Choline (a B vitamin)

I.U. per 100-gram (3.5 oz) portion		I.U. per 100-gram (3.5 oz) portion	
2200	Lecithin	1490	Egg yolk
550	Liver	504	Whole eggs
406	Wheat germ	340	Soybeans
300	Rice germ	257	Blackeyed peas
245	Garbanzo beans	240	Brewer's yeast
223	Lentils	201	Split peas
170	Rice bran	162	Peanuts, roasted
156	Oatmeal	145	Peanut butter
143	Bran	139	Barley
122	Ham	112	Brown rice

104	Veal		102	Rice polishings
94	Whole wheat cereal		86	Molasses
77	Pork		75	Beef
75	Green peas		48	Cheddar cheese
66	Sweet potatoes		42	Green beans
29	Potatoes		23	Cabbage
22	Spinach		20.5	Textured vegetable protein
15	Milk		12	Orange juice
5	Butter			

Inositol (a B vitamin)

I.U. per 100-gram (3½ oz) portion			I.U. per 100-gram (3½ oz) portion	
2220	Lecithin		770	Wheat germ
500	Navy beans		460	Rice bran
454	Rice polishings		390	Barley, cooked
370	Rice germ		370	Whole wheat
270	Brewer's yeast		270	Oatmeal
240	Blackeyed peas		240	Garbanzo beans
210	Oranges		205	Soy flour
200	Soybeans		180	Peanuts, roasted
180	Peanut butter		170	Lima beans
162	Green peas		150	Molasses
150	Grapefruit		150	Split peas
130	Lentils		120	Raisins
120	Cantaloupe		119	Brown rice
117	Orange juice		110	Whole wheat flour
96	Peaches		95	Cabbage
95	Cauliflower		88	Onions
67	Whole wheat bread		66	Sweet potatoes
64	Watermelon		60	Strawberries
55	Lettuce		51	Beef liver
46	Tomatoes		33	Eggs
13	Milk		11	Beef, round

Vitamin B-17 (Amygdalin)

For certain nutrients, there are few foods sources that contain appreciable quantities. In these cases we list those foods that are best sources, rather than relative nutrient amounts.

Foods containing more than 500 milligrams per 100-gram portion:

Wild blackberries	Apple seeds	Cherry seeds
Elderberries	Apricot seeds	Nectarine seeds
Peach seeds	Fava beans	Bamboo sprouts
Pear seeds	Mung beans	Alfalfa leaves
Plum seeds	Bitter almonds	
Prune seeds	Macadamia nuts	

Foods containing between 100 and 500 milligrams per 100-gram portion:

Boysenberries	Raspberries	Garbanzo beans
Currants	Alfalfa sprouts	Blackeyed peas
Gooseberries	Buckwheat	Kidney beans
Huckleberries	Flax seed	Lentils
Loganberries	Millet	Lima beans
Mulberries	Squash seed	
Quince	Mung bean sprouts	

Foods containing below 100 milligrams per 100-gram portion:

Commercial blackberries	Peas	Cashews
Cranberries	Lima beans	Beet tops
Black beans	Sweet potatoes, yams	

Para-Aminobenzoic Acid (PABA)
(a B vitamin)

Good sources include:

Mushrooms	Sunflower seeds	Whole milk
Liver	Wheat germ	Eggs
Bran	Oats	
Cabbage	Spinach	

Pangamic Acid (Vitamin B-15)

Good sources include:

Apricot kernels	Corn grits	Oat grits
Yeast	Wheat germ	Sunflower seeds
Liver	Wheat bran	Pumpkin seeds
Rice bran		

Vitamin C (Ascorbic Acid)

I.U. per 100-gram (3.5 oz) portion		I.U. per 100-gram (3.5 oz) portion	
1300	Acerola	369	Peppers, red chili
242	Guavas	204	Peppers, red sweet
186	Kale leaves	172	Parsley
152	Collard leaves	139	Turnip greens
128	Peppers, green sweet	113	Broccoli
102	Brussels sprouts	97	Mustard greens
79	Watercress	78	Cauliflower
66	Persimmons	61	Cabbage, red
59	Strawberries	56	Papayas
51	Spinach	50	Oranges and juice
47	Cabbage	46	Lemon juice
38	Grapefruit and juice	36	Elderberries

36	Calf liver	36	Turnips
35	Mangoes	33	Asparagus
33	Cantaloupes	32	Swiss chard
32	Green onions	31	Beef liver
31	Okra	31	Tangerines
30	New Zealand spinach	30	Oysters
29	Lima beans, young	29	Blackeyed beans
29	Soybeans	27	Green peas
26	Radishes	25	Raspberries
25	Chinese cabbage	25	Yellow summer squash
24	Loganberries	23	Honeydew melon
23	Tomatoes	23	Pork liver

Vitamin D

I.U. per 100-gram (3.5 oz) portion		I.U. per 100-gram (3.5 oz) portion	
500	Sardines, canned	350	Salmon
250	Tuna	150	Shrimp
90	Sunflower seeds	90	Butter
50	Liver	50	Eggs
40	Milk, fortified	40	Mushrooms
30	Natural cheeses		

Vitamin E (Tocopherol)

I.U. per 100-gram (3.5 oz) portion		I.U. per 100-gram (3.5 oz) portion	
216	Wheat germ oil	90	Sunflower seeds
88	Sunflower seed oil	72	Safflower oil
48	Almonds	45	Sesame oil
34	Peanut oil	29	Corn oil
22	Wheat germ	18	Olive oil
18	Peanuts	14	Soybean oil

13	Peanuts, roasted	11	Peanut butter
3.0	Bran	3.6	Butter
3.2	Spinach	3.0	Oatmeal
2.9	Asparagus	2.5	Salmon
2.5	Brown rice	2.3	Rye, whole
2.2	Rye bread, dark	1.9	Pecans
1.9	Wheat germ	1.9	Rye and wheat crackers
1.4	Whole wheat bread	1.0	Carrots
0.99	Peas	0.92	Walnuts
0.88	Bananas	0.83	Eggs
0.72	Tomatoes	0.29	Lamb

Vitamin K

I.U. per 100-gram (3.5 oz) portion

650	Turnip greens	200	Broccoli
129	Lettuce	125	Cabbage
92	Beef liver	89	Spinach
57	Watercress	57	Asparagus
35	Cheese	30	Butter
25	Pork liver	20	Oats
19	Green peas	17	Whole wheat
14	Green beans	11	Pork
11	Eggs	10	Corn oil
8	Peaches	7	Beef
7	Chicken liver	6	Raisins
5	Tomatoes	3	Milk
3	Potatoes		

Bioflavonoids (Vitamin P)

Goods sources include:

Grapes	Black currants	Peppers
Rose hips	Plums	Papaya

Prunes
Oranges
Lemon juice
Apricots

Parsley
Grapefruit
Cabbage

Cantaloupe
Tomatoes
Cherries

Minerals

Calcium

I.U. per 100-gram (3.5 oz) portion

1093	Kelp
750	Cheddar cheese
296	Dulse
246	Turnip greens
234	Almonds
203	Parsley
187	Dandelion greens
151	Watercress
128	Tofu
121	Buttermilk
120	Yogurt
119	Wheat bran
114	Buckwheat, raw
106	Ripe olives
99	English walnut
93	Spinach
73	Pecans
69	Peanuts
68	Romaine lettuce
66	Rutabaga
60	Black currants
56	Green snap beans
51	Dried prunes
50	Cooked dry beans

I.U. per 100-gram (3.5 oz) portion

925	Swiss cheese
352	Carob flour
250	Collard leaves
245	Barbados molasses
210	Brewer's yeast
200	Corn tortillas (lime added)
186	Brazil nuts
129	Goat's milk
126	Dried figs
120	Sunflower seeds
119	Beet greens
118	Whole milk
110	Sesame seeds, hulled
103	Broccoli
94	Cottage cheese
73	Soybeans, cooked
72	Wheat germ
68	Miso
67	Dried apricots
62	Raisins
59	Dates
51	Globe artichokes
51	Pumpkin and squash seeds

49	Common cabbage	48	Soybean sprouts
46	Hard winter wheat	41	Oranges
39	Celery	38	Cashews
38	Rye grain	37	Carrots
34	Barley	32	Sweet potatoes
32	Brown rice	29	Garlic
28	Summer squash	27	Onions
26	Lemons	26	Fresh green peas
25	Cauliflower	25	Lentils, cooked
22	Sweet cherries	22	Asparagus
22	Winter squash	21	Strawberry
20	Millet	19	Mung bean sprouts
17	Pineapple	16	Grapes
16	Beets	14	Cantaloupe
14	Jerusalem artichokes	13	Tomatoes
12	Eggplant	12	Chicken
11	Orange juice	10	Avocado
10	Beef	8	Bananas
7	Apples	3	Sweet corn

Magnesium

I.U. per 100-gram (3.5 oz) portion		I.U. per 100-gram (3.5 oz) portion	
760	Kelp	490	Wheat bran
336	Wheat germ	270	Almonds
267	Cashews	258	Blackstrap molasses
231	Brewer's yeast	229	Buckwheat
225	Brazil nuts	220	Dulse
184	Filberts	175	Peanuts
162	Millet	160	Wheat grain
142	Pecan	131	English walnut
115	Rye	111	Tofu
106	Beet greens	90	Coconut meat, dry
88	Soybeans, cooked	88	Spinach

88	Brown rice	71	Dried figs
65	Swiss chard	62	Apricots, dried
58	Dates	57	Collard leaves
51	Shrimp	48	Sweet corn
45	Cheddar cheese	41	Parsley
40	Prunes, dried	38	Sunflower seeds
37	Common beans, cooked	37	Barley
36	Dandelion greens	36	Garlic
36	Raisins	35	Fresh green peas
34	Potatoes with skin	34	Crab
33	Bananas	33	Sweet potatoes
30	Blackberries	25	Beets
25	Broccoli	24	Cauliflower
23	Carrots	22	Celery
21	Beef	20	Asparagus
19	Chicken	18	Pepper, green
17	Winter squash	16	Cantaloupe
16	Eggplant	14	Tomato
13	Cabbage	13	Grapes
13	Milk	13	Pineapple
13	Mushrooms	12	Onions
11	Oranges	11	Iceberg lettuce
9	Plums		

Phosphorus

I.U. per
100-gram (3.5 oz) portion

1753	Brewer's yeast	1276	Wheat bran
1144	Pumpkin and squash seeds	1118	Wheat germ
		837	Sunflower seeds
693	Brazil nuts	592	Sesame seeds, hulled
554	Soybeans, dried	504	Almonds
478	Cheddar cheese	457	Pinto beans, dried
409	Peanuts	400	Wheat

380	English walnuts	376	Rye grain
373	Cashews	352	Beef liver
338	Scallops	311	Millet
290	Barley, pearled	289	Pecans
267	Dulse	240	Kelp
239	Chicken	221	Brown rice
202	Garlic	175	Crab
152	Cottage cheese	150	Beef or lamb
119	Lentils, cooked	116	Mushrooms
116	Fresh peas	111	Sweet corn
101	Raisins	93	Milk
88	Globe artichoke	87	Yogurt
80	Brussels sprouts	79	Prunes, dried
78	Broccoli	77	Figs, dried
69	Yams	67	Soybean sprouts
64	Mung bean sprouts	63	Dates
63	Parsley	62	Asparagus
59	Bamboo shoots	56	Cauliflower
53	Potato, with skin	44	Green beans
44	Pumpkin	42	Avocado
40	Beet greens	39	Swiss chard
38	Winter squash	36	Carrots
36	Onions	35	Red cabbage
51	Spinach	33	Beets
31	Radishes	29	Summer squash
28	Celery	27	Cucumber
27	Tomatoes	26	Bananas
26	Persimmon	26	Eggplant
26	Lettuce	24	Nectarines
22	Raspberries	20	Grapes
20	Oranges	205	Eggs
17	Olives	16	Cantaloupe
10	Apples	8	Pineapple

Sodium

I.U. per 100-gram (3.5 oz) portion		I.U. per 100-gram (3.5 oz) portion	
3007	Kelp	2400	Green olives
2132	Salt (1 teaspoon)	1428	Dill pickles
1319	Soy sauce (1 tablespoon)	828	Ripe olives
747	Sauerkraut	700	Cheddar cheese
265	Scallops	229	Cottage cheese
210	Lobster	147	Swiss chard
130	Beet greens	130	Buttermilk
126	Celery	122	Eggs
110	Cod	71	Spinach
70	Lamb	65	Pork
64	Chicken	60	Beef
60	Beets	60	Sesame seeds
52	Watercress	50	Whole milk
49	Turnips	47	Carrots
47	Yogurt	45	Parsley
43	Artichoke	34	Dried figs
30	Lentils, dried	30	Sunflower seeds
27	Raisins	26	Red cabbage
19	Garlic	19	White beans
15	Broccoli	15	Mushrooms
13	Cauliflower	10	Onions
10	Sweet Potatoes	9	Brown rice
9	Lettuce	6	Cucumber
5	Peanuts	4	Avocado
3	Tomatoes	2	Eggplant

Potassium

I.U. per 100-gram (3.5 oz) portion		I.U. per 100-gram (3.5 oz) portion	
8060	Dulse	5273	Kelp
920	Sunflower seeds	827	Wheat germ
773	Almonds	763	Raisins
727	Parsley	715	Brazil nuts
674	Peanuts	648	Dates
640	Figs, dried	604	Avocado
603	Pecans	600	Yams
550	Swiss chard	540	Soybeans, cooked
529	Garlic	470	Spinach
450	English walnuts	430	Millet
416	Beans, cooked	414	Mushrooms
407	Potatoes, with skin	382	Broccoli
370	Bananas	370	Meats
369	Winter squash	366	Chicken
341	Carrots	341	Celery
322	Radishes	295	Cauliflower
282	Watercress	278	Asparagus
268	Red cabbage	264	Lettuce
251	Cantaloupe	249	Lentils, cooked
244	Tomatoes	243	Sweet potatoes
234	Papaya	214	Eggplant
213	Peppers, green	208	Beets
202	Peaches	202	Summer squash
200	Oranges	199	Raspberries
191	Cherries	164	Strawberries
162	Grapefruit juice	158	Grapes
157	Onions	146	Pineapple
144	Milk	141	Lemon juice
130	Pears	129	Eggs
110	Apples	100	Watermelon
70	Brown rice, cooked		

Iron

I.U. per 100-gram (3.5 oz) portion		I.U. per 100-gram (3.5 oz) portion	
100.3	Kelp	17.3	Brewer's yeast
16.1	Blackstrap molasses	14.9	Wheat bran
11.2	Pumpkin and squash seeds	9.4	Wheat germ
7.1	Sunflower seeds	8.8	Beef liver
6.2	Parsley	6.8	Millet
4.7	Almond	6.1	Clam
3.8	Cashews	3.9	Dried prunes
3.5	Raisins	3.7	Beef, lean
3.4	Brazil nuts	3.4	Jerusalem artichokes
3.2	Swiss chard	3.3	Beet greens
3.1	English walnuts	3.1	Dandelion greens
2.9	Pork	3.0	Dates
2.4	Sesame seeds, hulled	2.7	Cooked dry beans
2.3	Eggs	2.4	Pecans
2.1	Peanuts	2.1	Lentils
1.9	Tofu	1.9	Lamb
1.6	Brown rice	1.8	Green peas
1.5	Chicken	1.6	Ripe olives
1.2	Salmon	1.3	Mung bean sprouts
1.1	Currants	1.1	Broccoli
1.1	Cauliflower	1.1	Whole wheat bread
1.0	Strawberries	1.0	Cheddar cheese
0.9	Blackberries	1.0	Asparagus
0.8	Pumpkin	0.8	Red cabbage
0.7	Bananas	0.8	Mushroom
0.7	Carrots	0.7	Beets
0.7	Sweet potatoes	0.7	Eggplant
0.6	Figs	0.6	Avocado
0.6	Corn	0.6	Potatoes
0.5	Nectarines	0.5	Pineapple
		0.5	Winter squash

0.5	Brown rice, cooked	0.5	Tomatoes
0.4	Oranges	0.4	Cherries
0.4	Summer squash	0.3	Papaya
0.3	Celery	0.3	Cottage Cheese
0.3	Apples		

Copper

I.U. per 100-gram (3.5 oz) portion		I.U. per 100-gram (3.5 oz) portion	
13.7	Oysters	2.3	Brazil nuts
2.1	Soy lecithin	1.4	Almonds
1.3	Hazelnuts	1.3	Walnuts
1.3	Pecans	1.2	Split peas, dry
1.1	Beef liver	0.8	Buckwheat
0.8	Peanuts	0.7	Cod liver oil
0.7	Lamb chops	0.5	Sunflower oil
0.4	Butter	0.4	Rye grain
0.4	Pork loin	0.4	Barley
0.4	Gelatin	0.3	Shrimp
0.3	Olive oil	0.3	Clams
0.3	Carrots	0.3	Coconut
0.3	Garlic	0.2	Millet
0.2	Whole wheat	0.2	Chicken
0.2	Eggs	0.2	Corn oil
0.2	Ginger root	0.2	Molasses
0.2	Turnips	0.1	Green peas
0.1	Papaya	0.1	Apples

Black pepper, thyme, paprika, bay leaves, and active dry yeast are also high in copper.

Manganese

I.U. per 100-gram (3.5 oz) portion		I.U. per 100-gram (3.5 oz) portion	
3.5	Pecans	2.8	Brazil nuts
2.5	Almonds	1.8	Barley
1.3	Rye	1.3	Buckwheat
1.3	Split peas, dry	1.1	Whole wheat
0.16	Carrots	0.15	Broccoli
0.14	Brown rice	0.14	Whole wheat bread
0.13	Swiss cheese	0.13	Corn
0.11	Cabbage	0.10	Peaches
0.8	Walnuts	0.8	Fresh spinach
0.7	Peanuts	0.6	Oats
0.5	Raisins	0.5	Turnip greens
0.5	Rhubarb	0.4	Beet greens
0.3	Brussels sprouts	0.3	Oatmeal
0.2	Cornmeal	0.2	Millet
0.19	Gorgonzola cheese	0.09	Butter
0.06	Tangerines	0.06	Peas
0.05	Eggs	0.04	Beets
0.04	Coconut	0.03	Apples
0.03	Oranges	0.03	Pears
0.03	Lamb chops	0.03	Pork chops
0.03	Cantaloupe	0.03	Tomatoes
0.02	Milk	0.02	Chicken breasts
0.02	Green beans	0.02	Apricots
0.01	Beef liver	0.01	Scallops
0.01	Halibut	0.01	Cucumbers

Cloves, ginger, thyme, bay leaves, and tea are also high in manganese.

Zinc

I.U. per 100-gram (3.5 oz) portion		I.U. per 100-gram (3.5 oz) portion	
148.7	Fresh oysters	6.8	Ginger root
5.6	Ground round steak	5.3	Lamb chops
4.5	Pecans	4.2	Split peas, dry
4.2	Brazil nuts	3.9	Beef liver
3.5	Nonfat dry milk	3.5	Egg yolk
3.2	Whole wheat	3.2	Rye
3.2	Oats	3.2	Peanuts
3.1	Lima beans	3.1	Soy lecithin
3.1	Almonds	3.0	Walnuts
2.9	Sardines	2.6	Chicken
2.5	Buckwheat	2.4	Hazelnuts
1.9	Clams	1.7	Anchovies
1.7	Tuna	1.7	Haddock
1.6	Green peas	1.5	Shrimp
1.2	Turnips	0.9	Parsley
0.9	Potatoes	0.6	Garlic
0.5	Carrots	0.5	Whole wheat bread
0.4	Black beans	0.4	Raw milk
0.4	Pork chops	0.4	Corn
0.3	Grape juice	0.3	Olive oil
0.3	Cauliflower	0.2	Spinach
0.2	Cabbage	0.2	Lentils
0.2	Butter	0.2	Lettuce
0.1	Cucumber	0.1	Yams
0.1	Tangerines	0.1	String beans

Chromium

The values listed below show the total chromium content of these foods, and do not indicate the amount that may be biologically active as the Glucose Tolerance Factor (GTF). Those foods marked with an * are high in GTF.

I.U. per 100-gram (3.5 oz) portion		I.U. per 100-gram (3.5 oz) portion	
112	Brewer's yeast*	57	Beef round
55	Calf liver*	42	Whole wheat bread*
38	Wheat bran	30	Rye bread
30	Fresh chili	26	Oysters
24	Potatoes	23	Wheat germ
19	Peppers, green	16	Hen's eggs
15	Chicken	14	Apples
13	Butter	13	Parsnips
12	Cornmeal	12	Lamb chop
11	Scallops	11	Swiss cheese
10	Bananas	10	Spinach
10	Pork chop	9	Carrots
8	Navy beans, dry	7	Shrimp
7	Lettuce	5	Oranges
5	Lobster tails	5	Blueberries
4	Green beans	4	Cabbage
4	Mushrooms	3	Beer
3	Strawberries	1	Milk

Selenium

I.U. per 100-gram (3.5 oz) portion		I.U. per 100-gram (3.5 oz) portion	
144	Butter	141	Smoked herring
123	Smelts	111	Wheat germ

103	Brazil nuts	89	Apple cider vinegar
77	Scallops	66	Barley
66	Whole wheat bread	65	Lobster
63	Bran	59	Shrimps
57	Red swiss chard	56	Oats
55	Clams	51	King crab
49	Oysters	48	Milk
43	Cod	39	Brown rice
34	Top round steak	30	Lamb
27	Turnips	26	Molasses
25	Garlic	24	Barley
19	Orange juice	19	Gelatin
19	Beer	18	Beef liver
18	Lamb chop	18	Egg yolk
12	Mushrooms	12	Chicken
10	Swiss cheese	5	Cottage cheese
5	Wine	4	Radishes
4	Grape juice	3	Pecans
2	Hazelnuts	2	Almonds
2	Green beans	2	Kidney beans
2	Onions	2	Carrots
2	Cabbage	1	Oranges

Iodine

I.U. per 100-gram (3.5 oz) portion

90	Clams	65	Shrimp
62	Haddock	56	Halibut
50	Oysters	50	Salmon
37	Sardines, canned	19	Beef liver
16	Pineapple	16	Tuna, canned
14	Eggs	11	Peanuts
11	Whole wheat bread	11	Cheddar cheese
10	Pork	10	Lettuce

9	Spinach		9	Green peppers
9	Butter		7	Milk
6	Cream		6	Cottage cheese
6	Beef		3	Lamb
3	Raisins			

Nickel

I.U. per 100-gram (3.5 oz) portion

700	Soybeans, dry		500	Beans, dry
410	Soy flour		310	Lentils
250	Split peas		175	Green peas
153	Green beans		150	Oats
132	Walnuts		122	Hazelnuts
100	Buckwheat		90	Barley
90	Corn		90	Parsley
38	Whole wheat		35	Spinach
30	Fish		27	Cucumbers
26	Liver		25	Rye bread
25	Pork		25	Carrots
24	Eggs		22	Cabbage
20	Tomatoes		20	Onions
16	Potatoes		16	Beef
16	Apricots		16	Oranges
15	Cheese		15	Watermelon
14	Lettuce		13	Apples
12	Whole wheat bread		12	Beets
12	Pears		8	Grapes
8	Radishes		6	Pine nuts
6	Lamb		3	Milk

Molybdenum

I.U. per 100-gram (3.5 oz) portion		I.U. per 100-gram (3.5 oz) portion	
155	Lentils	135	Beef liver
130	Split peas	120	Cauliflower
110	Green peas	109	Brewer's yeast
100	Spinach	100	Wheat germ
77	Beef kidney	75	Brown rice
70	Garlic	60	Oats
53	Eggs	50	Rye bread
45	Corn	42	Barley
40	Fish	36	Whole wheat
32	Whole wheat bread	32	Chicken
31	Cottage cheese	30	Beef
30	Potatoes	25	Onions
25	Peanuts	25	Coconut
25	Pork	24	Lamb
21	Green beans	19	Crab
19	Molasses	16	Cantaloupe
14	Apricots	10	Raisins
10	Butter	7	Strawberries
5	Carrots	5	Cabbage
3	Whole milk	1	Goat's milk

Vanadium

I.U. per 100-gram (3.5 oz) portion		I.U. per 100-gram (3.5 oz) portion	
100	Buckwheat	80	Parsley
70	Soybeans	64	Safflower oil
42	Eggs	41	Sunflower seed oil
35	Oats	30	Olive oil
15	Sunflower seeds	15	Corn

14	Green beans	11	Peanut oil
10	Carrots	10	Cabbage
10	Garlic	6	Tomatoes
5	Radishes	5	Onions
5	Whole wheat	4	Lobster
4	Beets	3	Apples
2	Plums	2	Lettuce
2	Millet		

REFERENCES

While writing this book, we have consulted the following list of publications. Some of the authors are named in the book as the sources of our information. Readers may find this list of references useful for learning more about good nutrition.

Abou-Saleh MT, Coppen A. The biology of folate in depression: Implications for nutritional hypotheses of the psychoses. Journal of Psychiatric Research 1986;20:91-101.
Abrams SA. Nutritional rickets: An old disease returns. Nutrition Reviews 2002;60:111-15.
Agnew N, Hoffer A. Nicotinic acid modified lysergic acid diethylamide psychosis. Journal of Mental Science 1955;101:12-27.
Akhondzadeh S, Mohammadi MR, Khademi M. Zinc sulfate as an adjunct to methylphenidate for the treatment of attention deficit hyperactivity disorder in children: A double blind and randomized trial. BMC Psychiatry 2004;4:9.
Allison JR. The relation of hydrochloric acid and vitamin B complex deficiency in certain skin diseases. Southern Medical Journal 1945;38:235-41.
Alpert JE, Fava M. Nutrition and depression: The role of folate. Nutrition Reviews 1997;55:145-49.
Altschul R, Hoffer A, Stephen JD. Influence of nicotinic acid on serum cholesterol. Man. Archives of Biochemistry and Biophysics 1955;54:558-59.
Ames BN, Elson-Schwab I, Silver EA. High-dose vitamin therapy stimulates variant enzymes with decreased coenzyme-binding affinity (increased K_m) : Relevance to genetic disease and polymorphism. A J Clin Nutrition 2002;75:616-58.
Anderson J, Brosnan J, Hoffer J, Johnston J, et al. Report of the Expert Advisory Committee on Amino Acids. Ottawa, ON: Health and Welfare, Canada, 1990.

Andrès E, et al. Vitamin B12 (cobalamin) deficiency in elderly patients. Canadian Medical Association Journal 2004;171:251-59.

Angell M. The Truth about the Drug Companies. New York, NY: Random House, 2004.

Atkinson SA, Ward WE. Clinical nutrition 2. The role of nutrition in the prevention and treatment of adult osteoporosis. Canadian Medical Association Journal 2001;165:1511-14.

Barrie S. Heidelberg pH capsule gastric analysis. In Pizzorno J, Murray MT (eds.). Textbook of Natural Medicine. 2nd ed. New York, NY: Churchill Livingstone, 1999:173-76.

Beal CB, Brown JE. A rapid screening test for gastric achlorhydria. American Journal of Digestive Diseases 1968;13:113-22.

Beasley JD, Swift JJ. The Kellogg Report. The Impact of Nutrition, Environment & Lifestyle on the Health of Americans. Annandale-on-Hudson, NY: The Institute of Health Policy and Practice, The Bard College Center, 1989.

Bekaroglu M, et al. Relationships between serum free fatty acids and zinc, and attention deficit hyperactivity disorder: A research note. Journal of Child Psychology & Psychiatry 1996;37:225-27.

Benjamin H, et al. Inhibition of benzo[a]pyrene-induced mouse forestomach neoplasia by dietary soy sauce. Cancer Research 1991;51:2940-43.

Benjamin H, et al. Reduction of benzo[a]pyrene induced forestomach neoplasms in mice given nitrite and dietary soy sauce. Food Chemical Toxicology 1988;26:671-78.

Benjamin J, Levine J, Fux M, Aviv A, Levy D, Belmaker RH. Inositol treatment for panic disorder: A double-blind placebo-controlled crossover trial. American Journal of Psychiatry 1995;152:1084-86.

Benton D, Cook R. The impact of selenium supplementation on mood. Biological Psychiatry 199;29:1092-98.

Benton D. Dietary sugar, hyperactivity and cognitive functioning: A methodological review. Journal of Applied Nutrition 1989;41:13-22.

Benton D, Cook R. Vitamin and mineral supplements improve the intelligence scores and concentration of six-year-old children. Personality and Individual Differences 1991;12: 1151-58.

Benton D, Cook R. The impact of selenium supplementation on mood. Biological Psychiatry 1991;29:1092-98.

Birdsall TC. 5-hydroxytryptophan: A clinically-effective serotonin precursor. Alternative Medicine Review 1998;3:271-80.

Blockmans D, et al. Combination therapy with hydrocortisone and fludrocortisone does not improve symptoms in chronic fatigue syndrome: A randomized, placebo-controlled, double-blind, crossover study. American Journal of Medicine 2003;114:736-41.

Bolton EC, Mildvan AS, Boeke JD. Inhibition of reverse transcription in vivo by elevated manganese ion concentration. Molecular Cell 2002;9:879-89.

Boman B. L-tryptophan: A rational anti-depressant and a natural hypnotic ? Australian and New Zealand Journal of Psychiatry 1988;22:83-97.

Bowen P, et al. Tomato sauce supplementation and prostate cancer: Lycopene accumulation and modulation of biomarkers of carcinogenesis. Experimental Biology and Medicine 2002;227:886-93.

Bown SR. Scurvy. How a Surgeon, a Mariner, and a Gentleman Solved The Greatest Medical Mystery of the Age of Sail. Toronto, ON: Thomas Allen Publishers, 2003.

Braverman ER, Pfeiffer CC. The Healing Nutrients Within. New Canaan, CT: Keats Publishing, 1987.

Braverman ER, Pfeiffer CC, Blum K, et al. The Healing Nutrients Within. 2nd ed. New Canaan, CT: Keats Publishing, 1997:246-47, 247-58, 290-303.

Brody S, et al. A randomized controlled trial of high dose ascorbic acid for reduction of blood pressure, cortisol, and subjective responses to psychological stress. Psychopharmacology (Berl) 2002;159:319-24.

Burke KE, Combs GF Jr, Gross EG, Bhuyan, KC, Abu-Libdeh H. The effects of topical and oral L-selenomethionine on pigmentation and skin cancer induced by ultraviolet irradiation. Nutrition and Cancer 1992;17:123-37.

Butterworth CE, Hatch KD, Macaluso M, Cole P, Sauberlich HE, Soong Seng-Jaw, Borst M, Baker VV. Folate deficiency and cervical dysplasia. Journal of the American Medical Association 1992;267:528-33.

Butterworth RF, et al. Thiamine deficiency in AIDS. Lancet 1991;338:1086.

Caldwell AE. Origins of Psychopharmacology from CPZ to LSD. Springfield, IL: C.C. Thomas, 1970.

Campbell JD. Hair analysis: A diagnostic tool for measuring mineral status in humans. Journal of Orthomolecular Psychiatry 1985;14:276-80.

Campbell JD. Hair tissue mineral analysis: A review. Townsend Letter for Doctors 1993 May;118:436-44.

Cannell JD. Vitamin D and Mental Illness. www.cholecalciferol-council.com

Canner PL, Berge KG, Wenger NK, Stamler J, Friedman L, Prineas, RJ, Friedewald W. Fifteen year mortality in coronary drug project patients: Long term benefit with niacin. Journal of the American College of Cardiology 1986;8:1245-55.

Capper WM, Butler TJ, Kilby JO, et al. Gallstones, gastric secretion, and flatulent dyspepsia. Lancet 1967;1:413-15.

Carner MWP. Vitamin deficiency and mental symptoms. British Journal of Psychiatry 1990;156:878-82.

Cater RE 2nd. Helicobacter (aka Campylobacter) pylori as the major causal factor in chronic hypochlorhydria. Medical Hypotheses 1992;39:367-74.

Cater, RE 2nd. The clinical importance of hypochlorhydria (a consequence of chronic helicobacter infection): Its possible etiological role in mineral and amino acid malabsorption, depression, and other syndromes. Medical Hypotheses 1992;39:375-83.

Challem J. Too much iron . . . or too little vitamin E. The Nutrition Reporter 1993;4:1,4.

Cheraskin E, Ringsdorf WM, Sisley EL. The Vitamin C connection. New York, NY: Harper and Row, 1983.

Cheraskin E, Ringsdorf WM, Sisley EL. The Vitamin C Controversy: Questions and Answers. Wichita, KS: Bio-Communications Press, 1988.

Cheraskin E. The skin in health and disease. Journal of Orthomolecular Medicine 2001;16:94-98.

Cheraskin E. Vitamin C and the skin. Natural Medicine Online www.nat-med.com 1999 Dec; 2:11

Choi S-W, Mayer J. Vitamin B12 deficiency: A new risk factor for breast cancer? Nutrition Reviews 1999;57:250-60.

Cleave TL. The Saccharine Disease. New Canaan, CT: Keats Publishing, 1975.

Cleave TL, Campbell GD, Painter NS. Diabetes, Coronary Thrombosis and the Saccharine Disease. Bristol, UK: Wright & Sons Ltd, 1960.

Clemetson CAB. Elevated blood histamine caused by vaccinations and vitamin C deficiency may mimic the shaken baby syndrome. Medical Hypotheses 2004;62:533-36.

Colborn T, Clement C. Chemically-induced alterations in sexual and functional development: The wildlife/human connection. Advances in Modern Environmental Toxicology, Vol. 21. Princeton, NJ: Princeton Scientific Publishing, 1992.

Commentary. Oral cobalamin for pernicious anemia: Medicine's best kept secret? Journal of the American Medical Association 1991;265:94-95.

Coppen A, Bolander-Gouaille C. Treatment of depression: Time to consider folic acid and vitamin B-12. Journal of Psychopharmacology 2005;19;59-65.

Cott A. Orthomolecular approach to the treatment of learning disabilities. Journal of Orthomolecular Psychiatry 1971;3:95-105.

Cott A. Dr Cott's Help for Your Learning Disabled Child. New York, NY: Times Books, 1985.

Cott A. Orthomolecular approach to the treatment of children with behavioral disorders and learning disabilities. Journal of Applied Nutrition 1973;25:15-24.

Cromwell PE, Abadie BR, Stephens JD, Kyler M. Hair mineral analysis: Biochemical imbalances and violent criminal behavior. Psychological Reports 1989;64:259-66.

Crook WG. Can Your Child Read? Is He Hyperactive? Jackson, TN: Professional Books, 1977.

Crook WG. Detecting Your Hidden Allergies. Jackson, TN: Professional Books, 1988.

Crook WG. Solving the Puzzle of Your Hard-to-Raise Child. New York, NY: Random House, 1987.

Curhan GC, et al. A prospective study of the intake of vitamins C and B6, and the risk of kidney stones in men. Journal of Urology 1996;155:1847-51.

Curhan GC, et al. Intake of vitamins B6 and C and the risk of kidney stones in women. Journal of the American Society of Nephrology 1999;10:840-45.

Cutler P. Iron overload in psychiatric illness. American Journal of Psychiatry 1991:148: 1.

Cutler RG. Carotenoids and retinol: Their possible importance in determining longevity of primate species. Proceedings of the National Academy of Sciences of the United States of America 1984;81:7627-31.

Daly R, Palmer K. A drugged nation. Who's testing, who's telling. Toronto Star 2004 Monday, December 6.

Davis DR. The Harrell study and seven follow-up studies: A brief review. Journal of Orthomolecular Medicine 1987;2:111-15.

de Witte TJ, Geerdink PJ, Lamers CB. Hypochlorhydria and hypergastrinaemia in rheumatoid arthritis. Annals of the Rheumatic Diseases 1979;38:14-17.

Di Cyan E. Vitamin E and Aging. New York, NY: Pyramid Books, 1972.

Diplock AT. Safety of antioxidant vitamins and b-carotene. American Journal of Clinical Nutrition 1995;62(suppl):1510S-16S.

Docherty JP, et al. A double-blind, placebo-controlled, exploratory trial of chromium picolinate in atypical depression: Effect on carbohydrate craving. Journal of Psychiatric Practice 2005;11:302-14.

Dommisse J. Subtle vitamin B-12 deficiency and psychiatry: A largely unnoticed but devastating relationship? Medical Hypotheses 1991;34:131-40.

Dommisse J. Case report: The psychiatric manifestations of B12 deficiency. Primary Psychiatry 1996;3,4:50-55.

Eaton KK, Gaier HC, Howard M, et al. Gastric acid production, pancreatic secretions and blood levels of higher alcohols in patients with fungal-type dysbiosis of the gut. Journal of Nutritional & Environmental Medicine 2002;12:107-12.

Egger J, Wilson J, Carter CM, Turner MW, Soothill JF. Is migraine food allergy? A double-blind controlled trial of oligoantigenic diet treatments. Lancet 1983;2:865-68.

Eisenberg DM, Kessler RC, Foster C, Norlock FE, Calkins DR, Delbanco TL. Unconventional medicine in the United States. New England Journal of Medicine 1993; 328:246-52.

Embry AF. Vitamin D supplementation in the fight against multiple sclerosis. J. Orthomolecular Medicine 2004;19:27-38.

Erasmus U. Fats and Oils. Vancouver, BC: Alive, 1986.

Feldman M, Barnett C. Fasting gastric pH and its relationship to true hypochlorhydria in humans. Digestive Diseases and Sciences 1991;36:866-69.

Finn R. Food allergy – fact or fiction: A Review. Journal of the Royal Society of Medicine 1992;85:560-63.

Finnegan J. The Facts about Fats. Malibu, CA: Elysian Arts, 1992.

Foster HD. Fluoride and its antagonists: Implications for human health. Journal of Orthomolecular Medicine 1994;8:149-53.

Foster HD. Health, Disease and the Environment. Boca Raton, FL: CRC Press, 1992.

Foster HD. What Really Causes Aids. Victoria, BC: Trafford, 2002. www.hdfoster.com

Fux M, Levine J, Aviv A, Belmaker RH. Inositol treatment of obsessive-compulsive disorder. American Journal of Psychiatry 1996;153: 1219-21.

Freeland-Graves JH. Manganese: An essential nutrient for humans. Nutrition Today 1988 Nov/Dec:13-19.

Gaby AR. Commentary: Seizure disorder (epilepsy). Nutrition & Healing 1997; 4(4):1,10-11.

Gaby AR. Does high-dose vitamin E kill people? Townsend Letter for Doctors & Patients 2005;259/260:115-16.

Gaby AR, Wright JV. Nutrients and Bone Health. Wright/Gaby Nutrition Institute, August 1988.

Galler JR. Human Nutrition. New York, NY: Plenum Press, 1984.

Gelber D, Levine J, Belmaker RH. The effect of inositol treatment on bulimia nervosa and binge eating. International J of Eating Disorders 2001;29:345-48.

Genaro Pde S, Martini LA. Vitamin A supplementation and risk of skeletal fracture. Nutrition Reviews 2004;62:65-67.

Gerrard JW. Understanding Allergies. Springfield, IL: C.C. Thomas, 1973.

Gray AS. Fluoridation: Time for a new base line? Journal of the Canadian Dental Association 1987;10:763-65.

Gray C. British MD's face growing pressure from alternative medicine, government. Canadian Medical Association Journal 1990;143:132-43.

Goodhart RS, Shils ME. Modern Nutrition in Health and Disease. Philadelphia, PA: Lea & Febiger, 1974.

Gupta NP, Kumar R. Lycopene therapy in idiopathic male infertility – a preliminary report. International Urology and Nephrology 2002;34:369-72.

Hackman RM. Chromium and cholesterol. Townsend Letter for Doctors 1991 Oct:744 –48.

Hahn LJ, Kloiber R, Vimy MJ, Takahashi Y, Lorscheider FL. Dental silver tooth fillings: A source of mercury exposure revealed by whole-body image scan and tissue analysis. Journal of the Federation of American Societies for Experimental Biology 1989;3:2641-46.

Hall RH. Food for Naught: The Decline in Nutrition. New York, NY: Harper and Row, 1974.

Hanson M. Amalgam – Hazards in your teeth. Journal of Orthomolecular Psychiatry 1983;12:194-201.

Harris WS. Are omega-3 fatty acids the most important nutritional modulators of coronary heart disease risk? Current Atherosclerosis Reports 2002;6:447-52.

Hart JT. Subclinical rickets, an unexplained deficiency syndrome. International Journal of Biosocial Research 1981;6:38-43.

Hartung EF, Steinbrocker O. Gastric acidity in chronic arthritis. Annals of Internal Medicine 1935;9:252-57.

Hattersley JG. The answer to crib death. Journal of Orthomolecular Medicine 1993;8: 229-45.

Hayashida T. Correspondence – selenium deficiency and hypothyroidism. Journal of Orthomolecular Medicine 1994;9:186.

Heaney R. Editorial. New England Journal Medicine 1993;328:503-05.

Hemingway DC. Pantothenic acid and muscular function. Journal of Orthomolecular Medicine 1990;5:167-68.

Hemingway DC. Good nutrition lowers health care costs. Journal of Orthomolecular Medicine 1992;7:67-71.

Henkin Y, Johnson KC, Segrest JP. Rechallenge with crystalline niacin after drug-induced hepatitis from sustained-release niacin. Journal of American Medical Association 1990;264:241-43.

Herbert V, Jacobs E. Destruction of vitamin B-12 by ascorbic acid. Journal of the American Medical Association 1974;230:241-42.

Heseker H, Kubler W, Pudel V, et al. Psychological disorders as early symptoms of a mild-to-moderate vitamin deficiency. Annals of the New York Academy of Sciences 1992;669:352-57.

Hickey S, Roberts H. Ascorbate. The Science of Vitamin C. 2004; www.lulu.com

Hileman B. Fluoridation of water. Chemical & Engineering News 1988 Aug 1:26-42.

Hippchen LJ. An exploratory study of the use of nutritional approaches in the treatment of suicide prone persons. Journal of Orthomolecular Psychiatry 1981;10:147.

Hippchen LJ. Ecologic, Biochemical Approach to Treatment of Delinquents and Criminals. New York, NY: Van Nostrand Reinhold Co., 1978.

Hoffer A. A vitamin B-3 dependent family. Schizophrenia 1971;3:41-46.

Hoffer A. Ascorbic acid and kidney stones. Canadian Medical Association Journal 1985;132:320.

Hoffer A. Children with learning and behavioral disorders. Journal of Orthomolecular Psychiatry 1976;5:228-30.

Hoffer A. Chronic schizophrenic patients treated ten years or more. Journal of Orthomolecular Medicine 1994;8:7-37.

Hoffer A. Common Questions on Schizophrenia and Their Answers. New Canaan, CT: Keats Publishing, 1988.
Hoffer A. Five California schizophrenics. Journal of Schizophrenia 1967;1:209-20.
Hoffer A. Hong Kong veterans study. Journal of Orthomolecular Psychiatry 1974;3:34-36.
Hoffer A. Hyperactivity, allergy and megavitamins. Canadian Medical Association Journal 1974;111:905-07.
Hoffer A. Niacin Therapy in Psychiatry. Springfield, IL: C.C. Thomas, 1962.
Hoffer A. Orthomolecular Medicine for Physicians. New Canaan, CT: Keats Publishing, 1989.
Hoffer A. Orthomolecular nutrition at the zoo. Journal of Orthomolecular Psychiatry 1983;12:116-28.
Hoffer A. Safety, side effects and relative lack of toxicity of nicotinic acid and nicotinamide. Schizophrenia 1969;1:78-87.
Hoffer A. Vitamin B-3 (Niacin) Update. New Roles for a Key Nutrient in Diabetes, Cancer, Heart Disease and Other Major Health Problems. New Canaan, CT: Keats Publishing, 1990.
Hoffer A. Vitamin and mineral supplements increase intelligence. Nutrition Health Review 1989 Fall.
Hoffer A. Vitamin B-3 dependent child. Schizophrenia 1971;3:107-13.
Hoffer A, Foster HD. Feel Better, Live Longer with Vitamin B-3. In press, 2006.
Hoffer A, Osmond H. The Hallucinogens. New York, NY: Academic Press, 1967.
Hoffer A, Pauling L. Hardin Jones biostatistical analysis of mortality data for cohorts of cancer patients with a large fraction surviving at the termination of the study and a comparison of survival times of cancer patients receiving large regular oral doses of vitamin C and other nutrients with similar patients not receiving those doses. Journal of Orthomolecular Medicine 1990;5:143-54.
Hoffer A, Walker M. Smart Nutrients. Garden City Park, NY: Avery Publishing Group, 1994.
Hoffer A, Walker M. Orthomolecular Nutrition. New Canaan, CT: Keats Publishing, 1978.
Hoffer A, Osmond H, Callbeck MJ, Kahan I. Treatment of schizophrenia with nicotinic acid and nicotinamide. Journal of Clinical and Experimental Psychopathology 1957;18: 131-58.
Hoffer A, Osmond H, Smythies J, Schizophrenia: A new approach. II. Results of a year's research. Journal of Mental Science 1954;100:29-45.
Hoffer A, Pauling L. Healing Cancer. Toronto, ON: CCNM Press, 2004.
Hoffer A. Healing Schizophrenia. Toronto, ON: CCNM Press, 2004.
Hoffer A. Healing Children's Attention and Behavior Disorders. Toronto, ON: CCNM Press, 2004.
Hoffer M. Fueling Body, Mind and Spirit. Toronto, ON: Sumach Press, 2003.

Holub BJ. EPA/DHA (omega-3) fatty acids for human health: New evidence. Canadian College of Naturopathic Medicine, Toronto, Ontario, October 17, 2005.

Horrobin DF. Schizophrenia as a prostaglandin deficiency disease. Lancet 1977;1:936-37.

Horrobin DF. Clinical Uses for Essential Fatty Acids. St. Albans, UK: Eden Press, 1983.

Horrobin DF. Gamma linolenic acid: An intermediate in essential fatty acid metabolism with potential as an ethical pharmaceutical and as a food. Review of Contemporary Pharmacotherapy 1990;1:1-45.

Horrobin DF, Oka M, Manku MS. The regulation of prostaglandin E 1 formation: A candidate for one of the fundamental mechanisms involved in the actions of vitamin C. Medical Hypothesis 1979;5: 849-58.

Horrobin D. Are large clinical trials in rapidly lethal diseases usually unethical? The Lancet 2003;361;695-97.

Houston M, Fox B. Is vitamin E deadly? Why the study saying so was wrong. www,nutraceuticalreport. com/articles.cfm?dispart=55

Hughes J, Norman RW. Diet and calcium stones. Canadian Medical Association Journal, 1992;146:137-42.

Huggins HA. Mercury: A factor in mental disease. Journal of Orthomolecular Psychiatry 1982;11:3-16.

Hunter AGW. Fortification of foods with folic acid and vitamin B12: Definitive action is overdue. Annals Royal College of Physicians and Surgeons (Canada) 2000;33:172-75.

Hurwitz A, Brady DA, Schaal SE, et al. Gastric acidity in older adults. Journal of the American Medical Association 1997;278:659-62.

Ipatova OM, et al. Biological activity of linseed oil as the source of omega-3 alpha-linolenic acid. Biomeditsinskaia Khimiia 2004;50:25-43.

Irving JA, et al. Element of caution: A case of reversible cytopenias associated with excessive zinc supplementation. Canadian Medical Association Journal 2003;169:129-31.

Joffe PM, Jolliffe N. The gastric acidity in alcohol addicts. With observations of the relation of the B vitamins to achlorhydria. American Journal of Medical Sciences 1937: 501-11.

Johnstone EC, et al. Disabilities and circumstances of schizophrenic patients – A follow-up study. The British Journal of Psychiatry 199;Suppl 23:1159.

Kaplan BJ, M^{C}Nicol N, Conte RA, Moghadam HK. Dietary replacement in preschool-aged hyperactive boys. Pediatrics 1989;83:7-17.

Kassarjian Z, Russell RM. Hypochlorhydria: A factor in nutrition. Annual Review of Nutrition 1989;9:271-85.

Kaufman W. Common Form of Niacinamide Deficiency Disease: Aniacinamidosis. New Haven, CT: Yale University Press, 1943.

Kaufman W. Niacinamide: A most neglected vitamin. Journal International Academy of Preventive Medicine 1983;8:5-25.

Kelly GS. Hydrochloric acid: Physiological functions and clinical implications. Alternative Medicine Review 1997;2:116-27.

Kelly G. Peripheral metabolism of thyroid hormones: A review. Alternative Medicine Review 2000;5:306-33.

King CE, Leibach J, Toskes PP. Clinically significant vitamin B12 deficiency secondary to malabsorption of protein-bound vitamin B12. Digestive Diseases and Sciences 1979;24:397-402.

Kinrys G. Hypomania associated with omega3 fatty acids. Archives of General Psychiatry 2000;57:715-16.

Kotkas L. B_{12} and folic acid in treatment of some psychiatric illnesses. Annual Meeting of the Canadian Schizophrenia Foundation, June 4th, 1978.

Kozielec T, Starobrat-Hermelin B. Assessment of magnesium levels in children with attention deficit hyperactivity disorder (ADHD). Magnesium Research 1997;10:143-48.

Kozielec T, Starobrat-Hermelin B. The effects of magnesium physiological supplementation on hyperactivity in children with attention deficit hyperactivity disorder (ADHD). Positive response to magnesium oral loading test. Magnesium Research 1997;10:149-56.

Krilanovic N. No Sugar Added. Santa Barbara, CA: November Books, 1982.

Kunin RA. Manganese and niacin in the treatment of drug-induced dyskinesias. Journal of Orthomolecular Psychiatry 1976;5:4-27.

Larsen HL. Folic Acid: Don't be without it. www.yourhealthbase.com

Larkin M. Vitamins reduce risk of vision loss from macular degeneration. Lancet 2001;358:1347.

Lawson S. The Trials and tribulations of vitamin C. Journal of Orthomolecular Medicine 2003;18:173-86.

Lee KW, et al. Effects of dietary fat intake in sudden death: Reduction of death with omega-3 fatty acids. Current Cardiology Reports 2004;6:371-78.

Lee SH, et al. Vitamin C-induced decomposition of lipid hydroperoxides to endogenous genotoxins. Science 2001;292:2083-86.

Leung, L-H. Systemic lupus erythematosis: A combined deficiency disease. Medical Hypotheses 2004;62:922-24.

Leung L-H. A stone that kills two birds: Pantothenic acid in the treatment of acne vulgaris and obesity. Journal of Orthomolecular Medicine 1997;12:99-114.

Levine J, Gonzalves M, Barbam J, Stier S, Eliizur A, Kofam O, Belmaker, RH. Inositol six grams daily may be effective in depression but not in schizophrenia. Hum Psychopharmacology 1993;8;49-53.

Levine J, Gonzalves M, Barbam J, Stier S, Eliizur A, Kofam O, Belmaker, RH. A double-blind controlled trial of inositol treatment of depression. American Journal of Psychiatry 1995;152:792-94.

Levine J, Barak Y, Benjamin J, Bersudsky Y, Kofman O, Belmaker RH. Therapeutic potential of inositol treatment in depression, panic, dementia and lithium side effects. In Montgomery S, Halbreich U (eds.). Pharmacotherapy of Mood, Anxiety and Cognition. New York, NY: American Psychiatric Press, 2000:159-66.

Levine SA, Kidd PM. Antioxidant Adaptation: Its Role in Free Radical Pathology. San Leandro, CA: Allergy Research Group, 1986.

Lim LS, et al. Vitamin A intake and the risk of hip fracture in postmenopausal women: The Iowa Women's Health Study. Osteoporosis International 2004;15:552-59.

Logan A. Neurobehavioral aspects of omega-3 fatty acids: Possible mechanisms and therapeutic value in major depression. Alternative Medicine Review 2003;8:410-25.

Logan AC, Beaulne TM. The treatment of small intestinal bacterial overgrowth with enteric-coated peppermint oil: A case report. Alternative Medicine Review 2002;7:410-17.

Lowry F. Prescription of Health. Report to the Pharmaceutical Inquiry of Ontario, July 1990.

Lukaski HC, et al. Body temperature and thyroid hormone metabolism of copper deficient rats. Nutritional Biochemistry 1995;6:445-51.

Machlin LJ. Introduction. Annals of the New York Academy of Sciences 1992;669:1-6.

Mandell M, Scanlon LW. Dr Mandell's 5 Day Allergy Relief System. New York, NY: Thomas Y. Crowell, 1979.

Marlowe M, Medeiros D, Moon C, Errera J, Medeiros L. Hair minerals, diet and behavior of Prader-Willi syndrome youth. Journal of Orthomolecular Medicine 1987;2: 146-53.

Marlowe M, Errera J, Stellern J, Beck D. Lead and mercury levels in emotionally disturbed children. Journal of Orthomolecular Science 1983;12:260-67.

Martin W. Soy and breast cancer. Townsend Letter for Doctors 1993 April: 328-29.

McCarron DA, Morris CD, Henry HJ, Stanton JL. Blood pressure and nutrient intake in the United States. Science 1984;224:1392-98.

McGinnis WR. Oxidative stress in autism. Personal communications, 2004.

McGrath J. Hypothesis: Is low prenatal vitamin D a risk-modifying factor for schizophrenia? Schizophrenia Research 1999;40:173-77.

McGrath J, Saari K, Hakko H, et al Vitamin D supplementation and risk of schizophrenia. Schizophrenia Research 2004:67:237-45.

McLachlan DRC, Kruck TP, Lukiw WJ, Krishnan SS. Would decreased aluminum ingestion reduce the incidence of alzheimers disease? Canadian Medical Association Journal 1991;145:793-804.

McLeod MN, Gaynes BN, Golden RN. Chromium potentiation of antidepressant pharmacotherapy for dysthymic disorder in 5 patients. Journal of Clinical Psychiatry 1999;60:237-40.

Messman T. Interview with Robert Witaker. www.newstarget.com/011353.html

Meyers S. Use of neurotransmitter precursors for treatment of depression. Alternative Medicine Review 2000;5:64-71.

Miller ER, Pastor-Barriuso R, Dalal D, et al. Meta-analysis: High-dosage vitamin E supplementation may increase all cause mortality. Annals Internal Medicine 2005;142:37-46.

Miller JW. Vitamin B12 deficiency, tumor necrosis factor-α, and epidermal growth factor: A novel function for vitamin B12? Nutrition Reviews 2002;60:142-44.

Mitchell WA Jr. Foundations of Natural Therapeutics: Biochemical Apologetics of Naturopathic Medicine. Tempe, AZ: Southwest College Press, 1997:105-108.

Mitchell J. Dairy tales. There's more myth than truth to the fears fueling the growing dairy phobia. Globe and Mail, 1993.

Monograph – 5-Hydroxytryptophan. Alternative Medicine Review 1998;3:224-26.

Monograph – L-Arginine. Alternative Medicine Review 2005;10:139-47.

Monograph – L-Carnitine. Alternative Medicine Review 2005;10:42-50.

Monograph – L-Glutamine. Alternative Medicine Review 2001;4:406-10.

Monograph – L-Taurine. Alternative Medicine Review 2001;6:78-82.

Monograph – Methylcobalamin. Alternative Medicine Review 1998;3:461-63.

Moore RD, Webb GD. The K Factor. New York, NY: Macmillan Publishing, 1986.

Morello G. Treating epilepsy effectively. American Journal of Natural Medicine 1996;3(8):14-20.

Moss WW. Cancer Therapy. The Independent Consumers Guide to Non-Toxic Treatment & Prevention. New York, NY: Equinox Press, 1992.

Mullin GE, Greenson JK, Mitchell MC. Fulminant hepatic failure after ingestion of sustained-release nicotinic acid. Annals of Internal Medicine 1989;111:253-55.

Murray MF. Tryptophan depletion and HIV infection: A metabolic link to pathogenesis. Lancet Infectious Diseases 2003;3:644-52.

Murray MF. Niacin as a potential AIDS preventive factor. Medical Hypotheses 1999;53:375-79.

Murray MF. Nicotinamide: An oral antimicrobial agent with activity against both Mycobacterium tuberculosis and Human Immunodeficiency Virus. Clinical Infectious Diseases 2003;36:453-60.

Murray MT. The Healing Power of Foods. Rocklin, CA: Prima Publishing, 1993.

Murray MT. Encyclopedia of Nutritional Supplements. Rocklin, CA: Prima Publishing, 1996.

Murray MT. Indigestion, antacids, achlorhydria and H. pylori. The American Journal of Natural Medicine 1997;4:11-14, 16-17.

Murray MT. The Complete Book of Juicing. Rocklin, CA: Prima Publishing, 1998.

National Headache Foundation. www.headaches.org/consumer/generalinfo/factsheet.html

Newbold HL. Mega Nutrients for Your Nerves. New York, NY: Peter Wyden Publishing, 1975.

Newbold HL. Vitamin B-12: placebo or neglected therapeutic tool? Medical Hypotheses 1989;28:155-64.

Nicolson A. Seize The Fire. Heroism, Duty, and the Battle of Trafalgar. New York, NY: Harper-Collins Publishers, 2005.

Nolan KR. Copper toxicity syndrome. Journal of Orthomolecular Psychiatry 1983;12: 270-82.

Null G, Dean C, Feldman M, Rasio D. Death by medicine. Journal Orthomolecular Medicine 2005;20:21-34.

Obarzanek E, et al. Individual blood pressure responses to changes in salt intake: Results from the DASH-Sodium Trial. Hypertension 2003;42:459-67.

OH RC, Brown DL. Vitamin B12 deficiency. American Family Physician 2003;67:979-86.

Oski FA. Don't Drink Your Milk: The Frightening New Medical Facts about the Worlds Most Overrated Nutrient. Syracuse, NY: Mollica Press Ltd., 1977.

Ozgocmen S, et al. Vitamin D deficiency and reduced bone mineral density in multiple sclerosis: Effect of ambulatory status and functional capacity. Journal of Bone and Mineral Metabolism 2005;23:309-13.

Papakostas GI, et al, Serum folate, vitamin B12, and homocysteine in major depressive disorder. J Clin Psychiatry 2004;65:1096-98.

Passwater RA. Selenium as Food and Medicine. New Canaan, CT: Keats Publishing, 1980.

Passwater RA. L-glutamine: The surprising brain fuel. Health Express 1981;2:8-11.

Patrick L. Beta-carotene: The controversy continues. Alternative Medicine Review 2000;5:530-45.

Pauling L. Are recommended daily allowances for vitamin C adequate? Proceedings of the National Academy of Sciences USA 1974;71:4442-46.

Pauling L. How to Live Longer and Feel Better. New York, NY: W. H. Freeman, 1986.

Pauling L. Orthomolecular psychiatry. Science 1968;160:265-71.

Pauling L. Vitamin C and the Common Cold. San Francisco, CA: W.H. Freeman, 1970.

Pfeiffer CC. Mental and Elemental Nutrients. New Canaan, CT: Keats Publishing, 1975.

Pfeiffer CC. Zinc and other micro-nutrients. New Canaan, CT: Keats Publishing, 1978.

Pfeiffer CC, LaMola S. Zinc and manganese in the schizophrenias. Journal of Orthomolecular Psychiatry 1983;12:215-34.

Petersdorf RG, et al. Harrisons Principles of Internal Medicine. 10th ed. New York, NY: McGraw Hill, 1983.

Phillpott WH. Ecologic, orthomolecular and behavioral contributors to psychiatry. Orthomolecular Psychiatry 1968;3:356-70.

Phillpott WH. Maladaptive reactions to frequently used foods and commonly met chemicals and chronic factors in many chronic physical and chronic emotional illnesses. In A Physicians Handbook on Orthomolecular Medicine. Williams RJ, Kalita DK (eds.) New Canaan, CT: Keats Publishing, 1979.

Philpott WH, Kalita DK. Brain Allergies: The Psychonutrient Connection. New Canaan, CT: Keats Publishing, 1980.

Pleva J. Mercury poisoning from dental amalgams. Journal of Orthomolecular Psychiatry 1983;12:184-93.

Plummer N. The unseen epidemic: The linked syndromes of achlorhydria and atrophic gastritis. Townsend Letter for Doctors & Patients 2004;252:89-94.

Powell DW. Urine Indican Test (Obermeyer Test). In Pizzorno J, Murray MT (eds.). Textbook of Natural Medicine. 2nd ed. New York, NY: Churchill Livingstone, 1999:245-46.

Prasad AS. Trace Elements in Human Health and Disease. Vol 1: Zinc and Copper. New York, NY: Academic Press, 1976.

Prousky, J. Orthomolecular treatment of anxiety disorders. Townsend Letter for Doctors & Patients 2005;259/260:82-87.

Prousky J, Seely D. The treatment of migraines and tension-type headaches with intravenous and oral niacin (nicotinic acid): Systematic review of the literature. Nutrition Journal 2005;4:3.

Prousky J. Niacinamide's potent role in alleviating anxiety with its benzodiazepine-like properties: A case report. Journal of Orthomolecular Medicine 2004;19:104-10.

Prousky J. The Gastro-Test: A simple in-office test for the determination of gastric pH & gastroesophageal reflux disease. Townsend Letter for Doctors & Patients 2004;250:60-63.

Prousky J, Sykes E. Two case reports on the treatment of acute migraine with niacin. Its hypothetical mechanism of action upon calcitonin-gene related peptide and platelets. Journal of Orthomolecular Medicine 2003;18:108-10.

Prousky J, Seely D. A case report on the successful use of inositol hexaniacinate for the treatment of achlorhydria: Its possible mechanism of action upon the central nervous system and parietal cell-adenosine triphosphate-dependent K^+/H^+ pump. Townsend Letter for Doctors & Patients 2003;235/236:72-75.

Prousky J, Seely D. Follow-up report on the use of inositol hexaniacinate for the treatment of achlorhydria. Is a vitamin B-3 dependency the cause of this patient's gastrointestinal symptoms? Townsend Letter for Doctors & Patients 2003;238:70-71.

Prousky J, Kerwin C. Niacin (Nicotinic Acid) a putative treatment for hypochlorhydria: Re-analysis of two case reports. Journal of Orthomolecular Medicine 2002;17:163-69.

Prousky J. Is vitamin B3 dependency a causal factor in the development of hypochlorhydria and achlorhydria? Journal of Orthomolecular Medicine 2001;16;225-37.

Randolph TG, Moss RW. An Alternative Approach to Allergies. New York, NY: Harper and Row, 1980.

Rao AV, et al. Serum and tissue lycopene and biomarkers of oxidation in prostate cancer patients: A case-control study. Nutrition and Cancer 1999;33:159-64.

Rao AV. Biologically active phytochemicals in human health. NFH Nutraceutical Science Mini-Symposium and Continuing Education Seminar, Toronto, Ontario, October 15, 2005.

Rapp D. Allergies and the Hyperactive Child. New York, NY: Cornerstone Library, 1979.

Rappaport EM. Achlorhydria: Associated symptoms and response to hydrochloric acid. New England Journal of Medicine 1955:252:802-05.

Rath M, Pauling L. Solution to the puzzle of human cardiovascular disease: Its primary cause is ascorbate deficiency leading to the deposition of lipoprotein(a) and fibrinogen/fibrin in the vascular wall. Journal of Orthomolecular Medicine 1991;6:125-34.

Reed B. Food, Teens and Behavior. Manitowoc, WI: Natural Press, 1983.

Regland B, Abrahamsson L, Blennow K, et al. Vitamin B12 in CSF: Reduced CSF/serum B12 ratio in demented men. Acta neurologica Scandinavica 1992;85:276-81.

Rejnmark L, et al. No effect of vitamin A intake on bone mineral density and fracture risk in perimenopausal women. Osteoporosis International 2004;15:872-80.

Reuler JB, Broudy VC, Cooney TG. Adult scurvy. Journal of American Medical Association 1985;253:805-07.

Richards E. Vitamin C and Cancer: Medicine or Politics? London: Macmillan, 1991.

Riggs L. The Medical Post 1990 April 10.

Rimland, B. Recent research in infantile autism. Journal of Operational Psychiatry 1972;3: 35; rpt. Autism Research Review International 1993;2.

Rimland, B. The Feingold diet: An assessment of the reviews by Mattes, Kavale and Forness and others. Journal of Learning Disabilities 1983;6:331-33.

Rimland B, Callaway E, Dreyfus P. The effect of high doses of vitamin B-6 on autistic children: A double-blind crossover study. American Journal of Psychiatry 1978;135:472-75.

Rimm EB, Stampfer MJ, Ascherio A, Giovannucci E, Colditz GA, Willett WC. Vitamin E consumption and the risk of coronary heart disease in men. New England Journal of Medicine 1993;328:1450-56.

Rios J. Passe MM. Evidence-based use of botanicals, minerals, and vitamins in the prophylactic treatment of migraines. Journal of the American Academy of Nurse Practitioners 2004;16:251-56.

Rivers JM. Safety of high-level vitamin C ingestion. Annals of the New York Academy of Sciences 1987; 498:445-54.

Rogers LL, Pelton RB. Effect of glutamine on IQ scores of mentally deficient children. Texas Reports on Biology and Medicine 1957;15:84-90.

Ross H. Fighting Depression. New York, NY: Larchmont Books, 1975.

Rowen R. Alaska Governor Appoints Alternative Doctor. Health Action 1992/1993 Winter.

Rudin DO. The major psychoses and neuroses as omega-3 essential fatty acid deficiency syndrome: Substrate pellagra. Biological Psychiatry 1981;16:837-50.

Rudin DO, Felix C. The Omega-3 Phenomenon. New York, NY: Rawson Associates, 1987.

Russell TL, Berardi RR, Barnett JL, et al. Upper gastrointestinal pH in seventy-nine healthy, elderly, North American men and women. Pharmaceutical Research 1993;10:187-96.

Sacks FM, et al. DASH-Sodium Collaborative Research Group. Effects on blood pressure of reduced dietary sodium and the Dietary Approaches to Stop Hypertension (DASH) diet. DASH-Sodium Collaborative Research Group. New England Journal of Medicine 2001;344:3-10.

Sakimoto K. The cause of the eosinophilia-myalgia syndrome associated with tryptophan use. New England Journal of Medicine 1990;323:992-93.

Saltzman JR, et al. Effect of hypochlorhydria due to omeprazole treatment or atrophic gastritis on protein-bound vitamin B12 absorption. Journal of the American College of Nutrition 1994;13:544-45.

Saul AW. Vitamin E: A cure in search of recognition. J Orthomolecular Medicine 2003;18:205-12.

Schauss AG. Chromium picolinate and bariatric Medicine. International Journal of Biosocial Medical Research 1991;13:152-63.

Schauss AG. Diet, Crime and Delinquency. Berkeley, CA: Parker House, 1980.

Schauss, AG. Zinc status and eating disorders. International Journal of Biosocial Medical Research 1991;13:153-56.

Schnare DW, et al. Evaluation of a detoxification regimen for fat stored xenobiotics. Medical Hypotheses 1982;9:265-82.

Schoenthaler SJ, Doraz WE, Wakefield JA. The impact of a low food additive and sucrose diet on academic performance in 803 New York city public schools. International Journal of Biosocial Research 1986;8:185-95.

Schrauzer GN, Shrestha KP. Lithium in drinking water and the incidences of crimes, suicides, and arrests related to drug addictions. Biological Trace Element Research 1990;25:105-13.

Schrauzer GN, Shrestha KP, Flores-Arce MF. Lithium in scalp hair of adults, students, and violent criminals. Effects of supplementation and evidence for interactions of lithium with vitamin B12 and with other trace elements. Biological Trace Element Research 1992;4:161-76.

Seligman H, et al. Thiamine deficiency in patients with congestive heart failure receiving long-term furosemide therapy: A pilot study. American Journal of Medicine 1991;91:151-55.

Seligman T. The highs and lows of lithium therapy. Journal of Naturopathic Medicine 1998;8:40-44.

Seppanen K, et al. Effect of supplementation with organic selenium on mercury status as measured by mercury in pubic hair. Journal of Trace Elements in Medicine and Biology 2000;14:84-87.

Sharp GS, Fister HW. The diagnosis and treatment of achlorhydria: Ten-year study. Journal of the American Geriatrics Society 1967;15:786-92.

Shine I. Serendipity and St. Helena. New York, NY: Pergamon Press, 1970.

Shriqui C. Issues related to the long-term treatment of schizophrenia. Schizophrenia Management 1993 February:1.

Siblerund RL. The Relationship between Mercury from Dental Amalgam and Mental Health. American Journal of Psychotherapy 1989;43:575-87.

Simons FER, Chad ZH, Sampson HA, Tarlo SM, Chandra RK. Food allergy and intolerance: New directions. Annals of The Royal College of Physicians and Surgeons of Canada 1993;26:29-32.

Simopoulos AP. Genetic variation and nutrition. Nutrition Reviews 1999;57:S10-S19.

Simpson LO. Myalgic encephalomyelitis (ME): A haemorheological disorder manifested as impaired capillary blood flow. Journal of Orthomolecular Medicine 1997;2:69-76.

Singer P, Wirth W. Can n-3 PUFA reduce cardiac arrhythmias? Results of a clinical trial. Prostaglandins, Leukotrienes, and Essential Fatty Acids 2004;71:153-59.

Slanger A. Management of gastric achlorhydria and hypochlorhydria. Geriatrics 1966;21:193-98.

Slagle P. The Way Up from Down. New York, NY: Random House, 1987.

Smith L. Foods for Healthy Kids. New York, NY: McGraw Hill, 1981.

Smith M. Canadian tests link anorexia to deficiency of zinc in diet. Vancouver Sun 1993 February 27.

Soilu-Hanninen M. 25-hydroxyvitamin D levels in serum at the onset of multiple sclerosis. Multiple Sclerosis 2005;11:266-71.

Soothill J. Food intolerance. The Practitioner 1989;233:596-602.

South-Paul JE. Osteoporosis: Part I. Evaluation and assessment. American Family Physician 2001;63:897-904.

Stampfer MJ, Hennekens CH, Manson J, Colditz GA, Rosner B, and Willett WC. Vitamin E consumption and the risk of coronary disease in women. New England Journal Medicine 1993;328:1444-49.

Stever Y, et al. Iron treatment in children with attention deficit hyperactivity disorder. A preliminary report. Neuropsychobiology 1997;35:178-80.

Stiles RS, et al. Double-masked, placebo-controlled, randomized trial of lutein and antioxidant supplementation in the intervention of atrophic age-related macular degeneration: The Veterans LAST study (Lutein Antioxidant Supplementation Trial). Optometry 2004;75:216-30.

Stone I. The Healing Factor: Vitamin C against Disease. New York, NY: Grosset and Dunlap, 1972.

Swank RL, Pullen MH. The Multiple Sclerosis Diet Book. New York, NY: Doubleday, 1977.

Taylor EW. Selenium and viral diseases. Facts and hypotheses. Journal of Orthomolecular Medicine 1997;12:227-39.

Tilson MD. Decreased hepatic copper levels: A possible chemical marker for the pathogenesis of aortic aneurysms in man. Archives of Surgery 1982;117:1212-13.

Tretjak Z, et al. PCB reduction and clinical improvement by detoxification: an unexploited approach? Human & Experimental Toxicology 1990;9:235-44.

Truss CO. The Missing Diagnosis. Birmingham, AL: Self-Published, 1983.

Truss CO. The role of Candida albicans in human illness. Journal of Orthomolecular Psychiatry 1981;10:228-38.

Tsuru S, et al. Current status of occult iron deficiency in Japan and improvement by intake of heme iron: An analysis based on serum ferritin levels, 1984-2004. Journal of Orthomolecular Medicine 2005;20(suppl. issue):143-59.

Turkel N. Nusbaum I. Medical Treatment of Down Syndrome and Genetic Diseases. Southfield, MI: Ubiotica, 1985.

Turkel H. Medical Amelioration of Down Syndrome Incorporating the Orthomolecular Approach. Journal of Orthomolecular Psychiatry 1975;4:102-15.

Turkel H. Treatment of a mucopolysaccharide type of storage disease with the ëU' series. Journal of Orthomolecular Psychiatry 1981;10:239-48.

Urberg M, Zemel MG. Evidence for synergism between chromium and nicotinic acid in the control of glucose tolerance in elderly humans. Metabolism 1987;36:896-99.

van Tiggelen CJM, Peperkamp JPC, Tertoolen JFW. Vitamin B12 levels of cerebrospinal fluid in patients with organic mental disorders. Journal of Orthomolecular Psychiatry 1983;12:305-11.

van Tiggelen CJM, Peperkamp JPC, Tertoolen JFW. Assessment of vitamin B12 status in CSF. American Journal of Psychiatry 1984;141:136-37.

Vance DE, Ehmann WD, Markesbery WR. Trace element imbalances in hair and nails of alzheimer's disease patients. Neurotoxicology 1988;9:197-208.

Vieth R. Vitamin D nutrition and its potential health benefits for bone, cancer and other conditions. Journal of Nutritional & Environmental Medicine 2001;11:275-91.

Vieth R. Randomized comparison of the effects of the vitamin D3 adequate intake versus 100 mcg (4000 IU) per day on biochemical responses and the wellbeing of patients. Nutrition Journal 2004;3:8.

Waler MM. Phosphates as a cause of hyperactivity. Health Express 1981;2:15-17.

Weber CW, Nelson WG, de Vaquera MV, Pearson PB. Trace elements in hair of healthy and malnourished children. Journal of Topical Pediatrics 1990;36:230-34.

Weeks BS. Vitamin A and beta-carotene. Journal of Orthomolecular Medicine 2003;18:131-45.

Werbach MR, Moss JM. Textbook of Nutritional Medicine. Tarzana, CA: Third Line Press, Inc., 1999.

Whitaker R. Mad in America. Cambridge, MA: Perseus Publishing, 2004.

Williams RJ. Alcoholism: The Nutritional Approach. Austin, TX: University of Texas Press, 1958.

Wisner RM, et al. Human contamination and detoxification: Medical response to an expanding global problem. The Environmental Physician 1992 Spring:6,8,10.

Wright JV. Dr. Wright's Guide to Healing with Nutrition. Expanded ed. New Canaan, CT: Keats Publishing, Inc., 1990.

Wright JV. Treatment of childhood asthma with parenteral vitamin B12, gastric re-acidification, and attention to food allergy, magnesium and pyridoxine: Three case reports with background and an integrated hypothesis. Journal of Nutritional Medicine 1990;1:277-82.

Wright JV. Clinical tip 20. High "BUN," normal creatinine: Low stomach acid. Nutrition & Healing 1998;5(9):11.

Wright JV. Subclinical Rickets: Unexplained deficiency syndrome. Nutrition Healing 1999 Feb.

Xiao YF, et al. Inhibitory effect of n-3 fish oil fatty acids on cardiac Na+/Ca2+ exchange currents in HEK293t cells. Biochemical and Biophysical Research Communications 2004; 321:116-23.

Young SN. Tryptophan availability in humans: Effects on mood and behavior. Nato ASI: Series H20, 1988:267-74.

Young SN. Use of tryptophan in combination with other antidepressant treatments: A review. Journal of Psychiatry and Neuroscience 1991;16:241-46.

Young SN, Ghadirian AM. Folic acid and psychopathology. Progressive neuro-pyschopharmacology and biological psychiatry 1989;13:841-63.

Young SN, Teff KL. Tryptophan availability: 5HT synthesis and 5HT function. Progressive Neuro-Pyschopharm ocology & Biological Psychiatry 1989;13 373-79.

Zamm AV. Candida albicans therapy: Is there ever an end to It? Dental mercury removal: An effective adjunct. Journal of Orthomolecular Medicine 1986;1:261-66.

Zamm AV. Dental mercury: A factor that aggravates and induces xenobiotic intolerance. Journal of Orthomolecular Medicine 1991;6:67-78.

Zamm AV. Removal of dental mercury: Often an effective treatment for the very sensitive patient. Journal of Orthomolecular Medicine 1990;5:138-42.

Zimmermann M. Burgerstein's Handbook of Nutrition. New York, NY: Georg Thieme Verlag, 2001.

INDEX

Abdominal bloating, 101–103, 170, 294–295
Abundance, of high-tech foods, 45–46, 93
Acne
   low stomach acid and, 102, 103, 116
   pantothenic acid for, 180
   from vitamin B-12, 189
Acquired immune deficiency syndrome. See AIDS
Adaptation, 85–86
Addiction
   to additives, 31–33
   hypoglycemia and, 50
   to sugar, 29–31, 45, 58–59
Additives
   addiction to, 31–33
   autoimmune diseases and, 57–58
   chemical, 37–40, 45, 46
   cosmetic, 38, 46, 57
   environmental contaminants as, 57
   flavor, 46, 94
   in high-tech diet, 56–57
   learning/behavior disorders and, 58–59
   mental/emotional disorders and, 59
   nutrient, 39–40

   sugar as, 29–31
   trace, 38–39, 57
ADHD (attention deficit hyperactivity disorder)
   iron for, 220–221
   magnesium for, 216
   nutritional supplements for, 279–283
   zinc for, 227–228
   See also Behavioral disorders
Adrenal dysfunction (burn out), 179–180
Adrenochrome
   schizophrenia and, 165–166
   vitamin B-3 and, 163–164
Agricultural era, 35
AIDS (acquired immune deficiency syndrome)
   glutamine for, 259
   selenium for, 235–238
   vitamin B-1 for, 158, 159
   vitamin B-3 for, 172–173
Alcoholism
   glutamine for, 258
   vitamin B-1 for, 158
   vitamin B-3 for, 173
Aliveness, of natural food, 91
Alkaloids, 29
Allergic reactions

complex foods and, 47
monotonous diet and, 44–45
in ulcerative colitis/Crohn's
disease, 64
varied diet and, 91–92
See also Food allergies
Alopecia
betaine hydrochloride for,
297–298
low stomach acid and, 116
Aluminum
overview, 243–244
toxicity of, 244–245
Alzheimer's disease
aluminum and, 244
fluoride and, 215
mercury and, 246
Amalgams, mercury, 245–248
*The American Journal of
Epidemiology*, 194
American Psychiatric Association,
169
Ames, Bruce, 135, 181
Amino acids
antibodies and, 110
deficiency, 109–110
effect of heat on, 34
inhibitory, 259–262
overview, 249–250
Amygdalin (vitamin B-17), 311
Anemia
iron and, 111, 218–219
liver extract for, 119
low stomach acid and, 105, 107
vitamin B-12 deficiency and,
186–187
*Annals of the New York Academy of
Sciences*, 131
Anti-aging
folic acid for, 184
vitamin C for, 148–149
Antibiotics
mercury and, 247

yeast infections and, 52
Antibodies, 106, 110
Antioxidant activity
selenium and, 154, 234
of vitamin C, 147–148
of vitamin E, 153–154
Antioxidant Adaptation (Levine &
Kidd), 234
Antisocial behavior
high-additive diet and, 58–59
milk consumption and, 67
Anxiety disorders
inhibitory amino acids for, 260
niacinamide for, 171–172, 283–290
Anxiety Disorders: Grand Rounds
(Prousky & Hoffer), 172
*Anxiety: Orthomolecular Diagnosis
and Treatment* (Prousky), 172
Aortic aneurysms, 223
Apoplexy, 210–212
Appendicitis, 53, 64
Arginine
optimum dosage/safety of, 256
therapeutic uses, 254–256
Arteriosclerosis
folic acid for, 183
high-sugar diet and, 51–52
vitamin B-6 for, 178
vitamin C and, 149
Artifacts, 41, 73
Artificial flavors, 46
Ascorbate: The Science of Vitamin C,
147
Ascorbates, 156
Ascorbic acid. *See* Vitamin C
Atherosclerosis
high-fat diet and, 55
high-sugar/low-fiber diet and, 53
milk consumption and, 67,
69–70
poor quality fat and, 56
Athletic performance, 255–256
Atrophic gastritis, 105

Attention deficit hyperactivity disorder. *See* ADHD
Autism
   milk consumption and, 72–73
   vitamin B-6 for, 177–178
Autoimmune gastritis, 105

B vitamins
   content of common foods, 303–312
   deficiency of, 60–61
   See also specific B vitamins
Back pressure, 63–64
Bacterial growth
   gastrointestinal, high-sugar diet and, 65
   low stomach acid and, 108–109
Bad foods, 301
Bakin, Rita, 225
Baking soda test, 103–104
Balanced diet, 97–98
   See also Naturopathic nutrition
Beasley, J.D., 15
Behavioral disorders
   high-additive diet and, 58–59
   milk consumption and, 67, 72–73
   vitamin B-3 for, 89, 173, 279–283
   See also ADHD (attention deficit hyperactivity disorder)
Belmaker, C., 190
Benton, David, 233–234, 275–276
Benzodiazepines
   amino acids and, 260
   niacinamide and, 172
Beri beri, 158
Beta-carotene
   overview, 195–196
   therapeutic uses, 196–200
Betaine hydrochloric acid
   for alopecia, 297–298
   for bowel changes, 298
   for low stomach acid, 118–119
   See also Hydrochloric acid (HCl)

Bile, 101, 119
Bioflavonoids (Vitamin P), 314–315
Bioindividuality, 15–16, 87–88
Biological age *vs.* chronological age, 7–8
Biological Psychiatry, 234
Biosphere 2 environmental project, 74–75
Biotin (B vitamin), 309
Bipolar disorder
   lithium for, 241, 242
   tryptophan for, 251
Bitter taste, 28–29
Bland taste, 29
Bloating
   low stomach acid and, 101–103, 170
   niacin for, 294–295
Blood lipids. *See* Cholesterol levels
Blood pressure
   calcium/magnesium for, 216–217
   sodium/potassium for, 208–210
Blumberg, J., 130
Breakfast, 16–18
Breast cancer, 70, 186
The British Journal of Psychiatry, 167
Bulimia
   B vitamins deficiency and, 60–61
   zinc deficiency and, 224–225
Burkett, D., 53
Burn out (adrenal dysfunction), 179–180

Cadmium, 242–243
Calcium
   absorption of, 212–213
   blood pressure and, 209, 216–217
   content of common foods, 315–316
   food sources of, 111
   low stomach acid and, 110–111
   optimum dosage, 217
   for osteoporosis, 213–215
   safety of, 217–218

Calcium ascorbate, 156
Califano, Joseph, 15
Cameron, Ewan, 151, 152
Canada's Food Guide to Healthy Eating, 182
Canadian Medical Association Journal, 134
Cancer
   breast, 70, 186
   colon, 53, 64
   folic acid for, 183
   glutamine for, 259
   magnesium for, 216
   milk consumption and, 67, 70
   prostate, 199–200
   selenium for, 235
   serum copper to zinc ratio and, 223
   skin, 153–154
   stomach, 62–63, 105
   vitamin A for, 196–197
   vitamin B-3 for, 173
   vitamin B-12 for, 186
   vitamin C and, 145, 150–153
   vitamin D-3 for, 206
   vitamin E for, 194
Cancer and Vitamin C (Pauling & Cameron), 151
Candida yeast infections. *See* Yeast infections
Canned foods, 91
Cardiac arrhythmia, 266
Cardiac mortality, 266–267
Cardiovascular disease
   arginine for, 254–255
   high-fat diet and, 55
   See also Heart disease
Carnitine
   optimum dosage/side effects of, 257
   therapeutic uses, 256–257
Carotene. *See* Vitamin A
Carpal tunnel syndrome, 178

Case Studies In Natural Medicine (Werbach), 298
Castano, F., 71–72
Cataracts
   vitamin A for, 197
   vitamin B-2 for, 161
Cathcart, Roger, 144, 156
Centaurium minus (common or red centaury), 121
Cerebral function, 229
Cerebral hemorrhage, 210–212
Cervical dysplasia, 198
Challem, Jack, 183, 220
Chelation therapy, 248
Chemical additives
   artificial flavors, 46
   toxic effects of, 37–40, 45
   See also Additives
Chemical contaminants, 57
Chemical environment, 12–14
Chemical era
   additives, 37–40, 45, 46
   fermentation and sugar, 36–37
   food intake during, 35
   nutritional deficiency in, 37
Children
   attention deficit disorder in, 216, 220–221, 227–228, 279–283
   Down syndrome in, 278–279
   hyperactivity in, 60–61
   learning/behavior disorders in. *See* Behavioral disorders; Learning disorders
Cholesterol levels
   bile and regulation of, 101
   copper deficiency and, 223
   low-fat/low-sugar diets for, 55–56
   vitamin B-3 for, 131, 165
Choline (B vitamin), 309–310
Chromium
   content of common foods, 325
   optimum dosage, 232

overview, 231
safety of, 232–233
therapeutic uses, 231–232
Chronic disease, 85–86
Chronic fatigue syndrome, 186–187
Chronological age *vs.* biological age, 7–8
Cleave, T.L., 50, 64
Clemetson, C.A.B., 154–155
Cobalamin. *See* Vitamin B-12
Colic, 69
Colitis. *See* Ulcerative colitis
Colon, diseases of, 53, 63–65, 206
Common cold, 228
Complex foods, 47
Conant Sloan, B., 228
Congestive heart failure, 159
Constipation, 52–53, 63–64
Constituent fractions of food, 37, 41
Cook, R., 233–234, 276
Cooked era, 34
Copper
  accumulation of, 60
  content of common foods, 322
  optimum dosage/safety of, 228–229
  overview, 222–224
Coronary disease. *See* Heart disease
Coronary Drug Study, 131
Cosmetic additives, 38, 46, 57
Costs
  of high-tech diet, 78–79
  reducing healthcare, 123–125
Cott, Allan, 279
Criminal behavior
  high-additive diet and, 58–59
  lithium for, 241
  milk consumption and, 67
Crohn's disease
  glutamine for, 258
  high-sugar/low-fiber diet and, 64
  vitamin E for, 194
Cutler, Paul, 220

Dairy products
  additional nutrient deficiencies, 69
  allergic reactions to, 66–67
  atherosclerosis and, 69–70
  cancer and, 70
  diarrhea/iron deficiency from, 69
  lactase deficiency, 67–69
  milk allergies, 44–45, 66–67
  multiple sclerosis and, 70–71
  natural standards of, 96
  psychiatric/behavioral disorders and, 72–73
  tooth decay and, 71–72
DASH (Dietary Approaches for Stopping Hypertension) diet, 209
Dead food, 41–42
Dental amalgams, 245–248
Dental caries
  fluoride prevention, 239
  milk consumption and, 67
Depression
  chromium for, 231–232
  folic acid for, 185
  selenium for, 233–234
  tryptophan for, 250
Detoxification
  of toxic minerals, 248
  vitamin B-3 for, 173
Di Cyan, E., 193
Diabetes mellitus
  chromium for, 231
  saccharine disease and, 50
Diarrhea, 69
Digestive system, 99–100
  See also Stomach
Dioxins, 57
Diverticulosis, 53, 64
DNA damage, 145
Docosahexaenoic acid (DHA), 267–268
Don't Drink Your Milk (Oski), 66
Down syndrome, 278–279

Drug absorption, 109
Dubois, Rene, 147
Dyspepsia, 170–171

Eating disorders
  B vitamins deficiency and, 60–61
  zinc for, 224–225
Economic costs, of high-tech diet, 78–81
ECPO. *See* Enteric-coated peppermint oil
Eczema
  milk consumption and, 67
  selenium for, 234
Education, in good health, 13–14
Eicosapentaenoic acid (EPA), 267–268
Elderly population
  folic acid for, 184
  low stomach acid and, 106–107
  zinc deficiency in, 112
Ellis, John Marion, 178
Emotional disorders, 59
Endogenous foods, 93–94
Enstrom, James, 148
Enteric-coated peppermint oil (ECPO), 121
Environmental contaminants, 57
Environmental irritants, 106
Eosinophilia-myalgia syndrome (EMS), 251–252
Epidermolysis bullosa, 225–227
Erectile dysfunction, 255
Esophagus, diseases of, 62–63
Essential fatty acids
  for cardiac disease, 266–267
  destruction of, 56
  in endogenous foods, 93–94
  in exogenous foods, 46
  for GLA affected conditions, 264–265
  for mental disorders, 267
  oil quality, 269

  overview, 263–264
  for prostaglandin affected conditions, 265–266
  side effects of, 269
Exogenous foods, 46, 56

The Facts about Fats (Finnegan), 269
Fat, 54–56
Fatigue, 186–187, 216
Feast or famine cycle, 18
Feel Better and Live Longer with Vitamin B-3 (Foster & Hoffer), 89, 163
Felix, C., 264, 265, 267–268
Ferguson, Brian, 79
Fermentation, 36–37
Fiber
  deficiency in. *See* Low-fiber diet
  for peptic ulcers, 62
  protection provided by, 38
  small intestine/colon and, 63–65
Finnegan, J., 269
5-Hydroxytryptophan (5-HTP)
  optimum dosage, 251
  safety of, 251–252
  therapeutic uses, 250
Flavor additives, 46, 94
Fluoride
  Alzheimer's disease and, 215
  optimum dosage/safety of, 240
  therapeutic uses, 239–240
Folic acid (B vitamin)
  for anti-aging, 184
  for arteriosclerosis, 183
  for cancer, 183
  content of common foods, 307–308
  deficiency from low stomach acid, 113
  for depression, 185
  food sources of, 113
  for neural tube defects, 181–183

optimum dosage/safety of, 185
overview, 181
for psychiatric disorders, 184
Folkers, Karl, 178
Food allergies
dairy products, 66–73
low stomach acid and, 105, 108
overview, 65–66
processed protein, 73
See also Allergic reactions
Food for Naught: The Decline in Nutrition (Hall), 37
Food groups, 96–97
Food supply, 85–86
Foster, Harold D., 89, 162, 210, 215, 235–238
Fresh foods, 91
Frozen foods, 91
Fruit, 96
Fuelling Body, Mind and Spirit: A Balanced Approach to Healthy Eating (Hoffer), 16

GABA
inhibitory amino acid, 259–260
optimum dosage, 261
side effects of, 261–262
therapeutic uses, 260–261
Gaby, Alan, 195, 214
Gall bladder disease, 53, 64
Gamma linolenic acid (GLA)
affected conditions, 264–265
Gastric atrophy, 105
Gastrointestinal diseases
esophagus/stomach, 62–63
glutamine for, 258
milk and, 66–67
mouth, 61
small intestine/colon, 63–65
General anxiety disorder (GAD), 287–289
Genetic inheritance, 12–14
Gentiana lutea (gentian), 120–121

GERD (gastroesophageal reflux disease), 101, 295
Gerrard, J., 67–69
Glucose tolerance factor (GTF) chromium, 231–233
Glutamine
optimum dosage, 259
overview, 257–258
therapeutic uses, 258–259
Glutathione peroxidase, 235–237
Glycine
inhibitory amino acid, 259–260
optimum dosage/side effects of, 261
therapeutic uses, 260–261
Godfrey, J.C., 228
Godfrey, Paul, 185
Gold, 242–243
Goldberger, Joseph, 236
Grains, 97, 157, 231–232
Gray, C., 134

Hair analysis, 104
Hall, Ross Hume, 37–38
Harrell, C.F., 276
Hart, J.T., 203
Hayashida, T., 235
Headaches
vitamin B-2 for, 161
vitamin B-3 for, 171
Healing Cancer: Complementary Vitamin and Drug Treatments (Pauling & Hoffer), 89, 151
Healing Children's Attention and Behavior Disorders (Hoffer), 282
Healing Schizophrenia: Complementary Vitamin and Drug Treatments (Hoffer), 165
Healing wounds, 258–259
Health
basic elements of, 12–14
criteria for, 20
evaluation of, 20–22
four steps to optimum, 22–23

Health, Disease and the Environment (Foster), 210
Healthcare
    high-tech diet costs, 78–79
    integrative, 125
    irresponsibility of, 79–81
    reducing costs, 123–125
Heaney, R., 135, 214
Heart disease
    essential fatty acids for, 266–267
    high-fat/high-sugar diet and, 55
    iron for, 220
    low-fiber diet and, 53
    vitamin A for, 197
    vitamin B-6 for, 178
    vitamin E for, 193–194
Heat, effect of, 34
Hegsted, David Mark, 130
Helicobacter pylori, 62, 106
Heme iron, 112, 119, 219
Hemingway, D.C., 79–80, 180
Hemochromatosis, 218, 220
Hemorrhoids, 53, 63
Herbal bitters, 120–121
Herpes, 241
Hiatus hernia, 62
Hickel, Walter J., 125
High blood pressure, 207–210, 216–217
High-additive diet
    autoimmune diseases and, 57–58
    environmental contaminants in, 57
    learning/behavior disorders and, 58–59
    mental/emotional disorders and, 59
    overview, 56–57
High-fat diet
    function of fat, 54
    poor quality fat, 56
    too little fat, 54–55
    too much fat, 55–56
High-sugar diet
    arteriosclerosis and, 51–52, 55–56
    saccharine disease and, 50–51
    simple and free sugars, 49–50
    yeast infections and, 52
High-tech diet
    abundant, 45–46, 93
    artifact/dead/stale, 41–42
    artificially flavored/exogenous, 46
    complex, 47
    good health and, 12–14
    healthcare costs of, 78–79
    monotonous/toxic, 42–45
    nutritional deficiency in, 37
    senses as indicators in, 32–33
    sugar in, 29–31
Histamine, 105, 171
HIV (human immunodeficiency virus)
    glutamine and, 259
    manganese for, 229–230
    selenium for, 235–238
    vitamin B-3 for, 172–173
Hoffer, Miriam, 16
Homocysteine, 183
Horrobin, D.F., 263, 264
Horwitt, M.K., 162–163
Hospitals, malnutrition and, 75–76
How To Live Longer and Feel Better (Pauling), 148
Huggins, H., 245
Human immunodeficiency virus. *See* HIV
Huntington's Disease, 136
Hydrochloric acid (HCl)
    deficiency symptoms, 101–103
    digestion and, 100–101
    low. *See* Low stomach acid
    See also Betaine hydrochloric acid
Hydrolysis, 109–110
Hyperactivity
    B vitamins deficiency and, 61, 89
    high-additive diet and, 58–59

Hypercholesterolemia, 53
Hypertension, 208–210
Hypoascorbemia, 141
Hypochlorhydria. *See* Low stomach acid
Hypoglycemia, 50–51
Hypothyroidism
   copper deficiency and, 223
   selenium for, 235
   zinc deficiency and, 227

Idiopathic thrombocytopenic purpura (ITP), 150
Improved I.Q. (intelligence quotient), 275–277
Indican (urine) test, 104
Indigestion, 117–118
Infertility, male
   arginine for, 255
   vitamin A for, 199
Inflammatory conditions, 206
Inhibitory amino acids, 259–262
Injectable Vitamin C and the Treatment of Viral and Other Diseases, 147
Injuries, glutamine for, 258–259
Inoculations, 154–155
Inositol (B vitamin)
   content of common foods, 310
   therapeutic uses/optimum dosage, 190
Inositol hexaniacinate (IHN), 120
Integrative healthcare, 125
Intelligence
   glutamine for, 258
   nutritional supplements for, 275–277
Intoxication, mercury, 245–248
Intrinsic factor (IF) secretion, 108
Iodine, 326–327
Iron
   content of common foods, 321–322
   food sources of, 112
   for heart disease, 220
   for iron-deficiency anemia, 218–219
   low stomach acid and, 111–112
   for mental disorders, 220
   milk allergy and, 69
   optimum dosage, 221
   overview, 218
   safety of, 221–222
Islets of Langerhans, 51

Johnston, E.C., 167
Journal of Child Psychology & Psychiatry, 227
Journal of Clinical Psychiatry, 232
The Journal of Nutrition, 238
Journal of Orthomolecular Medicine, 145, 235
Journal of the American Medical Association, 80, 182

K factor, 208–209
The K Factor (Moore & Webb), 208
Kaufman, William, 170, 192
The Kellogg Report: The Impact of Nutrition, Environment and Lifestyle on the Health of Americans (Beasley & Swift), 15
Kidd, P.M., 234
Kidney stones, 144
Kryptopyrrole (KP)
   Vitamin B-6 and, 176–177, 225
   zinc deficiency and, 225
Kupk, R., 238

Labeled foods, 30
Lactase deficiency, 67–69
Lactose intolerance, 66–67
The Lancet, 70, 197, 275–276
Laxative, vitamin C as, 150
Lead toxicity, 242–243
Learning disorders

high-additive diet and, 58–59
vitamin B-3 for, 89, 173, 279–283
Leukemia, 67, 70
Leung, D. Lit-Hung, 180
Levine, S.A., 234
Lewis, Nolan D.C., 166
Lind, James, 142, 170
Lithium
   optimum dosage/safety of,
      241–242
   overview, 240
   therapeutic uses, 241
Liver
   extract, 119, 219
   function of, 119
Low stomach acid
   amino acid deficiency and,
      109–110
   B vitamins deficiency and,
      113–114
   calcium deficiency and, 110–111
   causes of, 105–106
   diagnosing, 103–104
   disorders associated with,
      107–109
   elderly population and, 106–107
   folic acid deficiency and, 113
   iron deficiency and, 111–112
   maldigestion from, 117–118
   questionnaire, 103
   skin conditions and, 116
   symptoms of, 101–103
   treatments
      enteric-coated peppermint oil,
         121
      HCl supplements, 118–119, 298
      herbal bitters, 120–121
      liver extract, 119
      niacin/inositol hexaniacinate,
         120
      nutritional supplements,
         121–122
      overview of, 116–117
   vitamin B-3, 170–171, 294–297
   vitamin C, 150
   vitamin B-6 deficiency and, 114
   vitamin B-12 deficiency and, 115
   vitamins A and E deficiencies, 115
   zinc deficiency and, 112
Low-fiber diet
   additional diseases from, 53–54
   constipation and, 52–53
   diseases of small intestine/colon
      and, 63–65
Lupus
   nutritional deficiency and, 58
   pantothenic acid for, 180
Lycopene, 199–200

Machlin, L.J., 129, 131
Macular degeneration, 197
Magnesium
   absorption of, 212–213
   for ADHD, 216
   blood pressure and, 209, 216–217
   for cancer, 216
   cerebral hemorrhage and, 210–211
   content of common foods,
      316–317
   deficiency disorders, 215–216
   optimum dosage, 217
   for osteoporosis, 213–215
   safety of, 217–218
Magnesium Research, 216
Maladaptation, 85–86
Maldigestion
   low stomach acid and, 117–118
   niacin for, 295–297
Malic acid, 244, 248
Malnutrition
   POW case study, 272–275
   studies of, 75–78
Manganese
   content of common foods, 323
   optimum dosage/safety of, 230
   therapeutic uses, 229–230

Manning, Roger, 161–164
Marks, John, 146, 159–160, 175–176, 179, 195
McCarron, D., 217
McGinnis, Woody, 177
McGrath, J., 205
McLachlan, D.R.C., 244
The Medical Post (on vitamins), 133
Medical Treatment of Down 'Syndrome (Turkel), 278
The Medical Tribune, 239
Medicine, irresponsibility of, 79–81
Megadoses, nutrient, 143
Men's conditions, 199–200
Mental disorders
　essential fatty acids for, 267
　high-additive diet and, 59
　iron for, 220
　vitamin D-3 for, 205
　See also Psychiatric disorders
Mental retardation, 276–277, 278–279
Mercury toxicity, 245–248
Migraine headaches
　vitamin B-2 for, 161
　vitamin B-3 for, 171
Milk allergies, 44–45, 66–67
　See also Dairy products
Miller, J., 186
Minerals
　absolutely essential
　　calcium and magnesium, 212–218
　　chromium, 231–233
　　iron, 218–222
　　manganese, 229–230
　　selenium, 233–238
　　sodium and potassium, 207–212
　　zinc and copper, 222–229
　diets deficient in, 59–60
　non-essential toxic
　　aluminum, 243–245

　　detoxification, 248
　　mercury, 245–248
　　overview of, 242–243
　overview, 207
　possibly essential
　　fluoride, 239–240
　　lithium, 240–242
Mixed carotenoids, 195–200
Molybdenum, 328
Monotonous diet
　allergic reactions and, 44–45
　nutritional deficiency in, 42–44
Mood disturbances, 241
Moore, R.D., 208
Mouth, diseases of, 61
Multiple sclerosis
　milk consumption and, 67, 70–71
　nutritional deficiency and, 58
　vitamin D-3 for, 204–205
The Multiple Sclerosis Diet Book (Swank), 71
Murray, John, 153
Murray, M.F., 172–173
Muscle spasms, 216
Muscular dystrophy, 58
Mycobacterium tuberculosis, 173

National Institutes of Health Office for the Study of Unconventional Medical Practices, 133–134
Natural food qualities, 90–95
Natural nutritional standards
　in balanced diet, 97–98
　of food groups, 96–97
　overview, 95–96
Naturopathic nutrition
　for anxiety disorders, 283–290
　defined, 10
　naturally flavored/simple, 94–95
　non-toxic/scarce/endogenous, 92–94
　reducing healthcare costs with, 123–125

for schizoaffective disorders,
    290–294
  standards for, 95–97
  whole/alive/fresh/varied, 90–92
Nephrosis, 67
Neural mediated hypotension
  (NMH), 211
Neural tube defects (NTDs), 181–183
*The New England Journal of
  Medicine*, 133–134
New York Newsday, 193
The New York Times (on vitamins),
  133
Newsweek (on vitamins), 133
Niacin
  for low stomach acid, 114,
    294–297
  See also Vitamin B-3
Niacinamide
  benzodiazepines and, 172
  for general anxiety disorder,
    287–289
  for panic attacks, 289–290
  for panic disorder/social phobia,
    286–287
  for severe anxiety, 283–286
  See also Vitamin B-3
Nickel content of common foods, 327
Nicotinamide. *See* Vitamin B-3
Non-verbal intelligence, 276
Nursing homes, malnutrition in,
  75–76
Nutrient additives, 39–40
Nutrient dependencies
  defined, 130, 135–136
  in POW malnutrition, 272–275
Nutrients and Bone Health (Gaby &
  Wright), 214
The Nutrition Reporter, 183
Nutrition Reviews, 186, 202
Nutritional deficiency
  autoimmune diseases and, 57–58
  in chemical era, 37

  defined, 130
  in monotonous diets, 42–44
Nutritional education
  in good health, 13–14
  importance of, 79–81
  regarding bioindividuality, 87–88
Nutritional supplements
  for Down syndrome, 278–279
  finding optimum dosage, 136–137
  improved I.Q. and, 275–277
  for low stomach acid, 121–122

Obesity
  B vitamins deficiency and, 60–61
  high-sugar diet and, 50
  pantothenic acid for, 180
  zinc deficiency and, 224–225
Omega-3 fatty acids
  functions of, 264
  for mental disorders, 267
  substrate pellagra and, 266
Omega-6 fatty acids, 264, 268
Optimum absorption, 99–100
  See also Stomach
Optimum adaptation, 128
Optimum dosage
  arginine, 256
  calcium/magnesium, 217
  chromium, 232
  fluoride, 240
  folic acid, 185
  inhibitory amino acids, 261
  inositol, 190
  iron, 221
  lithium, 241–242
  manganese, 230
  nutritional supplements, 136–137
  pantothenic acid, 180
  phenylalanine/tyrosine, 253
  selenium, 238
  sodium/potassium, 212
  vitamin A, 200–201
  vitamin B-1, 159

vitamin B-2, 161
vitamin B-3 (niacin), 173–174
vitamin B-6, 179
vitamin B-12, 189
vitamin C, 155–156
vitamin D-3, 206
vitamin E, 194
zinc/copper, 228
Optimum nutrition, 87–88
Oral cancer, 194
Orthomolecular medicine
   for anxiety disorders, 283–290
   basic principles of, 89–90
   defined, 10
   reducing healthcare costs, 123–125
   for schizoaffective disorders, 290–294
Oski, Frank, 66
Osteomalacia, 204
Osteoporosis
   calcium/magnesium for, 213–215
   fluoride for, 239–240
   vitamin A for, 200
   vitamin D-3 for, 204, 214
Osteoporosis International, 202
Over consumption, 92–93

PABA (para-aminobenzoic acid), 312
Panacea diets, 15–16
Pangamic acid (vitamin B-15), 312
Panic attacks/disorder, 286–287, 289–290
Pantothenic acid (vitamin B-5)
   content of common foods, 305–306
   optimum dosage, 180
   therapeutic uses, 179–180
Passwater, Richard A., 235
Pathogen overgrowth, 108–109
Pauling, Linus, 89, 136, 142–143, 147, 148, 149, 151

PCBs (polychlorinated biphenyls), 57
Pellagra
   essential fatty acids for, 265–266
   low stomach acid and, 114
   vitamin B-3 for, 130, 164–165, 236
Peppermint oil, enteric-coated, 121
Peptic ulcer
   high-tech diet and, 62
   milk consumption and, 67
Pernicious anemia, 105, 107, 185, 186–187
Pesticides, 57
Pfeiffer, Carl C., 176, 184, 222–224
Phenylalanine
   optimum dosage/side effects of, 253–254
   therapeutic uses, 252–253
Phenylketonuria, 252
Phosphates, 58–59
Phosphorus content of common foods, 317–318
Physical costs, of high-tech diet, 78–81
Porteous, George, 273–275
Potassium
   cerebral hemorrhage and, 210–212
   content of common foods, 320
   for hypertension, 208–210
   optimum dosage, 212
   overview, 207–208
Potassium ascorbate, 156
Preventive vitamin paradigm, 129–131
Principles of Medicine (Harrison), 225
Prisoner of war (POW) malnutrition, 272–275
Proceedings of the National Academy of Science, 74
Processed foods
   chemical additives in, 37–40
   processed protein, 73

sugar in, 29–31
See also High-tech diet
Prostaglandin affected conditions, 265–266
Prostate cancer
  vitamin A for, 199–200
  vitamin D-3 for, 206
Proteins
  effect of heat on, 34
  processed, 73
Psychiatric disorders
  folic acid for, 184
  milk consumption and, 72–73
  vitamin B-1 for, 159
  vitamin B-12 for, 187–188
  vitamin E for, 194
  See also Mental disorders
Psychosis, 245
Psychosocial costs, of high-tech diet, 78–81
Pure diet
  high-tech diet *vs.*, 40–41
  nutritional variety in, 43–44
  See also Naturopathic nutrition
Pyridoxine. *See* Vitamin B-6
Pyrroluria, 176

Questionnaire, low stomach acid, 103

Rath, M., 149
Raw era, 33
Recommended daily allowances (RDAs)
  inadequacy of, 130
  variation in, 88–89
Rectangular diet, 16–18
Relative hypoglycemia, 50
Respiratory disturbances, 66–67
Restless leg syndrome, 221
Rheumatoid arthritis
  milk consumption and, 67
  nutritional deficiency and, 58
Riboflavin. *See* Vitamin B-2

Rickets, 203–204
Riggs, L., 239–240
Rimland, Bernard, 177–178, 279
Rimm, E., 193
Roberts, Gwilym, 275–276
Rose, Colin, 74–75
Rowento, R., 125
Rudin, D., 264, 265–266, 267–268

Saccharine disease
  diseases of small intestine/colon and, 63–65
  high-sugar diet and, 50–51
The Saccharine Disease (Cleave), 50
Safety
  arginine, 256
  calcium/magnesium, 217–218
  chromium, 232–233
  fluoride, 240
  folic acid, 185
  iron, 221–222
  lithium, 242
  manganese, 230
  selenium, 238
  tryptophan/5-HTP, 251–252
  vitamin A, 201–202
  vitamin B-1 supplements, 159–160
  vitamin B-3 (niacin), 175–176
  vitamin B-6, 179
  vitamin C supplements, 144–145
  vitamin D-3, 206
  vitamin E, 195
  zinc/copper, 228–229
Sakimoto, K., 252
Salonen, J., 220
Salty taste, 29
Saul, Andrew, 146
Scarcity of food, 92–93
Schauss, A.G., 224
Schizoaffective disorders, 290–294
Schizophrenia
  adolescent, 277–278

kryptopyrrole syndrome and, 176–177, 225
milk consumption and, 72
nutrition and, 59
vitamin B-3 for, 89, 165–170
Schrauzer, G.N., 241
Scurvy, 141–142, 145
Selenium
   antioxidant activity of, 154, 234
   for cancer, 235
   content of common foods, 325–326
   for depression, 233–234
   for HIV/AIDS infection, 235–238
   optimum dosage, 238
   safety of, 238
   for skin conditions, 234
   for thyroid function, 235
Selenium as Food and Medicine (Passwater), 235
Selye, Hans, 106
Senses
   in food selection, 12–13, 14–15
   in high-tech diet, 32–33
   survival reflex and, 28–29
Serotonin
   syndrome, 252
   tryptophan/5-HTP and, 250
   vitamin B-12 and, 187
Sgoutas, D.S., 193–194
Shine, I., 51
Shrestha, K.P., 241
Shute, Evan, 153–154, 191, 192, 194
Shute, Wilfred, 191, 192, 194
Shwartzendruber, D., 246
Siblerud, R.L., 247
Silica, 244–245, 248
Silver toxicity, 242–243
Simplicity, of natural diet, 94–95
Sizman, Moses M., 178
Skin disorders
   low stomach acid and, 116–117
   selenium for, 234

vitamin C and, 153–154
Slagle, P., 252–253
Small intestine
   modern diet and diseases of, 63–65
   pathogen overgrowth in, 108–109
   pH level, 109
Smell
   survival reflex and, 12, 28
   zinc deficiency and, 59–60, 112
Smithells, R.W., 181
Social phobia, 286–287
Sodium
   cerebral hemorrhage and, 210–212
   content of common foods, 301, 319
   for hypertension, 208–210
   optimum dosage, 212
   overview, 207–208
Sodium ascorbate, 156
Sour taste, 29
Spies, T.D., 80
Staleness, of high-tech foods, 42
Stampfer, M., 183, 193
Starches, 34
Stomach
   cancer, 62–63, 105
   emptying problems, 108
   functions of, 100
   hydrochloric acid, 100–101
   low HCl. *See* Low stomach acid
   modern diet and diseases of, 62–63
Stone, Irving, 141
Stool analysis, 104
Storage, of high-tech foods, 41–42
Stoute, J.A., 145
Stress
   low stomach acid from, 106
   vitamin C for, 149
The Stress of Life (Selye), 106
Stroke
   cerebral hemorrhage and, 210–211
   essential fatty acids for, 266–267

high-fat diet and, 55
high-sugar/low-fiber diet and, 53
vitamin B-6 for, 178
Subclinical rickets, 203–204
Substrate pellagra, 266
Sugar(s)
    addiction, 29–31
    allergic reactions to, 44–45
    annual consumption of, 36–37
    diseases from. See High-sugar diet
    effect of heat on, 34
    elimination of, 22, 31
    learning/behavior disorders from, 58–59
    low-fat diet and, 55–56
    trace additives in, 39
    undigested, 64, 65
Sullivan, Jerome L., 220
The Summary, 192
Summers, A., 247
Survival reflex
    maladaptation and, 85–86
    natural nutrition and, 26–28
    senses and, 28–29
Swank, R.L., 71
Sweetness, 29
Swift, J.J., 15
Swinging gait, 180
Szent-Gyorgyi, A., 141

Tardive dyskinesia, 230
Taste
    epidermolysis bullosa and, 226
    survival reflex and, 28–29
    zinc deficiency and, 59–60, 224
Taurine
    inhibitory amino acid, 259–260
    optimum dosage, 261
    side effects of, 262
    therapeutic uses, 260–261
Tension-type headaches, 171
The Way Up From Down (Slagle), 253

Therapeutic uses
    calcium/magnesium, 213–217
    chromium, 231–232
    fluoride, 239–240
    folic acid, 181–185
    inositol, 190
    lithium, 241
    pantothenic acid, 179–180
    sodium/potassium, 207–212
    tryptophan/5-HTP, 250
    vitamin A, 196–200
    vitamin B-1, 158–159
    vitamin B-2, 160–161
    vitamin B-3, 164–173
    vitamin B-6, 177–178
    vitamin B-12, 186–189
    vitamin C, 147–155
    vitamin D-3, 203–206
    vitamin E, 192–194
    zinc/copper, 224–228
Therapeutic vitamin paradigm, 131–132
Thiamin. See Vitamin B-1
Thyroid function, 235
Time Magazine (on vitamins), 133
Tooth decay
    fluoride prevention, 239
    milk consumption and, 67
Townsend Letter for Doctors & Patients, 195
Toxicity
    aluminum, 244–245
    avoiding, 92
    cadmium/silver/gold/lead, 243
    of chemical additives, 37–40, 45
    detoxification, 248
    of high-tech foods, 45
    mercury, 245–248
    natural standards of, 97
    vitamin A, 201–202
Trace additives, 38–39, 57
Triangular diet, 16–17
Truss, O., 57–58

Tryptophan
    optimum dosage, 251
    safety of, 251–252
    therapeutic uses, 250
    vitamin B-3 and, 162–163
Turkel, Henry, 278–279
20-year rule, 50–51
Type A gastritis, 105
Type B gastritis, 105
Tyrosine
    optimum dosage, 253
    side effects of, 254
    therapeutic uses, 252–253

Ulcerative colitis
    glutamine for, 258
    low stomach acid and, 107
    low-fiber diet and, 53, 64
Ultraviolet light
    vitamin C and, 153
    vitamin D-3 and, 203
Universal healthcare, 78–79
Unsaturated fats, 34, 46, 56, 94
Urine (indican) test, 104

Vaccinations, 154–155
Vanadium content of common
    foods, 328–329
Variety, in food selection, 91–92
Vascular disease, 55, 71, 190
Vegetables, natural standards of, 96
Vieth, R., 205, 206
Vimy, Murray J., 245–246
Violent behavior, 241
    See also Behavioral disorders
Visual function, 197–198
Vitamin A (carotene)
    for cancer, 196–197
    for cataracts, 197
    content of common foods,
        302–303
    deficiency from low stomach
        acid, 115
    food sources of, 115
    for heart disease, 197
    for men's conditions, 199–200
    optimum dosage, 200–201
    for osteoporosis, 200
    overview, 195–196
    safety of, 201–202
    for vision, 197–198
    for women's conditions, 198–199
Vitamin B complex, 157
Vitamin B-1 (thiamin)
    content of common foods,
        303–304
    food sources of, 114
    low stomach acid and, 113–114
    optimum dosage, 159
    overview, 157
    safety of, 159
    therapeutic uses, 158–159
Vitamin B-2 (riboflavin)
    content of common foods, 304
    food sources of, 114
    low stomach acid and, 113–114
    optimum dosage, 161
    therapeutic uses, 160–161
*Vitamin B-3 and Schizophrenia:
    Discovery, Recovery, Controversy*
    (Hoffer), 131, 165
Vitamin B-3 (niacin)
    for anxiety disorders, 171–172
    for cholesterol, 131, 165
    content of common foods, 305
    for detoxification, 173
    food sources of, 114
    for headaches, 171
    history of, 161–164
    for HIV/AIDS infection, 172–173
    for low stomach acid, 120, 170–171
    low stomach acid and, 113–114
    for mental disorders, 59, 89, 131,
        135–136
    optimum dosage, 173–174
    for pellagra, 130, 164–165

for peptic ulcers, 62
POW malnutrition and, 273–275
prevention for diabetes, 51
safety of, 175–176
for schizophrenia, 89, 165–170, 277–278
side effects of, 174–175
Vitamin B-5. *See* Pantothenic acid
Vitamin B-6 (pyridoxine)
  content of common foods, 306–307
  food sources of, 114
  kryptopyrrole and, 176–177
  low stomach acid and, 114
  for mental disorders, 59, 176–177
  milk allergy and, 69
  optimum dosage, 179
  safety of, 179
  side effects of, 179
  therapeutic uses, 177–178
Vitamin B-12 (cobalamin)
  for breast cancer, 186
  for chronic fatigue syndrome, 186–187
  content of common foods, 308
  food sources of, 115
  intrinsic factor and, 108
  low stomach acid and, 115
  optimum dosage, 189
  for psychiatric disorders, 187–188
  side effects of, 189
Vitamin B-15 (pangamic acid), 312
Vitamin B-17 (amygdalin), 311
Vitamin C and Cancer: Discovery, Recovery, Controversy (Hoffer), 151
Vitamin C and the Common Cold (Pauling), 89, 143, 144
Vitamin C (ascorbic acid)
  anti-aging activity, 148–149
  antioxidant activity, 147–148
  arteriosclerosis and, 149
  ascorbates, 156
  benefits *vs.* risks, 145–147
  for cancer prevention/treatment, 150–153
  content of common foods, 312–313
  controversy, 142–143
  effect of heat on, 34
  for hardening of the arteries, 53
  for idiopathic thrombocytopenic purpura, 150
  interferon production and, 57–58, 71
  laxative effect, 150
  megadose controversy, 143
  optimum dosage, 155–156
  protection provided by, 38
  safety controversy, 144–145
  scurvy and, 141–142
  for skin disorders, 153–154
  stomach acid supplement, 150
  stress reduction, 149
  vaccinations/inoculations and, 154–155
  variation of optimum dosage, 88–89
Vitamin D-3
  for cancer, 206
  content of common foods, 313
  for inflammatory conditions, 206
  for mental disorders, 205
  for multiple sclerosis, 204–205
  optimum dosage, 206
  for osteomalacia, 204
  for osteoporosis, 204
  overview, 202–203
  for rickets/subclinical rickets, 203–204
  safety of, 206
Vitamin deficiency paradigm, 129–131
Vitamin E and Aging (Di Cyan), 193
Vitamin E (tocopherols)
  antioxidant activity of, 153–154
  content of common foods, 313–314